Learning
Mechanisms in *Smoking*

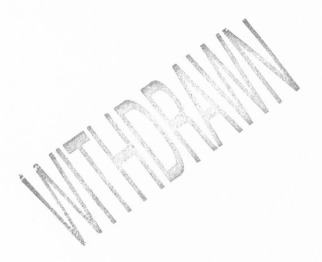

Learning Mechanisms in *Smoking*

William A. Hunt

Editor

AldineTransaction
A Division of Transaction Publishers
New Brunswick (U.S.A.) and London (U.K.)

First paperback printing 2007
Copyright © 1970 by The American Cancer Society

This book is printed on acid-free paper that meets the American National Standard for Permanence of Paper for Printed Library Materials.

Library of Congress Catalog Number: 2007022238
ISBN: 978-0-202-36147-5
Printed in the United States of America

Library of Congress Cataloging-in-Publication Data

Learning mechanisms in smoking / [edited by] William A. Hunt.
     p. cm.
  Includes bibliographical references and index.
  Originally published: Chicago: Aldine Pub. Co., 1970, in series: Modern applications of psychology.
    ISBN 978-0-202-36147-5 (alk. paper)
  1. Tobacco use. 2. Tobacco—Physiological effect. I. Hunt, William Alvin, 1903-

RC567.L38 2007
616.86'5—dc22   2007022238

Preface

WHEN the Committee on Tobacco Habituation of the American Cancer Society decided to recommend to the Society that it sponsor a conference on the role of learning in smoking behavior, it projected a small working group, to facilitate free interaction among the members. Moreover, the wish was expressed that the conference concentrate on the free interchange of ideas (rather than devoting itself to developing any specific program of either research or treatment), in the hope that such an interchange would provide a basis for future research planning and theoretical development. Put simply, the Committee desired to try a small mix of "learning people" and "smoking people," in the belief that innovative and cooperative approaches to the problems of smoking would be facilitated in the future.

The subcommittee appointed to plan and execute the actual conference kept these general goals firmly in mind. The membership was limited, although the limitation caused the committee much personal and corporate anguish and sometimes no little anxiety and guilt. There were many times during our deliberations when we looked around the table to address a question to the colleague whose experimental work was best suited to an answer, only to realize with regret that he was not present. But communication *was* facilitated, and the resulting exchange, while always gentlemanly, was certainly irreverent and frank. The few pages of discussion presented in this volume are the residue of some 300 pages of transcription that the editor was forced to review and condense. Whatever else may have been accomplished, there was talk, and in an atmosphere of friendly aggression that I think we all enjoyed.

Beyond these general goals, of course, lay the innumerable individual and specific motivations of each participant. I hesitate to speak for even as limited a group as the planning committee; for me there was the feeling that behavior modification (or contingency management), has outgrown the simple models that an earlier learning or conditioning theory offered and that it must return to its experimental source material for more modern and more sophisticated models. The current transition of interest in aversive conditioning—from the technological advantages and manipulative convenience of electric shock as an aversive stimulus to its appropriateness or contextual significance within the behavior system being manipulated—is a case in point. And there is every indication that modern learning theory can supply more complicated and suitable models once the communications gap can be lessened.

Irrespective of merit or social justification, however, no conference can be held and subsequently reported without a great deal of work on the part of a great number of people. Our basic gratitude must go to the Board of Directors of the American Cancer Society for its support in making the conference possible, and particularly to two members of the national staff, Drs. Sam Hall and Richard Mason, as the active agents of that support.

I should like to add my thanks to my colleagues on the planning committee: Vincent Dole, Murray Jarvik, Conan Kornetsky, Joseph Matarazzo, and Silvan Tomkins. They were unusually responsive and labored mightily to keep their chairman on the track. We are grateful as well to the participants and can only hope their efforts produced some personal hedonic reinforcement. Finally, and by no means least, our thanks are due to all our coworkers in the field, who, while they were not present, have by their dedicated labors provided the sound experimental and theoretical foundation that must be present before a profitable conference can be held.

A conference is one thing; the report of its proceedings is another. Closing thanks are therefore due to Captain Laurence Branch of the Army's Medical Service Corps for his editorial assistance in the preparation of the manuscript, to Greta Rowe for her secretarial endeavors, and to the pleasant, friendly people at Aldine Publishing Company for their encouragement.

William A. Hunt

Contents

Participants

Mitchel B. Balter, Ph.D., Chief, Special Studies Section, Psychopharmacology Research Branch, National Institute of Mental Health

Douglas A. Bernstein, Ph.D., Assistant Professor, Department of Psychology, University of Illinois—Urbana

Edgar F. Borgatta, Ph.D., Research Professor, Department of Sociology, University of Wisconsin

Charles B. Ferster, Ph.D., Professor, Department of Psychology, The American University

Enoch Gordis, M.D., Associate Professor, Rockefeller University

Dorothy Green, Ph.D., Chief, Program Research Section, National Clearinghouse for Smoking and Health

Winfred F. Hill, Ph.D., Professor, Department of Psychology, Northwestern University

William A. Hunt, Ph.D., Professor, Department of Psychology, Loyola University—Chicago

Murray E. Jarvik, M.D., Ph.D., Professor, Department of Pharmacology, Albert Einstein College of Medicine, Yeshiva University

Peter H. Knapp, M.D., Research Professor, Department of Psychiatry, School of Medicine, Boston University

Conan Kornetsky, Ph.D., Research Professor, Division of Psychiatry and Department of Pharmacology, School of Medicine, Boston University

Frank A. Logan, Ph.D., Professor, Department of Psychology, University of New Mexico

Elijah Lovejoy, Ph.D., Assistant Professor, Department of Psychology, University of California at Santa Barbara

Joseph D. Matarazzo, Ph.D., Professor, Department of Medical Psychology, School of Medicine, University of Oregon

Jack H. Mendelson, M.D., Chief, National Center for the Prevention and Control of Alcoholism, National Institute of Mental Health

David Premack, Ph.D., Professor, Department of Psychology, University of California at Santa Barbara

Charles R. Schuster, Ph.D., Associate Professor, Department of Psychiatry, University of Chicago.

Gene M. Smith, Ph.D., Assistant Professor, Department of Anaesthesia, Harvard Medical School, Massachusetts General Hospital

Janet Taylor Spence, Ph.D., Professor, Department of Psychology, University of Texas

Silvan S. Tomkins, Ph.D., Research Professor, Department of Psychology, Livingston College, Rutgers University

Part One
Reviews of Relevant Literature

The Modification of Smoking Behavior: An Evaluative Review[1]

DOUGLAS A. BERNSTEIN

CIGARETTE smoking is a widespread and pervasive phenomenon in the Western world, and while it has received the passing attention of researchers in various disciplines over a period of time, it has only been within the last fifteen years that the pace of published research on smoking has quickened. The primary impetus for this focus has been, of course, the alleged causal relationship between cigarette smoking and various physical disorders. A series of "health scares"—beginning in 1953 with a paper presented to the New York Dental Association (Day, 1959) and continuing to include, among others, the Royal College of Physicians Report on Smoking and Health (1962) and the 1964 report of the Advisory Committee to the Surgeon General, *Smoking and Health* (U.S. Public Health Service, 1964)—has resulted in a monumental outpouring of research on many aspects of smoking behavior. It is of some interest to note that within this body of research there is a relatively

1. Preparation of this manuscript was supported by United States Public Health Service Predoctoral Research Fellowship 5-F1-MH-32, 578-02. A condensed version has appeared in the *Psychological Bulletin*, 1969, 71(6), 418-440.

recent trend (since 1962) toward investigations designed to attack the problem of modification (i.e., elimination) of smoking behavior as opposed to studies aimed at correlating smoking with psychological or morphological characteristics.

Moreover, while the volume of modification-oriented research has increased dramatically during the past six years, there has been at the same time a tendency toward the use of psychological and sociological models upon which to base such research. Though the medical model is not being completely neglected, the drug studies typical of its approach are being overshadowed by more psychologically oriented techniques.

The most interesting and at the same time disturbing conclusion to be drawn from a survey of recent smoking literature is that the "health scares" have done far more to influence the research behavior of psychologists and sociologists than to change the smoking behavior of the general public.

In view of the consequent proliferation of research (National Clearinghouse for Smoking and Health, 1968), a review and critical evaluation of the work on smoking behavior, with special attention to attempts at modification published or reported since 1962, seems appropriate at this time.

It should be noted at the outset that the justifiability of causal statements linking smoking to disease is not at issue here. In an effort to resolve the question, hundreds of research projects have been completed (American Cancer Society, 1963; National Clearinghouse for Smoking and Health, 1967a), and many more are under way (National Clearinghouse for Smoking and Health, 1967b, 1968). For the present purposes the behavior of the American public in response to reports containing such causal statements is more relevant. The typical pattern immediately after a "health scare" involves a temporary drop in the price of tobacco stock, accompanied by reductions in tobacco sales, but followed within a period of months by recoveries that ultimately surpass prereport levels. This effect has been noted both in Great Britain and in the United States (Brown, C. T., 1964; Brecher and Brecher, 1964; Day, 1959; Janis and Mann, 1965; Straits, 1965; Toch, Allen, and Lazer, 1961; U. S. News and World Report, 1965) and is really not surprising, especially when viewed in historical perspective. Even with virtually absolute power, seventeenth-century rulers were unable to prevent their subjects from smoking, even when the death penalty (far more certain and immediate than cancer) was made contingent upon it.

The discontinuance of smoking in America is the exception, not the rule. National studies have found that less than 20 per cent of the smoking population ever quit (Haenszel, Shimkin, and Miller, 1956; Hammond and Percy, 1958), and other investigators have reported figures as low as 10 per cent (Cartwright, Martin, and Thompson, 1960). More recently Straits (1965) found that of the men surveyed in 2,000 Chicago households, only 24 per cent had ever tried to stop smoking, and of those only about one in three was successful. The question of why the majority of smokers do not quit in light of the available evidence is not an easy one, but Straits (1965) has, for conceptual purposes, neatly broken the non-quitters down into the uninformed, the unbelieving, the unmotivated, and those who are unable to quit. Of these subgroups the most fascinating and frustrating are the last two: those smokers who know of the alleged link between smoking and health and who believe it to be causal and yet will not or cannot modify their smoking behavior.

We already know that whatever factors influence individuals to start smoking, the effect is evident by the early teens (Haenszel et al., 1956; Straits, 1965; U. S. Public Health Service, 1964) and that the trend is in the direction of even earlier onset (Guilford, 1966). Once this behavior is established, however, the factors responsible for its long-term maintenance must be searched out.

SMOKING BEHAVIOR

Maintenance of smoking behavior

To find the factors that establish smoking behavior becomes more and more important as one moves from theoretical positions whose modification techniques emphasize original, underlying causes toward those that deal exclusively with observable behavior and its current reinforcers.

The issue is incredibly complex because, first, there is little reason to believe that one factor or even one set of factors is consistently responsible for the maintenance of all smokers' behavior; second, it may be the case that, even within the individual smoker, there is inconsistency such that from moment to moment, day to day, or even over phases in the life cycle, the factors that maintain smoking behavior are very different (Guilford, 1966). Cigarette smoking has been characterized as "not one behavior but a range of psychologically diverse behaviors each of which may be induced by a different combination of factors" (U.S. Public Health Service, 1964, 376). Theories of maintenance vary in their recognition of this complexity, with the result that some seek to explore and illuminate interacting "motivation systems," while others ignore them and attempt to deal with the problem in more global terms. Perhaps the most controversial of the latter type has been the view that the cigarette smoker's behavior is maintained by the addictive properties of nicotine.

Before this hypothesis is examined, it should be clear what is meant by the term "addictions," so that for both views the arguments may be compared in a meaningful way. The World Health Organization has defined drug addiction as a state of periodic or chronic intoxication produced by the repeated consumption of a drug (natural or synthetic). Its characteristics include: an overpowering desire or need (compulsion) to continue taking the drug and to obtain it by any means; a tendency to increase the dose; a psychic (psychological) and generally a physical dependence on the effects of the drug; detrimental effect on the individual and on society." It defines drug habituation as "a condition resulting from the repeated consumption of a drug. Its characteristics include: a desire (but not a compulsion) to continue taking the drug for the sense of improved well-being which it engenders; little or no tendency to increase the dose; some degree of psychic dependence on the effect of the drug, but absence of physical dependence and hence of an abstinence syndrome; detrimental effects, if any, primarily on the individual" (quoted in U. S. Public Health Service, 1964, 351).

These definitions are not the only ones in use, however, and the resulting misunderstanding accounts for much of the "addiction versus habituation" dispute. For example, addiction has been so broadly defined (De Jongh, 1951, 1954, cited in Van Proosdij, 1960) as to include any consistent behavior that is difficult to discontinue. In these terms, a daily cup of coffee, regular viewing of a particular television program, and "all sorts of other hobbies which have become habits increasingly difficult to break" (Van Proosdij, 1960, 36) would be considered addictions.

Between these extremes various other sets of criteria for addiction can be found. Tomkins (1965, cited in Guilford, 1966) lists five phenomenologically oriented ones: the absence of the addicting substance is always noted; awareness of this absence regularly instigates an intense negative affect, for which there is also awareness; the addict expects that only the addicting substance can reduce this negative affect; the addict expects that only the addicting substance will produce positive affects? these expectations are invariably confirmed. J.A.C. Brown (1963) adds yet another facet to the concept of addiction by noting that it leads to "ultimate moral deterioration" and that addicts usually have a history of previous maladjustment.

It should thus be clear that the problem of characterizing cigarette smoking as either a habit or an addiction can be very much one of semantics. Yet while some (e.g., Van Proosdij, 1960) question the value or meaningfulness of such a distinction, a clear understanding of the issue and its resolution, based upon common criteria, is crucial for the development of modification procedures. "Thus if tobacco smoking is an addiction *comparable to cocaine or morphine addiction,* then one line of treatment, presumably pharmacological, will be necessary, but if it turns out to be largely, or even entirely, a socially conditioned and psychologically motivated habit, we shall have to take another line altogether" (Brown, J. A. C., 1963, 187; italics added). It seems that, when *addiction* is required to meet a rigid pharmacological definition (the only one that has clear consequences for treatment of the smoker), the issue has already been largely resolved.

Cigarette smoking at least partially satisfies two of the World Health Organization's criteria for classification as an addiction. First, it is well known by most smokers, especially heavy smokers, that there is an "overpowering desire or need (compulsion)" to continue smoking; however, whether the smoker will obtain cigarettes "by any means" is open to serious question. Second, regardless of the position taken on the smoking-health issue, it is undeniable that cigarette smoking has some detrimental effect on the individual, whether it be in the form of increased blood pressure, reduced oxygen supply to the brain, increased work load for the heart, or any of the other recognized effects of the inhalation of tobacco smoke (Hammond, 1962). It is not clear, however, that there is also a detrimental effect on society and in view of the size and importance of the tobacco industry in America, it would not be wholly unrealistic to argue that smoking is, on one level, actually beneficial.

Thus far the addiction theory of smoking is not fully substantiated, but those espousing it have based their position primarily upon evidence relating to the remaining World Health Organization criteria—that smokers tend to "increase the dose" and that physical dependence upon nicotine is present.

There is little doubt that, in terms of number of cigarettes smoked per day, the average smoker does tend to increase the dose. Such an increase is made possible by the development of a growing, though self-limiting, tolerance for nicotine intake (Johnston, 1942; Winsor and Richards, 1935). It has been noted, however (Van Proosdij, 1960), that increasing the number of cigarettes smoked per unit time is not comparable to the per-dose increase practiced by the morphine addict. In the latter case, the unpleasant secondary effects of the drug forces the addict to increase the dose in order to avoid them, and this, in turn further aggravates the secondary effects, leading to further dose increase, and so on. In contrast, "a smoker lights up more and more cigarettes a day . . . because he craves for the soothing or pleasant effect of nicotine, but to satisfy that craving, there is no necessity to increase nicotine content of the tobacco" (Van Proosdij, 1960, 44). While it has been shown that, when switched to low-nicotine cigarettes, many smokers miss it, are not "satisfied," and seek cigarettes that contain more nicotine (Finnegan, Larson, and Haag, 1945), smoking low-nicotine cigarettes at a higher rate is not an adequate substitute. Thus it cannot be said that smokers tend to increase the dose in a way that satisfies the World Health Organization's criterion. Further, the development of increasing tolerance for nicotine is not in itself evidence that those who have developed such tolerance are nicotine addicts. Van Proosdij (1960) noted that *tolerance* and *addiction* have totally different meanings, though they are often used interchangeably; and Brown (1963, 188) points out that "while it is perfectly true that all drugs of addiction produce tolerance and habituation, it is wholly untrue to say that everything to which we develop tolerance and habituation must be a drug of addiction."

This raises the final World Health Organization criterion: "psychic and physical dependence." The existence of the former, as it is popularly defined, will not be disputed, but that of the latter seems open to debate. It has been noted that "Proof of physical dependence requires demonstration of a *characteristic* and *reproducible* abstinence syndrome upon withdrawal of a drug or chemical which occurs spontaneously, inevitably, and is not under the control of the subject" (U. S. Public Health Service, 1964, 352; italics added). In the case of abstinence from cigarette smoking, this effect simply has not been demonstrated. This is not to say that "withdrawal symptoms" have not been reported; they take a wide variety of forms, including gastric disorders, dry mouth, irritability, sleeplessness, headaches, weight gain, anxiety, tremors, nausea, swelling of hands and feet, drowsiness, impaired concentration, and restlessness (Bell, 1961; Bergler, 1946; Cain, 1964; Dale, 1964; Heise, 1962; Johnston, 1952; Knapp, 1962; Knapp, Bliss, and Wells, 1963; Larson, Haag, and Silvette, 1961; Straits, 1965).

However, there is no evidence to support the notion that a consistent, characteristic withdrawal syndrome occurs in all or even most individuals who discontinue smoking. Even in cases where similarity in symptoms exists, there may be widespread differences in terms of point of onset and duration of discomfort. In fact, many smokers—even those who smoke heavily—experience no withdrawal symptoms at all, though they may retain their desire to smoke (U. S. Public Health Service, 1964).

The variety of physical and emotional consequences that follow discontinuance of smoking behavior does not, therefore, constitute sufficient evidence for physical dependence upon nicotine. Moreover, it has not been demonstrated that the "withdrawal symptoms" reported differ in any significant way from those observed "in any emotional disturbance secondary to deprivation of a desired object or habitual experience"

(U. S. Public Health Service, 1964, 352). There is an obvious need for systematic research aimed at comparing the consequences of eliminating smoking behavior to those of some equally disruptive environmental modification, such as the prolonged use of image-distorting lenses.

In summary, it must be concluded that cigarette smoking satisfies the World Health Organization's definition of habituation far better than it does that of addiction. Further, the use of the term *addiction,* even when defined less rigorously, in the description of smoking behavior should be discouraged, in the hope that much of the confusion and misunderstanding surrounding the issue can then be eliminated.

This very brief look at maintenance is by no means exhaustive. There is no shortage of alternative theories relating to the issue, many of which are considered in an informative overview by Guilford (1966, 29–34). What can be concluded from the plethora of theoretical notions? Summarizing her review, Guilford (1966, 34) notes that "habituation to smoking is the result of a very complex system of physiological, social and psychological *needs* and that within any one individual, one or more, or even all, of these needs may exist" (italics added). In the same vein, the Surgeon General's Report (U. S. Public Health Service, 1964, 354) concluded that "The habitual use of tobacco is related primarily to psychological and social *drives*" (italics added). The terms *needs* and *drives* have been emphasized because they characterize the "internal" approach to the problem of maintenance of smoking behavior. It should be noted, however, that an attractive alternative, based primarily on environmental events, is available, though—for reasons to be considered later—it has not yet been extensively used as a rationale for treatment. On this view, cigarette smoking is maintained by the observable environmental stimuli (including those originating within the body wall) that elicit it and by those which it produces—that is, by a combination of respondent and operant conditioning. The word *observable* is, of course, crucial, since it distinguishes this learning-theory approach from those approaches that attempt to deal with inferred drive states and the like. Among the advantages of such a conceptualization is flexibility. Any environmental variable can be assigned a role in maintenance as long as it is somehow observable and potentially manipulable. The second requirement is as important as the first, since another major advantage to the approach is its testability. The implications for modification techniques are clear and direct and can result in procedures so closely related to their rationale that they are capable of validating or invalidating it. This circumstance is not always, or even often, available to other maintenance conceptualizations.

To paraphrase Guilford (1966), then, it might be said that habituation to smoking is the result of a very complex system of physiological, social, and other environmental stimuli; and that, for any one individual, some particular combination of them is relevant (i.e. functional).

The complexity of that system, however, results in formidable difficulties, even for such a relatively "simplistic" conceptualization, since even if all the stimuli relevant for even one individual could be enumerated, the problem of discontinuation would still be far from solved. Precise manipulation of one, let alone all, relevant reinforcement contingencies and all the discriminative and conditioned stimuli is not always possible or even desirable. Attempts to do so may run the risk of making the "cure" more disagreeable than the "disease." Thus it would hardly seem worthwhile to quit smoking if eating must be replaced by intravenous feeding and certain social contacts by isolation because they signal or elicit smoking behavior. Though some progress is being made, learning theory has not yet provided us with a practically useful and easily applicable set of behavior-modification procedures relevant to smoking. It does, however, represent the clearest, most systematic, and potentially fruitful approach to date.

Discontinuation of smoking behavior

Internal constructs and variables, which were noted as characteristic of most maintenance theories, are no less evident in theories and models of discontinuation; and while they are often not the same ones, they do share an inferred, rather than an observed, nature. Thus, most models of discontinuation involve some sort of "decision-making process" that is influenced both by internal and external variables. In the general "health belief model" cited by Swinehart and Kirscht (1966), a given health behavior (e.g. quitting smoking) is most likely to occur when the individual is *aware* of his susceptibility to a health problem, when the actual occurrence of that problem is *seen* as having serious consequences, when the health behavior is *believed* to be effective in reducing the threat, and when obstacles to the behavior are *thought* to be minimal. In their report, Swinehart and Kirscht noted that, because too few subjects were available who actually changed their smoking behavior, the model was not adequately tested.

A more elaborate decisional model has been suggested and tested by Straits (1965). On this view, a smoker's decision to quit would involve changes in one or more of three "subjective variables": the state of nature (smoking is harmful or it is not), personal or "Bernoullian Utilities" (the relative values the individual assigns to the consequences of possible courses of action), and the subjectively perceived probability that a given state of nature will occur (belief in a smoking-disease relationship). Now since the actual state of nature is unknown, the decision to continue smoking or to quit is made so as to maximize expected utility. Straits' data provided only mixed support for the model, which was acknowledged as empirically weak because of the difficulty involved in measurement of the subjective variables.

Of even greater interest than his decisional model is Straits' (1965, 1966) use of multiple discriminant analysis to predict successful attempts at quitting smoking. He found that the best predictor of attempting to quit was mention by the smoker of specific, existing health ailments or a doctor's advice to quit. Success in quitting was best predicted by presence of physical ailments, heavier consumption, and older age.

Theories of discontinuation based on "decision-making processes" and such other internal concepts as willpower (e.g., Angus, 1963; Ochsner, 1964) are hard pressed to account for the well-documented observation that even though smokers are as well informed (if not better informed) as nonsmokers about the alleged hazards of smoking and in addition believe the information to which they are exposed, they do not attempt or express a desire to attempt to change their behavior (Leventhal and Niles, 1964; McGrady, 1960; Straits, 1965). Evidence that such individuals reduce the resultant "cognitive dissonance" by various means (Baer, 1966; Cannell and McDonald, 1956; Janis and Terwilliger, 1962; Levin, 1959; Quinn, 1961) is not unequivocal and results contradicting dissonance theory have been reported (Feather, 1962, 1963; Lane, 1961; Straits, 1965). "From the findings regarding dissonance theory as applied to smoking behavior, we are forced to draw the conclusion that there are a great many smokers tolerating a large degree of dissonance" (Guilford, 1966, 39). Straits' suggestion that further research be aimed at determining the means by which smokers maintain such dissonance would seem less fruitful than Guilford's recognition that its presence indicates the need for new approaches to the problem.

The learning-theory conceptualization outlined earlier would seem to represent such a new approach. Its use in treatment later, will be considered subsequently; for the moment, let only its economy be noted. No new variables need be added to its view of smoking maintenance to account for quitting. Thus, cigarette smoking is discontinued when the majority of the strongest reinforcers that act to maintain it lose effectiveness or when they are outnumbered or overpowered by reinforcers which maintain incompatible responses (not smoking).

This section has outlined a few of the theoretical notions that have been advanced to account for the maintenance and discontinuation of cigarette smoking. With this rough outline in mind, consideration should now be given in some detail to the behavior modification techniques that have evolved from them.

MODIFICATION PROCEDURES

By way of introduction, it might be noted that there have been at least as many (if not more) suggested modification techniques as there are theories to support them. Indeed, many exist without benefit, or restriction, of a clear rationale; while others, supposedly based in theory, do not have clear implications for validation of the conceptualizations from which they arose. Modification techniques, like the theories considered in the previous section, vary widely in subtlety and in recognition of the complexity and intransigence of smoking behavior. From the least sophisticated of these this review will move toward those that reflect more systematic and individualistically oriented approaches.

Legislative action

In spite of historical precedents that would seem to contradict such action, several countries have attempted to legislate cigarette-smoking behavior out of existence. In Ceylon, Norway, Romania, and the U.S.S.R. selective prohibition of smoking in certain places and/or by certain persons (children) have been put into effect (American Cancer Society, 1964). In the United States, where some bans also exist, it has been suggested that cigarettes be outlawed in a manner reminiscent of the Eighteenth Amendment, but such suggestions have not received support from public-health authorities. Brecher and Brecher (1964, 9) note that the memory of the experience of Prohibition is too fresh and that "the failure of even the most stringent laws to stamp out illegal traffic in narcotics is a further reminder that a better way must be found to achieve public health goals in a free society." Some legislative alternatives, such as prohibiting or limiting tobacco advertising (Italy and Great Britain) or requiring that health warnings be printed on each pack of cigarettes (United States), have been implemented, but outright bans seem clearly impractical.

Another governmental approach has been the establishment of an increase in taxes on tobacco and tobacco products. In Argentina and West Germany such revenue is used to actively discourage tobacco consumption (American Cancer Society, 1964); and it has been suggested that a one-cent-per-pack tax on cigarettes in the United States could finance an anti-smoking propaganda campaign even more extensive than the appeals of the cigarette manufacturers (Brecher and

Brecher, 1964). Even where such tax revenue is not available, anti-smoking campaigns are common. The American Cancer Society (1964) noted that twenty countries in addition to the United States sponsor them.

The results of antismoking legislation, tobacco taxation, and anti-smoking campaigns have not been encouraging. There is no sign at present that selective bans and health warnings on cigarette packs have been effective in curtailing the continuing increase in cigarette consumption. In Great Britain, where tobacco taxes have been steadily increasing since 1962 (Brecher and Brecher, 1964), there has been no measurable change in the behavior of that country's smokers. Such suggestions as placing differentially higher taxes on cigarettes containing more tar and nicotine (Brecher and Brecher, 1964) are reasonable but would probably have little real effect.

Campaigns

Various types of national antismoking campaigns, while becoming more imaginative of late, have for the most part met with very little measurable success. Even when such campaigns have been focused on relatively small target populations of children or adults, the picture does not improve. Neither do precampaigns and postcampaign measures of smoking behavior and/or attitudes change (e.g. Baltimore City Health Department, 1963, 1964; Cartwright et al., 1960; Evans, 1967; Horne, 1963; Jeffreys, Norman-Taylor, and Griffiths, 1967; Monk, Tayback, and Gordon, 1965) nor can the observed change be attributed to the campaign alone because of methodological limitations (Estrin and Querry, 1965; Horn, 1964; Watne, Montgomery, and Pettit, 1964).

Campaigns usually consist of some combination of lectures, movies, pamphlets, letters, posters, exhibits, scientific articles, newspaper items, and advertisements—tactics that have been criticized for their impersonal and nonmotivational approach (American Cancer Society, 1964). An alternative that has become increasingly popular in recent years is the smoking-withdrawal clinic. The first of these was begun in Sweden in 1955 by Dr. Borje Ejrup. Since then the idea has spread mainly to the United Kingdom (Dalzell-Ward, 1964) and the United States (American Cancer Society, 1964). Basically such clinics involve "an interpersonal, two-ended linkage between a counselor (usually, though not always, a physician) and the individual desirous of breaking his smoking habit" (American Cancer Society, 1964, 76). "Treatment" techniques vary considerably, and subjects may be seen individually or in groups. In Ejrup's original clinics and in many of those that followed, various kinds of medication were employed as an aid to quitting. Efforts of this type will be considered before clinics employing only "nonmedical" techniques. A subsequent section will deal with efforts to validate claims for the usefulness of such drugs. Suffice it to say at this point that their use has become widespread, either as the sole agent of therapy or in combination with other means.

Clinics employing medication

Ejrup's therapy changed over the years from 1956 to 1960 such that various combinations of techniques were applied during the ten-day course of treatment. As a rule, however, the would-be quitter received "information and education" regarding his smoking behavior (including discussion of his problem with a physician), explanation of treatment techniques, and one or more drugs, including lobeline, meprobamate, nicotine, anticholinergics, amphetamines, and caffeine. Results of this treatment were classified as "good" if, on the day preceding the final treatment session a subject (S) had not smoked at all or had smoked one-fourth or less of his normal rate. Results not meeting this criterion were termed "poor." The percentage of Ss who stopped smoking entirely increased over time such that 43 per cent had done so in 1956, while the figure had reached 88 per cent in 1960. The quit rate over all 2271 Ss in all reported explications (Ejrup, 1964) is 60.3 per cent. Six months after treatment, 50 per cent of the patients who had been successfully treated had relapsed, and after a year 70 per cent (in some series) had done so.

Evaluation of Ejrup's clinics is difficult as is typically the case, they were in fact clinics, not controlled experiments (with one exception: see section on drug studies). The reported increasing success rate may have been owed to a number of uncontrolled variables—including, as Ejrup has noted, the factor of suggestion. The major mechanism operating to produce the increasing success rate may have been an ever more powerful placebo effect as more drugs and more impressive techniques were employed. More will be said to this point subsequently. For now, let it be noted that the relatively high and constant relapse rate tempts one to suspect that such a factor might have been prominent.

Bachman (1964; 1966) has reported results of ten eight-week antismoking "courses." These were run in groups, with a maximum enrollment of thirty per course, which consisted of weekly ninety-minute meetings. The first half of each meeting was devoted to a medical lecture on smoking, its effects, and its dangers. During the remainder of each session discussion of problems and questions about lecture topics took place. In addition, each participant was asked to change to a less enjoyable brand of cigarettes, to paste a "poison" label or skull-and-crossbones on each pack, to carry a card reading "Is smoking worth it?" to avoid various types of "smoking eliciting" situations, and to pray (if desired). After the first two courses were completed, the use of lobeline sulfate in a cherry-flavored pastille was instituted as a smoking deterrent. Participants were instructed to take a pastille whenever they had a "strong desire" to smoke, but never more often than once an hour. All Ss were asked to keep a daily record of their smoking behavior throughout the eight-week program. A total of 254 individuals (mean age: 40; mean rate/day: about 40) took part in these clinics. Of these, 164 attended six or more of the eight meetings. At the end of treatment, 158 (62 per cent) had stopped smoking completely; and of these, 137 were subjects who had been regular attenders. Only 21 of the 90 who had attended less than six meetings succeeded in stopping. Of the Ss taking lobeline, 50 per cent succeeded in quitting, while only 27.2 per cent of the nonlobeline Ss quit. Follow-up data was not clearly presented, but the general impression is that after periods ranging from two months to one year, 34 (77 per cent) of 44 quitters followed up from the first five courses were still not smoking. However, this figure is probably not an accurate indicator of long-term success, since time elapsed after treatment was not the same for all Ss. The relapse rate may have been due to the data for short-term follow-up Ss. There is some evidence in fact (Bachman, 1966) that the success rate after one year was closer to 63 per cent.

Edwards (1964a) ran an antismoking clinic in which fifty smokers (mean age: 43; mean rate/day: about 27) received either buffered lobeline sulphate or a placebo (double-blind design) along with four weekly individual discussion sessions. A total of fifteen lobeline and sixteen placebo Ss dropped out of treatment. All remaining Ss reduced their smoking significantly during the clinic contact period, and there was no difference between the performance of the two groups. Of ten Ss who had stopped smoking completely during treatment, only five were still abstinent three months later.

In another clinic, Edwards (1964b) used either hypnosis or lobeline therapy on forty volunteers (mean age: 44; mean rate/day: about 30). In addition to these techniques, all Ss were given the opportunity during four weekly sessions to discuss various problems related or unrelated to smoking. Smoking behavior was recorded by all Ss during both the study and the week following it. The twenty Ss who were given hypnosis were placed in a "light trance" during each session and given the suggestion that the pleasures of not smoking would begin to outweigh those of smoking and that cues for smoking would now become signals for not smoking. Ss treated with lobeline were enthusiastically told of the beneficial effects of the drug in terms of its abilty to produce reduced craving for cigarettes, but they were further informed that their active participation and determination were vital. At each session the drug prescription was renewed. By the fourth session eight Ss had dropped out of each group. Of those remaining, twelve (50 per cent) succeeded in quitting by the end of the treatment. There were no between-group differences, even when only the twenty-four regular attenders were included in the analysis. Moreover, after the first week, during which the major behavior changes were noted, no further significant decreases occurred. At follow-up inquiries both groups were smoking more (nonsignificant for regular attenders) than at the end of treatment, and again there were no between-group differences. Unfortunately no individual data for those who quit were presented, so that it is difficult to assess their posttreatment behavior. Noting the similarity between groups, the author concluded that suggestion seemed to be the operative factor in both treatments.

Hoffstaedt (1964a, 1964b) conducted a clinic that offered individual treatment, involving "common sense psychological handling and moral support," as well as lobeline (2 mg., 4–10 tablets/day) as a smoking deterrent for some Ss. Of the 146 Ss (median age: about 40) who began, 57 (39 per cent) had dropped out by the second session. Of those remaining, 68 had completed treatment (duration not specified) at the time the report was published and 40 (58.8 per cent) of these were not smoking when last seen. No follow-up data was reported.

A clinic procedure reported by Ross (1964) of the Rosswell Park Memorial Institute may more properly belong in the section on drug studies, but it is included here because drugs were not the sole method of treatment. Seven group clinics were run, sixty Ss in each replication. Each treated S was given lobeline sulphate tablets (5 mg., 2/day) and .5 mg. cinnamon-flavored lozenges to be taken ad lib (presumably as a substitute for cigarettes). Those who felt that increased appetite and consequent weight gain would be a problem were also given amphetamine (8 m., one/day). Untreated Ss received placebo medication corresponding to that given treated Ss. About two-thirds of the Ss in each group took their medication as prescribed. In addition to the medication, which was dispensed in a double-blind design, all Ss received health information on the hazards of smoking by way of both lectures and printed material, as well as pretreatment physical examination. Group meetings were held once a week for one month, and a follow-up was conducted six months later. Results, which were highly variable across replications, were presented only in terms of percentages quitting after the first day and after one week. At the end of one week, 75 to 80 per cent of the treated Ss and 45 to 90 per cent of the placebo Ss had stopped smoking. Overall success rate at follow-up varied between 16 and 20 per cent. Ss not responding to follow-up questionnaires (number not reported) were considered relapses.

A far more extensive report of Roswell Park clinic activity was presented by Plakun, Ambrus, Bross, Graham, Levin, and Ross (1966), although it is not completely clear whether the data they report represents new Ss. They presented the results of eight clinics consisting of 313 Ss. Pretreatment indoctrination (with the exception of one group, which received none) included the medical lecture and physical examination mentioned by Ross (1964), a medical and smoking history taking, and a psychological questionnaire. During the first week each S handed in a daily report on medication-taking behavior, smoking behavior, and side effects. Weekly summaries of these behaviors were handed in during the subsequent three weeks of treatment. Otherwise treatment was identical with that reported by Ross (1964). Again, results were presented in terms of status after one week of treatment. Significantly more treated Ss than placebo Ss (66 per cent versus 50 per cent) were not smoking at that point. In addition, it was found that first-day status (smoking versus nonsmoking) was the best predictor of seventh-day success. The last clinic in the series, which had no indoctrination procedure, was the least successful. Only 122 Ss were included in the follow-up, which occurred from one to four months after treatment. Only 42 per cent of those who had not been smoking after one week of treatment were still not smoking at follow-up.

Graff, Hammett, and Bash (1966) ran a clinic designed to study, among other things, the best available methods for helping smokers to give up their habit. The procedure involved ten weekly meetings, for which each S paid $25.000 (not necessarily in advance). At the first meeting the 111 Ss present were given a briefing on the aims of the project, after which they decided whether or not to participate. Only thirty-seven individuals decided favorably, and each was assigned to one of four treatments: group therapy, hypnotherapy, lobeline, or chlordiazepoxide. After the assignments were made, three more Ss dropped out, leaving thirty-four (mean age: 41; mean rate/day: 20–30), of whom only twenty-four finished all ten weeks. Subjects who had not volunteered were used as a no-treatment control group. One therapist conducted the group therapy, another the hypnotherapy, and a third the two drug treatments. The first two were "highly committed" to helping people quit smoking while the third "approximated the attitude of a busy general practitioner dispensing drugs while giving brief supportive therapy" (Graff et al., 1966, 40). Follow-up was conducted three months after treatment. Of the twenty-four Ss who stayed in the program, nineteen (79 per cent) stopped smoking. At follow-up, fifteen (62.5 per cent) were still not smoking. Hypnosis was by far the most successful initially (100 per cent quit during treatment), followed by group therapy (55 per cent), chlordiazepoxide (33 per cent), and lobeline (29 per cent). Similarly, relapse rate was lowest for hypnosis and highest for lobeline. These results fit fairly well into the typical pattern that has taken shape so far concerning clinic treatment. However, lethal design errors (Underwood, 1957) render this experiment meaningless as a procedure aimed at making group comparisons. Such errors will be discussed in more detail subsequently. For the present, it is enough to note that treatments involving more suggestion and attention (drug Ss received a total of one hour of contact, as opposed to ten hours for non-drug Ss) from a "therapist" appear to be more effective than those not having these properties.

Leone, Musiker, Albala, and McGurk (1967) ran 312 Ss (mean age: 41; mean rate/day: about 25) in a series of nine six-to-eight-week smoking-withdrawal clinics employing a combination of educative talks, group discussion, and in all but one case, lobeline (natural or synthetic) or placebo medication. Specific procedures varied somewhat over the series, but results did not differ across clinics; and smoking reduction for lobeline Ss was not significantly different from that for Ss receiving placebo. A total of 255 Ss attended at least three clinic sessions, of whom 102 (40 per cent) stopped smoking during treatment, and 14 (5 per cent) quit at some point after clinic activity was over. Follow-up at a point at least nine months after clinic contact found the number of quitters reduced to 57 (22 per cent).

Clinics not employing medication

Lawton (1962) used a "group therapeutic" approach with nineteen Ss (rate/day: 20–60) who were seen for nine ninety-minute meetings over a period of six weeks. During these sessions the group discussed the smoking habit, the problems attendant upon quitting, and related topics. At the ninth meeting twelve (75 per cent) of the sixteen regular attenders were not smoking. At the twelve-week follow-up, only eight (50 per cent) were still abstinent, and this figure dropped to three (18.7 per cent) after eighteen months. Four years later only two (12.5 per cent) were not smoking (Lawton, 1967).

In a later study, Lawton (1967) assigned volunteer Ss (mean rate/day: 20–30) to one. of four types of group procedures: an educative program of health information, group therapy similar to Lawton's 1962 technique, a combination of these two, or an intensified version of group therapy. This last condition was a variant on "five-day plan" procedures (see below). The Ss assigned to the combination condition first served as no-treatment controls during the eight weeks of initial treatment. The intensive-therapy group (which was not recruited and run until five months after all other Ss had been run) also acted as a control group before treatment. In addition to being asked to wait for treatment, however, these Ss were instructed to attempt to quit smoking on their own. Each group was to have consisted of twenty to twenty-five members, but attrition both prior to and during treatment was high (as few as nine Ss took part in one group). Only one control S quit smoking during the waiting period, and he was in the group that had not been instructed to quit. All group techniques resulted in significantly greater reduction in smoking than occurred during control periods, but there were no differences in effectiveness among treatment conditions. One week after treatment, an average of 25 per cent of the Ss in all groups were not smoking. After seven months this figure had dropped to 17 per cent and was still at that level fifteen months after treatment. Interpretation of these results is complicated by some design confounds, but the attempt to employ relevant control procedures is encouraging. More will be said on this point subsequently.

Results of the clinic that provided the basic procedure for Hoffstaedt's (1964a, 1964b) work are reported by Cruickshank (1963a, 1963b). In this case the technique involved seven weekly individual sessions that, after the initial history taking, apparently consisted of discussion of the problem and "moral support." Of thirty-two participating Ss, only ten agreed to try quitting; the others decided merely to "cut down." All Ss kept a record of their smoking behavior throughout the study. Hypnotherapy, involving suggestion that smoking would be unpleasant, was used with an unspecified number of Ss. In addition, some Ss received unknown and uncontrolled medication for "withdrawal symptoms" from their family doctors. At the seventh session eleven Ss (34 per cent of the total, but 100 per cent of those who tried to quit, plus one) were not smoking. At a five-months follow-up three quitters had relapsed, leaving a success rate of 60 per cent relative to those wanting to quit, or 18.7 per cent of all Ss, participating. Relapse was more marked for those who had "cut down."

In cooperation with the Seventh Day Adventists, McFarland (McFarland, Gimbel, Donald, and Folkenberg, 1964; McFarland, 1965), inaugurated the now famouŝ "five day plan" to help smokers to quit. During each of five daily ninety-minute to two-hour sessions a combination of medical, religious, and informational techniques are employed, including lectures, films, demonstrations, and discussions. In addition, Ss are instructed to carry out a variety of extrasession procedures, such as embarking upon a program of physical fitness and going on a special diet. The "buddy system" is encouraged. Often, 200 to 400 Ss attend the meetings, although there may be as few as 12. The results reported on 144 Ss who had completed treatment indicated that 72.2 per cent had quit; but at the three month follow-up only 33.9 per cent were still not smoking. Five-day plans, like other clinic procedures, seem to be relatively popular in spite of their limited and relatively short-term effectiveness.

Hess (1964) reported some preliminary results from a clinic program that employed "five-day plan" techniques plus several additional features, including instruction of participants in breaking other habits in addition to smoking in an effort to divert attention away from the habit of reaching for a cigarette. A total of sixty-three cases were reported upon. Of these, fifty completed the "plan" and twenty-five were not smoking at that time. Six weeks later eleven had relapsed or could not be contacted, yielding a success rate of 28 per cent.

Somewhat better results with a "five-day plan" clinic were reported by Dale (1964), who found that 85 per cent of 644 Ss reporting had stopped smoking at the end of treatment. Incomplete six-month follow-up data indicated that 60 per cent were still abstinent.

Thompson and Wilson (1966) conducted a five-day clinic with 298 Ss (mean age: 39). Of the 201 completing treatment, 72.6 per cent had not smoked in the twenty-four hours prior to the fifth session. A rather confused presentation of follow-up procedures seems to indicate that of 287 Ss contacted ten weeks after treatment, 84 (29.4 per cent were still successful, i.e. had not smoked for at least seven days prior to the follow-up call), and there is some evidence that long-term success was more frequent among those who had been regular clinic attenders. Ten months after treatment, of forty-nine Ss (of whom sixteen had been abstinent at ten weeks) who were contacted again, only eight were still not smoking. Some participants in this project had had "partners" who were also attempting to quit. Cross-partner checks on accuracy of reports resulted in agreement in over 90 per cent of the cases.

In a study designed to characterize "quitters" and "non-quitters" Guilford (1966) compared the success rate of 173 participants in two "five-day plan" clinics with a matched group of 175 Ss who were given no treatment. All Ss (mean age: 42; mean rate/day: 31) were paid for their participation and were again contacted three and six months after treatment ended. No immediate posttreatment data were given, but at the three-months follow-up the treated Ss had a success (91–100 per cent reduction) rate of 34 per cent compared to 23 per cent for untreated Ss. Three months later these figures were 28 per cent and 17 per cent respectively. Of further interest is the fiinding that while no group differences in success rate were found for males, treated females did significantly better than females who were untreated. K. A. Campbell (1965) ran a "smokers' clinic" in which 73 Ss (mean rate/day: about 24) attended ninety-minute educational/group-discussion sessions on five consecutive evenings. No immediate treatment results were reported, but questionnaires returned by 70 Ss four weeks after the end of the clinic indicated that 28 (40 per cent) had stopped smoking entirely, 30 (42.9 per cent) had reduced their smoking, three had quit initially but had relapsed, and nine (12.9 per cent) had remained unchanged. A "reunion" meeting was held three months after the clinic. Of the nineteen Ss attending, sixteen were not smoking.

Mausner (1966) conducted a clinic that consisted of seven group-discussion sessions over a period of three weeks and was initially attended by seventeen Ss (age: 18-22; rate/day: 10–20). At the final session only four Ss were in attendance, and of these only two were not smoking. Ten weeks later only one of these was still abstinent. Smoking-behavior measures on an untreated control group (N=16) indicated that three had quit at the follow-up. The unexplained presence of one control S who was apparently a nonsmoker at the beginning of the study reduces the control quit-frequency to two.

While this review by no means exhausts the clinic literature, or even considers the large number of clinics now in progress (National Clearinghouse for Smoking and Health, 1968), the results reviewed here are typical. Most clinic procedures result in an immediate quit rate of from 30 to 85 per cent, which begins to deteriorate substantially over time as soon as the formal meetings are terminated. Clinics are open to and have received considerable criticism (e.g. Hochbaum, 1964; Plakun et al., 1966) mainly on theoretical grounds. Further comment will be taken up in a subsequent section on evaluation.

Antismoking drugs

For the present let us consider efforts to assess the pharmacological activity of several "smoking deterrent" drugs, some of which, as noted earlier, have been employed as an integral part of smoking withdrawal clinic procedures. There is a wide variety of such preparations, including anticholinergics, stimulants, and several types of nicotine substitutes (Ford and Ederer, 1965). Noningested agents, such as mouthwashes and astringents, will not be included in this review. Let us begin by examining the research on the original and still most widely used of the nicotine substitutes: lobeline, which is available in several preparations (Rosenheim, 1962) and whose action, like the other substitutes, in some degree mimics the effect of nicotine.

The first test of this drug's ability to deter smoking was conducted in 1936 by J. L. Dorsey. His subjects were instructed to take an 8-mg. lobeline sulphate pill whenever they felt the urge to smoke. After the "acute discomfort" of quitting passed, treatment was discontinued. While no data were reported, Dorsey (1936) indicated that this treatment is often effective. No significant side effects were noted.

A year later Wright and Littaur (1937) administered lobeline sulphate (8 mg.) to twenty-eight smokers and five nonsmokers and administered a placebo (magnesium oxide) to control Ss. As in Dorsey's (1936) study, all Ss were told to take a pill when they felt the need for tobacco. Smokers taking lobeline reported a reduced desire to smoke, though once again no data were presented. Of greater interest was the observation that those Ss taking lobeline experienced such severe gastrointestinal side effects that none of them took more than three pills per day for more than three days. Placebo Ss experienced no side effects. Wright and Littaur (1937, 653) concluded that "the effects of ingestion of the drug are too unpleasant to warrant its use in the doses recommended."

In an effort to avoid such side effects, Rapp and Olen (1955) combined a reduced dose of lobeline (2 mg.) with 100 mg. of fast-acting and slow-acting antacids (the compound is known as Bantron). Two hundred Ss kept a record of their smoking for one week prior to the study and were then given a week's supply of lobeline capsules, placebo capsules, lobeline tablets, or placebo tablets (dosage instructions were not specified) and were told to continue to record during that week. They were also told that the drug would curb their desire to smoke. One month later all Ss again recorded a baseline week, followed by a week of medication that was the exact opposite in form and content of that taken earlier. More than 80 per cent of the Ss stopped smoking during the Bantron week. During non-Bantron and control weeks, less than 10 per cent of the Ss stopped.

The same general procedure was used in a further test with forty new Ss who received either lobeline (minus the antacids) or antacids (minus lobeline). The results indicated that lobeline sulphate alone was not significantly more effective than the antacids alone. Such discrepant results are difficult to understand unless there was a difference in instructions or other variables across studies.

Bartlett and Whitehead (1957) tested the Bantron compound in a double-blind trial against meprobamate and a placebo. All thirty-three Ss (who did not want to quite smoking) took all three preparations for one week each in four different orders. Treatment weeks were separated by a "recovery week" (no drugs) and a baseline recording week (which also preceded the first drug week). All pills were to be taken three times daily and although Ss were informed that the medication would probably reduce their smoking rate, they were instructed to go on smoking whenever they wished. Neither drug was found to be more effective than the placebo in reducing smoking rate and, in fact, no significant changes in rate occurred. In a second experiment, sixteen Ss who wished to stop smoking were given either meprobamate or a placebo, to be taken ad lib (up to eight times daily) and told that the drug would reduce their desire to smoke. Three Ss in each group stopped smoking, and there were no differences across groups in terms of the drugs' perceived effectiveness.

Miley and White (1958) tested a compound containing lobeline (1 mg.) and copper sulphate against both the copper sulphate alone and an antacid placebo. Their sixty Ss, all of whom wanted to quit smoking, were instructed to take two tablets every four hours (up to eight per day). No differences between groups were found, either in terms of number of Ss quitting (15) or number cutting down (30).

In a double-blind test of Bantron, Rapp, Dusza, and Blanchet (1959) found, as before (Rapp and Olen, 1955), some evidence for the effectiveness of lobeline. Their fifty Ss (25 per cent of whom wanted to quit smoking) first recorded their smoking behavior for one week and then were given a starch placebo, to be taken after meals for a second week. Three weeks after the end of the placebo period, a second baseline recording week occurred, followed by seven days of Bantron medication, taken on the same schedule as the placebo. A unique feature of this study involved asking all Ss to save and turn in their cigarette butts during baseline, placebo, and Bantron weeks in order to provide a measure of weight of tobacco smoked as well as the usual frequency data. Results indicated that Bantron reduced the number of cigarettes smoked by Ss who wanted to quit; and, while not doing so for the other Ss, it reduced the amount of tobacco they smoked (in terms of weight). Thus, while those not wanting to quit lit as many cigarettes as before, they tended to put them out sooner.

Scott, Cox, MacLean, Price, and Southwell (1962) evaluated another lobeline preparation, known as Lobidan (lobeline sulphate, 2 mg.; magnesium carbonate, 125 mg.; calcium phosphate, 180 mg.). The Ss (N=55; rate/day: at least 15) were seen every two weeks and were asked to keep records of their smoking over the six-week study. Most of them wanted to stop smoking (number not specified). For the first two weeks all Ss took placebo pills three times daily, and half of them continued in the same way for the second two weeks, while the other half took Lobidan on the same schedule. For the final two week period each S received the opposite of what he had had during the previous two weeks. All procedures with the exception of those of the first two weeks were double-blind. Only twenty-nine of those starting the program completed it, and of these twenty-three wanted to stop. During the initial placebo weeks many (number not specified) Ss decreased their smoking rate (relative to an estimated baseline). Results of the subsequent four weeks' treatment indicated that four Ss did better on Lobidan than on placebo and that six others performed exactly the opposite. All other Ss (N=19) showed no difference between Lobidan and placebo periods. Unfortunately, complete data on actual quitting or rate reductions overall were not presented.

Another study involving Lobidan was conducted by Merry and Preston (1963) with 90 Ss (age: 20–65) who expressed a desire to quit smoking. Each was interviewed once each week during the four weeks of the study, and each kept records of smoking behavior throughout. Ss were told to quit smoking and were given no aid for the first week. During the second week Ss received antacid placebos to be taken three times daily. Those Ss who were still smoking after the second week were paired off on the basis of original consumption rate and degree of reduction, with one member receiving two more weeks of placebo and the other getting two weeks of Lobidan. About half the Ss followed medication instructions exactly, but nearly all took at least two tablets per day. A total of seventy-six Ss completed treatment, twenty-three (30 per cent) of whom had stopped smoking; thirteen of these after only the first two weeks. There was no significant difference in terms of rate reduction between the Lobidan and placebo groups.

London (1963) tested lobeline sulphate (.5 mg.) in a cherry-flavored lozenge against a placebo (the same lozenge minus the lobeline). All seventy-four Ss who wanted to "curb their smoking" were seen individually once each week for four weeks. They were instructed to take one tablet every one to two hours for the first week, every three hours the second week, every four hours the third week, and every five to six hours during the final week. In addition, they were instructed to smoke when they desired to do so and to record their smoking behavior. Six lobeline Ss and five placebo Ss dropped out before the end of treatment. After four weeks five lobeline and no placebo Ss had stopped smoking. Only four placebo Ss succeeded even in reducing their rate by as much as 50 per cent as compared to 24 lobeline Ss who did so. However, failure to employ double-blind procedures and the possibility that interexperimenter differences existed (several doctors conducting separate procedures at various locations pooled their data for this report) casts considerable doubt upon the meaningfulness of these findings.

A "smoking deterrent study" (1963) that employed double-blind procedures to test Lobidan against a placebo began with eighty-one Ss (rate/day: at least 20) who wanted to stop smoking. The Ss were assigned to treatment groups (Lobidan: 43; placebo: 38) and instructed to take four tablets per day during the six weeks of the study. Results were reported for thirty-nine Lobidan and thirty-six placebo Ss. After two weeks, 12 per cent of the Lobidan Ss and 8 per cent of the placebo Ss were not smoking; but at the end of treatment, 10 per cent of each group were abstinent. There were no significant between-group differences in terms of the number of Ss reducing their rate. None of the quitters in either group had relapsed at the six-week follow-up.

Ejrup (1964) reports a series of studies using lobeline hydrochloride or nicotine as smoking deterrents. Unfortunately, only one of these employed control procedures (Ejrup and Wikander, 1959, cited in Ejrup, 1964), and even in that case (where lobeline was found to be superior to a placebo) the drugs were apparently used in conjunction with more complex clinic procedures, making clear interpretation of the results impossible.

In an uncontrolled four-week trial of Smokurb (the cherry-flavored lozenge used by London, 1963), Swartz and Cohen (1964) found that 32.6 per cent of their forty-nine volunteer Ss (rate/day: 7–60) stopped smoking, 34.7 per cent reduced their rate, and 32.6 per cent were unaffected.

In spite of the weight of generally negative evidence apparent in the above review, various forms of lobeline still enjoy widespread use, both commercially and in private practice (e.g. Perlstein, 1964, cited in Ford and Ederer, 1965; Hoffstaedt, 1964a). The dismal picture presented by lobeline research is not improved on examination of the available publications on other types of drugs. Tests of benzedrine sulphate (Miller M. M., 1941), methyphenidate (Ritalin) and diazepam (Valium) (Whitehead and Davies, 1964), and hydroxyzine (Turle, 1958) failed to establish the effectiveness of any of these as smoking deterrents.

In general it seems reasonable to conclude that suggestion is the primary and common "active ingredient" in all antismoking preparations tested so far. However, even though the specific effectiveness of these agents is not supported, their nonspecific activity has important implications for the development of future behavior-modification techniques. This point will be considered again subsequently.

OTHER BEHAVIOR-MODIFICATION TECHNIQUES

Having now considered antismoking clinics and smoking-deterrent drugs, let us turn to an examination of the wide variety of other techniques that have been used to attempt to bring about the modification of smoking behavior. Many of these have been recommended for years and seem to share at least two common characteristics. First, they attempt to provide an alternative response that can "take the place of smoking"; and second, they act to produce substantial changes in the smoker's environment in addition to the absence of cigarettes. In 1938 Furnas noted several such procedures, many of which still survive as components of more complex programs such as "five-day-plan" projects or in various "how-to" books (e.g. Cain, 1964; Heise, 1962; Shryock, 1965). These involve such diverse activities as chewing food a certain number of times before swallowing, keeping especially clean, avoiding profane language, changing diet, rising early, taking hot baths, taking cold showers, sending clothes to be cleaned, and performing deep-breathing exercises, to name just a few. Unfortunately there has been little or no research designed to assess the effectiveness of such techniques, with the exception of Kaufman (1954) and Mees (1966), but it seems fairly obvious that whatever traditional value they possess results primarily from suggestion and/or incompatibility with smoking behavior. Moreover, that effectiveness depends to a great extent upon continued occurrence of the new behavior— a requirement that is often inconvenient, fatiguing, or both. This is not to say that certain of these activities are utterly useless, but one should be clearly aware of their limitations.

Many other antismoking techniques have been proposed, often without benefit of substantiating data. Thus Beck (1953, 1955) recommends that the smoker attempt to quit only for a specified length of time, followed by normal smoking (which will by then be aversive) and further abstinence. This plan allows "pharmacological addiction" to subside while avoiding the anxiety that may result from an irrevocable decision to quit and in addition incorporates a sort of aversive conditioning paradigm. Horn (1964) recommends among other things "systematic tapering off" by first abstaining in some specific situations and then gradually increasing their number until none that permit smoking remain. Homme (1965), utilizing the Premack principle (Premack, 1965), advocates increasing the frequency of various "coverants" (covert operants) that are presumably incompatible with smoking, such as "smoking causes cancer," by emitting them just prior to performing some higher-probability behavior (excluding smoking). This notion has implications for long-term maintenance of behavior change and will be mentioned in that context subsequently. There now remain several other treatment methods for which some data are available. These include hypnosis, role-playing, and behavior therapy.

Clawson (1964) and Povorinskii (1962) used and apparently recommend hypnotic suggestion as a main treatment technique, but they did not actually present results. Moses (1964) combined discussion with hypnotic suggestion of reduced pleasure from smoking in seventy-five adult smokers seen over a period of three years. All but five of these were seen for only one session, and only one for as many as three. Results were reported for the fifty Ss who could be contacted after treatment. Of these, thirty-seven had stopped smoking after treatment, but twenty-eight relapsed after periods ranging from a few hours to thirty months. The remaining nine Ss were still abstinent two to five years after treatment. Thirteen Ss reported no change in smoking behavior after treatment.

Von Dedenroth (1964a, 1964b) used hypnotic suggestion in conjunction with a series of instructions given over a period of three weeks that led to gradual reduction and then elimination of smoking. These consisted of having Ss change to a less desirable brand of cigarettes, cut out smoking for increasing periods after meals and before retiring, and the like. When S was in a "trance state" during each of the four sessions, the suggestion was given that smoking would become less pleasurable and would in fact be unpleasant. In the first series of fifty adult Ss (Von Dedenroth, 1964a), forty-eight were reported to have quit after treatment and remained abstinent for from four to thirteen months. In a subsequent series (Von Dedenroth, 1964b) 145 of 150 smokers quit, 40 per cent of these after only three sessions. Unfortunately no follow-up data on these Ss were reported.

At least two of the available studies employed nonhypnotic suggestion as the main treatment technique. Gould (1953) administered lozenges containing benzocaine and a variety of spices to 349 Ss as a smoking deterrent. The Ss were instructed to place a lozenge on the tongue whenever they felt a desire to smoke (average dosage was six per day). Complete results were not reported, but in 77 per cent of the Ss, "Smoking appeal was effectively reduced" (Gould, 1953, 54).

In a study designed to assess the effect of a "doctor's" smoking behavior during an initial interview upon success of subsequent "drug" treatment, Poussaint, Bergman, and Lichtenstein 1966; (Lichtenstein, Poussaint, Bergman, Jurney, and Shapiro, 1967) administered placebo tablets to ninety-seven Ss (age: 21–54; rate/day: at least 20) who believed they were taking part in a double-blind evaluation of a nicotine substitute. They were asked to quit smoking after the first interview (during which, for half the Ss, the "doctor" smoked) and to begin taking two tablets daily for thirty days and one per day for an additional fifteen days. All Ss were told that half the participants would be receiving a placebo. They were instructed to record their smoking behavior and any side effects, and they were seen for five-minute sessions at weekly intervals. Results were analyzed after four weeks of treatment for the sixty-three Ss still remaining in contact. At that time all Ss had reduced their rates by an average of 80 per cent (there was no "doctor" effect). A total of fifteen Ss were not smoking at all at this point. Only forty Ss were available at the six-month follow-up. Of these, eight were not smoking at all and twelve more, who had smoked at a reduced rate during the study, had since relapsed. About half the Ss assessed at follow-up indicated that they had found the "drug" helpful in quitting. While several methodological difficulties impair interpretation of these data relative to the stated aims of the study, they do not invalidate the finding that suggestion alone resulted in dramatic behavioral changes, especially during the first four weeks of "treatment."

An interesting, though less direct, approach to smoking modification has been employed by Janis and Mann (1965). Their twenty-six Ss (age: 18–23; rate/day: at least 15) were assigned to one of two conditions: "role-players," who acted in five scenes, or "judges," who listened to tape recordings of a "role-player's" scenes. The scenes were all related to smoking and lung cancer and included such situations as being informed by a doctor of the presence of cancer and of the necessity of immediate surgery and termination of smoking. Neither role-players nor judges were led to believe that the procedures were aimed at modifying smoking behavior. Postexperimental measures indicated that role-players showed a marked increase in anti-smoking attitudes relative to judges. Two weeks later role-players reported an average decrease in smoking of 10.5 cigarettes per day, while the average decrease of the judges was only 4.8 per day.

Later Mann (1966) employed three types of role-playing and two verbalization conditions; he found that "emotional" role-playing was more effective in changing both smoking attitudes and smoking behavior than was "cognitive" role-playing (acting as a debater).

As has been the case with theorists of other persuasions, behaviorally oriented investigators have been interested in smoking as a modifiable behavior. While aversive conditioning and desensitization are the most commonly reported techniques, other approaches have also been employed. For example, Tighe and Elliot (1967) required each of twenty-five Ss (mean rate/day: 25) to place a cash deposit ($50–65.00) at the beginning of a twelve-to-sixteen-week quitting program, which consisted mainly of signing a statement containing (1) a pledge not to smoke for the duration of the program; (2) an agreement that portions of the deposit would be returned at specific intervals, contingent upon abstinence, and that smoking during the experimental period would result in loss of the remainder; (3) an agreement to permit a notice of participation in the project to appear in a student newspaper; and (4) an agreement to read a specified article on the effects of smoking. Three such programs were conducted over a two-year period (N per program: 5, 9, 11). A total of twenty-one Ss completed the program (i.e. reported no smoking). Postprogram follow-up assessment contacts, made at intervals ranging from three to seventeen months, indicated that nine Ss were still abstinent.

Wilde (1964) used cigarette smoke mixed with hot air as an aversive stimulus, the presentation of which was made contingent upon smoking in a laboratory situation. In addition, presentation of lightly mentholated room-temperature air plus the opportunity to eat a peppermint was made contingent upon Ss' putting out the cigarette and saying, "I want to give up smoking." After six to twenty trials, S was invited to light a cigarette which, though not followed by the aversive stimulus, was usually put out voluntarily after two or three inhalations. Between daily twenty-five-minute sessions Ss were instructed to try to recall the laboratory situation whenever they wanted a cigarette and to eat a peppermint or other substitute instead of smoking. If smoking did occur, Ss were told to hold the cigarette between the lips as long as was tolerable and then to extinguish it. Treatment continued until an S reported that he was not smoking and that there was no longer a need to exercise "excessive self-control." Results with seven Ss were reported. Three stopped smoking after one to two sessions, one reduced his rate by 95 per cent after one session, one switched to a pipe after twenty sessions, and two dropped out of treatment. The five Ss who remained in treatment eventually relapsed (Wilde, 1965).

Franks, Fried, and Ashem (1966) made presentation of hot air and cigarette smoke contingent upon smoking in a similar, though better controlled laboratory situation. Each S smoked under these conditions until the situation became unbearable and was reinforced with cool, mentholated air upon putting his cigarette out. All Ss received twelve individual treatment sessions (ten trials per session) over a period of four weeks. Of the twenty-three who began, only nine completed treatment. No immediate posttreatment data were presented, but the six-months follow-up indicated that four Ss were not smoking, one was smoking less, one had switched to a pipe, and two had not changed their smoking behavior. One S was lost to follow-up.

Greene (1964), using mentally retarded Ss (age: 16–25), punished smoking in a laboratory situation by presenting white noise over on-going music in connection with it. Ten experimental Ss and eleven controls (who were not punished) were given one trial (listened to one of five tapes) per day on four successive days but were not told that the procedure would change their smoking behavior. Results indicated that the contingency did not reduce smoking behavior (inhalations/minute) even in the experimental setting. Indeed, both groups increased their smoking rate in the laboratory. This surprising result was attributed to reinforcement provided by sounds coming from automatic recording equipment. When a second control group was run without such equipment, no increase in rate was found. It was noted that termination of white noise (for experimental Ss) may have negatively reinforced smoking. At any rate, no decrease in smoking resulted with this technique.

Raymond (1964) reported the successful use of aversion therapy in a case report on a fourteen-year-old boy. Apomorphine-induced nausea was paired with cigarette smoking in each of three treatment sessions. The S stopped smoking after treatment and, according to the report of his parents, had not relapsed a year later.

A portable aversive conditioning apparatus, originated by Whaley, Rosenkranz, and Knowles (in press), has been employed by Powell and Azrin (1968) outside the laboratory setting to punish smoking behavior with electric shock. A total of six male smokers (rate/day for Ss completing treatment: 30–50) volunteered to participate in the study, while fourteen others declined. Half of the participants dropped out of the experiment prior to its completion. The three remaining Ss showed progressive reductions in smoking as shock intensity was increased. Ultimately one S reduced his smoking nearly 100 per cent while the others reduced their rates by 30 per cent and 70 per cent. When the smoking-shock contingency was removed, all Ss returned immediately to their preexperimental levels. It is of some interest to note that the number of hours per day during which the shock apparatus was worn decreased with increasing shock intensity. Verbal reports of smoking behavior were supplemented in this study by an automatic counter that advanced each time a cigarette was withdrawn from the shock apparatus; for two Ss additional reports were kept by volunteer coworker/observers who made five to twelve randomly spaced, direct observations per day of smoking or nonsmoking behavior. Agreement between the counter and the observer reports was 93 per cent and 88 per cent for S_1 and S_2, respectively.

While the results of aversive control techniques have so far not been particularly encouraging, further research is under way in the area, and there is some evidence of efforts to upgrade the technology, and perhaps the efficiency, of the approach (Lublin, 1968; Whaley et al., in press).

Koenig and Masters (1965) compared the effectiveness of aversive conditioning, supportive counseling, and a variant on systematic desensitization (Wolpe, 1958). Each of seven therapists treated six Ss, two under each treatment condition. After one week of baseline recording, all forty-two volunteer Ss (rate/day: at least 20) were seen for nine individual treatment sessions over a period of six weeks, during which time they were asked to gradually reduce and finally eliminate smoking. In the desensitization condition Ss were asked to signal, not when anxiety occurred, but when they felt a desire to smoke. Aversion therapy involved randomly shocking 50 per cent of eighteen distinct smoking-behavior components occurring in the laboratory. Supportive counseling consisted of discussions of the smoking problem and the "underlying" reasons for it. Although no significant main effect of treatment was found, there was a significant effect of the therapists, indicating that the skill of individual therapists, regardless of the treatment they administered, is the effective variable in reducing smoking. Moreover, while most Ss showed a decrease in smoking regardless of treatment condition, nearly all had relapsed at the six-months follow-up.

Ober (1966) assigned sixty volunteer Ss (rate/day: at least 20) respectively to a self-control program, aversion therapy, transactional analysis therapy (Berne, 1964), or no treatment. Each of two therapists treated six to nine Ss under each treatment condition. Following one week of baseline recording, all Ss (except controls) were seen for ten fifty-minute group sessions over a period of four weeks; at these sessions they turned in daily records of their smoking behavior. Follow-up consisted of four weekly reports; they were mailed to the experimenter (E) and their accuracy was checked through the corroborative reports of at least one acquaintance of each S (correlation between reports of Ss and those of friends was + .94). All treatment groups reduced their smoking rates significantly more than did control Ss, but there were no significant treatment or therapist main effects, either after treatment or over the follow-up period. A total of twenty-five Ss (69 per cent of those treated) were not smoking at the end of treatment, but nine of these had relapsed by the end of the follow-up period.

Pyke, Agnew, and Kopperud (1966) assigned fifty-five volunteer Ss to (1) a combination of individual systematic desensitization, group discussion, anti-smoking literature, and feedback (making graphs of progress and getting information on performance relative to the group); (2) monitoring (making graphs) alone for the first eight weeks; or (3) monitoring alone during the first and eighth week only. Each treated S attended one individual desensitization session and one group session a week for ten weeks. After treatment, only the treated Ss had reduced their rate significantly, but four months later they had relapsed to pretreatment levels.

In a study only indirectly related to smoking R. F. Sibley (1966) compared the effectiveness of group aversive conditioning with that of an educative program. Three replications of the experiment were performed, one with volunteers and two with nonvolunteers. The aversive conditioning paradigm involved pairing inhalation of cigarette smoke with color slides depicting, for example, advanced cases of mouth cancer, removal of a cancerous lung, and the like. "Cognitive" treatment consisted of a paper-and-pencil teaching program designed to present evidence relating smoking to lung cancer. Both treatments were completed in one session. In the replication involving volunteers, both treatments resulted in significant reduction in smoking (relative to pretreatment estimates of rate) and did not differ with respect to effectiveness. Results of one of the nonvolunteer replications indicated that only the aversion condition was effective in changing behavior, while those of the other treatment showed no result for either group. In all three replications, behavior change was measured for only six days following treatment, and no further follow-up data are available.

C. S. Keutzer (1967) assigned smokers to one of various procedures: a coverant control procedure (Homme, 1965); a breath-holding technique (Mees, 1966); a negative practice condition; an attention-placebo; or no treatment, to form a control group. All Ss (except those in no treatment) were seen once a week for five weeks, but only three of these sessions involved treatment (the first and last were devoted to introduction and debriefing, respectively). Treatments were administered in groups (N per group: 33–40), and possibly because of a required deposit of $20 (refundable after treatment), only three Ss dropped out of the experiment. All treated groups reduced smoking significantly more than did untreated controls, but they did not differ from one another. Reduction of smoking behavior was found to be unrelated to ten variables of demographic, smoking-history, and personality items (including extroversion and neuroticism, IPAT anxiety, and internal versus external control).

Other investigations (Janis and Miller, 1968; Marston and McFall, 1968; Resnick, 1968b; Rutner, 1967; Tooley, 1968) have employed and compared various behaviorally oriented techniques, such as stimulus satiation, covert sensitization, contingency management, contract management, response substitution, behavior monitoring, counterconditioning, self-reinforcement, and role-playing. These studies have failed to provide a clear demonstration of the superiority of any of them (except relative to absence of treatment); they thus corroborate the evidence provided by Keutzer (1967), Koenig and Masters (1965), and Ober (1966).

In order to test the hypothesis that the results of most smoking-modification treatments are explicable mainly in terms of the effects of nonspecific factors contained within them, Bernstein (1968) conducted a series of three experiments employing a total of ninety-six volunteer Ss (age: 18–25; rate/day: at least 20) in which a group smoking-withdrawal clinic procedure (emphasizing social pressure) was compared with an attention-placebo condition, a no-contact group, and two notreatment groups, both of which were instructed to try to quit on their own (one with and one without the promise of future treatment). Both social pressure and placebo Ss showed significant reduction in smoking but did not differ from each other. Ss asked to quit on their own displayed consistent and significant gains (at least as large as those found in treated groups) only if future aid was not expected. No-contact Ss' smoking remained essentially unchanged. Follow-up results, collected over periods ranging from five to sixteen weeks after treatment, reflected the now familiar picture in which relapse is the rule rather than the exception; though, especially in the first two experiments, the social pressure condition was superior to the placebo "treatment" in terms of maintenance of treatment-period gains. Unaided quitters who had not expected help tended to maintain their posttreatment levels—though again the effect was less pronounced in the third study. Smoking reduction failed to correlate significantly with internal versus external control, extroversion, suggestibility, or emotionality.

DISCUSSION

Evaluation of modification techniques

Paul (1966) characterized the current state of affairs in research on behavior modification by quoting Colby's (1964) statement: "Chaos prevails." As the preceding sections noted, that condition is clearly reflected in the research literature relating to the modification of smoking behavior and, as Paul (1966, 2) noted for the more general case, seems to result from "formidable methodological and control problems . . . and from a lack of a feasible model for outcome research." These serious shortcomings seem a function of the investigators who execute smoking-research projects as well as of the theories on which those projects are based. An examination of the research presented in this paper allows assignment of the researchers to categories closely parallelling those set up by Straits (1965) to describe smokers.

There seem to be investigators who are apparently uninformed with respect to the minimum methodological and design standards necessary for the generation of meaningful data. Their errors include failure to employ control groups, simultaneous manipulation of more than one independent variable in the same condition, failure to equate groups on important environmental and task variables (Underwood, 1957), such as duration of treatment or frequency of experimenter contact, and lack of control over other experimenter variables (often a different therapist conducts each treatment).

Other researchers seem to appreciate the need for control in the design of experiments but are apparently uncertain as to how to incorporate it in their projects. Thus, a "no-treatment control group" is made up of those individuals who do not volunteer for treatment (Graff et al., 1966); Ss' pretreatment estimates of smoking rate are used as a basis for change scores (e.g. Poussaint) et al., 1966; Scott et al., 1962; Sibley, 1966); or no base rate data are reported at all (e.g. Hoffstaedt, 1964a, 1964b).

The final type of researcher might be termed "unable" to include adequate control in his designs. This failure is due to limitations imposed by his goals. Most of those who fit into this category conduct projects that are not experiments. Their efforts usually (but not always) involve clinic procedures, with the aim of taking a group of smokers and by some means turning them into nonsmokers. While this goal is admirable (given that the smokers wish to quit), reports of uncontrolled attempts to achieve it can serve only to provide researchable hypotheses, not to validate the procedures employed. Failure to make this crucial distinction has resulted in the proliferation of more and more clinics whose methods are either carbon copies of those reported in the literature or an amalgam of several diverse partially successful techniques.

Claims for success notwithstanding, this type of clinic activity tells us little or nothing about smoking behavior or the means by which it can be reliably modified. Thus, except for those smokers who are helped, most clinic procedures reported to date represent a great deal of wasted time and effort (Bernstein, 1968). This is not to say, of course, that smoking clinics are useless; on the contrary, once appropriate modification techniques are developed, clinics will probably prove to be the most efficient means of large-scale implementation. However, since those techniques are now simply not available, the present need is for controlled experimentation (either within or without the clinic framework), rather than uncontrolled use of nonvalidated notions that, regardless of their apparent effect on smoking behavior, tell us nothing about it.

With these general criticisms in mind, consideration should now turn to some more specific methodological problems that are particularly troublesome in smoking research. As noted above, a great many investigations either lack control groups or employ inappropriate ones. While this state of affairs is obviously undesirable, a difficult question remains: What is an appropriate control condition for use in smoking modification research? As Paul (1966) has shown, the answer might involve several control conditions, each designed to subtract a particular segment of nontreatment variance. It must be made clear that, especially in smoking research, several types of "no-treatment" groups are possible and that the differences between them may be crucial. Let us therefore consider conditions that might be included in future investigations.

First, since mere participation in a smoking experiment may profoundly affect behavior (Merry and Preston, 1963), a group of Ss who are entirely acceptable in terms of *E*'s criteria could be told that they are (for some innocuous reason) in fact unacceptable for treatment. They could then be contacted at times corresponding to contact with other control and treatment groups. This condition would correspond to the minimal contact and lack of participation awareness found in Paul's (1966) "contact control" group; it has already been employed by Ober (1966) and Bernstein (1968).

Second, since it can be argued that assessment of the effectiveness of a smoking-modification technique should be made not only relative to "no treatment" but also relative to smokers' unaided efforts, one should control for such efforts. Thus, an "effort control" group could be told that, while they are acceptable for treatment, they will be required to wait (for a period corresponding to that covered by treatment of experimental Ss) until it becomes available. In addition, they could be asked to quit smoking on their own during the waiting period. Merry and Preston (1963) and Lawton (1967) employed a variant of this procedure through the use of an "unaided quitting" period.

Since the expectation of aid following an unsuccessful independent effort will very probably have an effect on that effort, yet another control is desirable. In this "expectation control" condition, Ss would be asked to stop smoking on their own but without assurance of later help. This can be brought about by informing the Ss that determination is the key to quitting and that no one else can help them in this attempt. Obviously, exactly what is said to such Ss would be crucial, since one would not want to introduce surplus demand characteristics (Orne, 1962) on the one hand or generate hostility on the other. The difficulties involved in setting up such a condition, however, are far outweighed by the control gained, and thus an "expectation control" group should be employed if at all possible (especially if "effort control" is used). At present such a group has been included in only two studies (Bernstein, 1968; Guilford, 1966).

The last control procedure to be discussed here is an extremely important though, except in drug studies, a largely neglected one. This is the "attention-placebo" condition, which, by providing the same degree of therapist contact, attention, and interest present in experimental treatment conditions while at the same time excluding "active" treatment procedures, determines the extent of behavior change based on "nonspecific treatment effects, such as the expectation of relief, therapeutic relationship . . . , suggestion, and 'faith'" (Paul, 1966, 22). While the use of placebo control is commonplace in studies relating to the effects of drugs on smoking behavior, it has been generally ignored in nondrug investigations. This serious deficiency in research design may prove to be more damaging, in terms of the meaningfulness of published smoking-modification data, than all other errors taken together. A good deal of data is now available to indicate that an attention-placebo "treatment" can be at least as effective as clinic procedures in modifying smoking behavior (Bernstein, 1968; Keutzer, 1967). If findings such as these can be further substantiated, they have obvious and far-reaching implications for both past and future smoking research.

The problem of appropriate control has been considered in some detail both because it is a necessary condition for meaningful behavior-modification research and because its presence in smoking research is the exception rather than the rule. Other methodological problems particularly important for research in smoking modification must now be considered.

The need to avoid simultaneous manipulation of independent variables within the same treatment condition has already been noted. Once this aspect of design (and that of adequate control) is satisfactorily handled, however, other, no less troublesome obstacles relating to the nature and validity of generated data arise.

The requirement is easily spelled out: accurate information regarding the smoking behavior of Ss prior to, during, and following their participation in the experiment. This need necessitates the assessment of baseline smoking behavior for at least one week prior to the first treatment session, continuous assessment throughout treatment (except for no-contact controls), and systematic follow-up contact. As noted, even these basic conditions are often inadequately met, such that results are based on estimates of undetermined validity.

In many studies self-report data are supplemented by a monitoring system that requires each S to keep a record of each cigarette he smokes, but institution of recording procedures does not in itself guarantee accuracy. Such procedures are open to criticism on the grounds that, first, Ss may intentionally or unintentionally commit recording errors, and second, the measurement technique, being reactive, therefore may affect the behavior it is to assess. While there is some evidence that smokers' reports of present behavior are, when elicited within a survey context, quite accurate (Hoinville and Biggs, 1966; Todd and Laws, 1959) and that, even under experimental conditions, validity coefficients may be high (Ober, 1966; Thompson and Wilson, 1966), this evidence does not mean that the possibility of falsification, especially during and after treatment, can always be ruled out.

Probably the best presently available insurance against such falsification is careful attention to the instructions given to Ss prior to and following the baseline recording period. If it is not emphasized that accurate reporting is vital in the interest of science, Ss may report spuriously low rates in order to avoid "ruining the experiment." If, on the other hand, too much emphasis is placed on recording procedures, accurate reporting, or the acceptability of reporting residual smoking behavior, it may be interpreted as instruction to continue smoking (perhaps at a lower rate) or to report smoking behavior even if none occurs, in order to be "normal."

It has been argued (e.g., Hoinville and Biggs, 1966) that self-report measures seem adequate, in the sense that the errors generated are small enough that, especially when smokers are placed in broad cate-gories (e.g. quit, reduced, unchanged), serious consequences for data interpretation are unlikely. However, acceptance of this point of view and continued, unsupplemented use of measurement procedures that essentially trust S to be only slightly and unidirectionally inaccurate in his reports seems untenable, especially in view of the paucity of available research evidence to support the use of such procedures (Hoinville and Biggs, 1966; Ober, 1966; Thompson and Wilson, 1966; Todd and Laws, 1959).

Ultimately employment of recording procedures, manipulation of instructional variables, and the like must be replaced by techniques capable of accurate and nonreactive measurement of smoking behavior. Development of such techniques is now just beginning (e.g. Densen, Davidow, Bass, and Jones, 1967), and it must continue if this measure-ment gap is to be closed.

Moving beyond the validity of the data, appropriate means of report-ing them should also be considered. The basic metric in nearly every smoking study has been the number of cigarettes smoked per unit time, and while at least one supplementary measure—weight of tobacco smoked—has been suggested (Rapp et al., 1959), rate per day is probably more meaningful in terms of the goals of smoking modification procedures (presumably the interest lies in changing the frequency of smoking, not its duration). The ways in which these data are reported, however, vary widely across investigations, with the result that lack of comparability is common.

Perhaps the most frequent discrepancies occur in the calculation of "success rates." Experimenters are, of course, free to set up their own criteria for posttreatment "success"; and though uniformity would be convenient, adequate specification of those criteria can avoid mis-understanding. Difficulties arise, however, when some investigators report success rates based upon the number of Ss beginning treatment, while others consider in their analyses only those completing treatment. It seems more reasonable to take the latter course, since it allows for more precise evaluation of the treatment techniques themselves without including relatively less meaningful data (i.e. data for Ss not fully participating). Of course, full information with respect to excluded Ss should be provided, including data on the condition to which they were assigned, the point of discontinuation, and the reasons for doing so. These data, in addition to "success rates," should be included as part of a complete evaluation of any treatment procedure.

The methodological issues considered in this discussion are, for the most part, basic. Most of the errors committed in smoking research involve internal validity (Campbell, D.T., and Stanley, 1966). While the problems of appropriate control are less obvious than the others, they are certainly not obscure. It is to be hoped that future smoking-modification research efforts will reflect increased awareness of the problems involved, as well as recognition of and determination to avoid past errors.

Some theoretical considerations

The purpose of this brief section is simply to point out again that theories relating to the maintenance and modification of smoking behavior can be validated only if they are testable. Thus, they must be capable of generating hypotheses and predictions whose fate, when tested under rigorously controlled experimental conditions, has implications for the status of the theory. Most "smoking theories" do not have this capability, thereby resulting in self-perpetuating "experimentation" based on unverifiable hypotheses and the manipulation or correlation of nonmeasurable variables.

As noted, the most promising and scientifically useful approach to the problem of smoking behavior seems to be that offered by learning-theory conceptualizations. Its view of cigarette smoking as learned, modifiable behavior, functionally related to a large but finite number of stimulus classes, provides investigators with a wealth of testable hypotheses that relate observable behavior to observable antecedents and consequents. The formulation and testing of such hypotheses is now in its earliest stages, and the research available so far (Bernstein, 1968; Franks et al., 1966; Greene, 1964; Keutzer, 1967; Koenig and Masters, 1965; Lublin, 1968; Ober, 1966; Powell and Azrin, 1968; Pyke et al., 1966; Tighe and Elliott, 1967; Whaley et al., in press; Wilde, 1964)—while not uniformly well designed and executed (Keutzer, Lichtenstein, and Mees, 1968),—provides a rough theoretical and methodological framework upon which future investigators may build. Indeed, if anything useful is to be learned about smoking modification, research in this area must, like outcome research in psychotherapy and other behavior-modification areas, enter a long-overdue experimental era (Paul, in press).

Present status and directions for future research

After six years of intensified research on cigarette-smoking behavior, preceded by decades of less feverish efforts, very little useful knowledge has been contributed, beyond the rather elementary observations that smoking behavior is widespread and becoming more so, that it is very probably unsafe, and that it is incredibly resistant to long-term modification. Moreover, little evidence is available at this time to indicate that the majority of workers interested in the problem are attempting to modify their own research behavior such that the cycle of relatively meaningless, though self-perpetuating "experimentation" can be broken. Attempts to refine, build upon, and apply nonvalidated techniques are still common and in turn generate most of the research that follows.

This state of affairs is primarily the result of two major obstacles to progress. The most prominent of these is, as already noted, the deplorable condition of current research methodology in the area. A second, more subtle difficulty lies in the persistence of investigators in asking the wrong research questions. A careful review of the available literature should make the following assessment obvious: the basic problem in the modification of smoking behavior revolves about long-term maintenance of nonsmoking, not about production of immediate, short-term behavior change. The latter can be accomplished by a variety of "treatments" (including individual effort and placebo), but is followed in the majority of cases by a return to pretreatment rates.

Failure to attack the very difficult problem of long-term maintenance has brought research to a virtual standstill in terms of its capability to reliably influence smoking behavior much beyond the point at which the "experiment" ends. As shown, treatment-period results can be accounted for in terms of the fact that most if not all "treatments" employed so far contain certain common agents independent of and usually more potent than the "active" treatment procedures programmed by E. The most obvious of these unrecognized and/or uncontrolled agents are suggestion, social pressure, demand characteristics, and placebo effects. While the effectiveness of some treatment techniques is probably attributable mainly to one of these agents (e.g. placebo effects in drug studies; social presssure in group clinics), it would be difficult to analyze any treatment procedure and fail to identify a combination of factors participating in the observed behavior change.

Instead of despairing over this situation and attempting to develop "truly active" (though perhaps short-term) treatments for use in clinic settings and the like, efforts should be focused upon the distillation of techniques that, regardless of their specificity or nonspecificity, will reliably bring about initial behavior change. At the same time attention must be directed to the development of procedures designed to maintain nonsmoking on a long-term basis. Ideally such procedures would be a natural outgrowth of or actually incorporated in the short-term behavior-change techniques.

Perhaps this method would involve bringing the Ss' smoking behavior under the control of stimulus classes that, though made relevant within the experimental context, would maintain control independently during the postexperimental period. The suggestions made by Homme (1965), for example, may prove to be extremely useful in bringing about such autonomous control. Regardless of the specific tactics, the important point here is that a great deal may be discovered about the nature and modification of smoking behavior if meaningful research questions are asked. It is to be hoped that future investigators will recognize the necessity of doing so and will in addition appreciate and attempt to fulfill the methodological requirements that are prerequisites for obtaining unambiguously interpretable answers to the questions they pose.

This paper has considered the nature of the problem posed by cigarette-smoking behavior as well as the means by which its modification has been attempted. It became obvious that the problem is a major one and that there is a real need for the development of reliable modification techniques for use with individuals who wish to discontinue smoking.

It was noted that the theoretical underpinnings of most smoking-modification research are inadequate because they are not capable of generating treatment techniques that can validate or invalidate them; the design of and methodology employed in most smoking-modification research is so poor that the data generated are not meaningful; a crucial aspect of the problem—the need for long-term maintenance of nonsmoking—has been largely ignored, with the result that much current research is following a directionless, or at best circular, course.

Recommendations for upgrading research, in terms both of design and methodology, were made in the hope that the present state of knowledge with respect to the modification of smoking behavior can begin to expand.

Personality and Smoking: A Review of the Empirical Literature

GENE M. SMITH

STUDIES of the differences between smokers and nonsmokers have concentrated on many variables: disease; age; sex; race; socioeconomic status; intelligence; academic performance; religion; occupation; marital status; accident-proneness; personality; attitudes toward smoking; and smoking practices of parents, siblings, peers, and spouses. In addition, many speculative articles have discussed the "psychology of smoking." The present review deals only with *empirical* studies of relations between smoking and *personality*. (For a broader treatment, see Matarazzo and Saslow, 1960; Larson et al., 1961; and the report by the Advisory Committee to the Surgeon General, published by the U.S. Public Health Service, 1964.)

This review will attempt to answer three questions: What conclusions are justified by the empirical literature concerning the relations between smoking and personality? What value does this literature have? What changes in research strategy might enhance its future yield?

The studies reviewed here vary in quality and approach. Sample sizes range from 22 to 3,666. Methods of classifying pipe smokers, cigar smokers, and ex-cigarette smokers differ, as do the cut-off points used for distinguishing degrees of smoking—for example, mild, moderate, heavy, very heavy. In addition, numerous methods have been used to measure various aspects of personality,[1] and the populations sampled by different investigators vary widely. Despite these differences, some order does emerge, and some definitive conclusions can be drawn from the accumulated data. Indeed, where results are consistent in spite of differences in instruments and populations, the very heterogeneity of approach adds to the generality of meaning of the findings.

The literature relating smoking to personality is organized under seven categories: extraversion, antisocial tendencies, internal-external control, impulsiveness, orality, mental health, and miscellaneous. This choice is intuitive and arbitrary. It is defended here only on the grounds that for summarization some conceptual scheme was needed, and this one seemed appropriate.

Construction of tables

Before discussing the results summarized in Tables 1–6, a few comments will be made concerning the conventions followed in constructing the tables. Each entry identifies the author(s), year of publication, sample size, characteristics of the sample, procedure used to measure personality, direction of association[2] between personality and smoking, and an indication of whether that association reached the two-tailed 0.05 level of significance.

When a particular study yields separate and independent analyses of

1. The following personality questionnaires were used in one or more of the studies reviewed here; they are referred to by abbreviations: Cornell Medical Index (CMI), California Personality Inventory (CPI), Edwards Personal Preference Schedule (EPPS), Guilford-Zimmerman Temperament Survey (G-Z), James Test of Internal and External Control (JTIEC), Maudsley Personality Inventory (MPI), Minnesota Counseling Inventory (MCI), Minnesota Multiphasic Personality Inventory (MMPI), Neuropsychiatric Screening Adjunct (NSA), Saslow Psychosomatic Screening Inventory (SPSI), Sixteen Personality Factor Questionnaire (16 PF), Strong Vocational Interest Blank (SVIB), and Taylor Manifest Anxiety Scale (TMAS). In addition to these published questionnaires, numerous unpublished questionnaires were also used. These will be referred to hereafter as Special Questionnaires (SQ). The standard abbreviations are used to designate scales of the MMPI: Lie (L), Hypochrondriasis (H_s), Depression (D), Hysteria (H_y), Psychopathic Deviate (P_d), Masculine-Feminine (Mf), Paranoia (P_a), Psychasthenia (P_t), Schizophrenia (S_c), Hypomania (M_a), Social Introversion (Si).

2. Throughout this review the term "association" is used to refer to the findings themselves, rather than to the statistical test applied to those findings. Thus, smoking is said to be significantly associated with a particular aspect of personality, whether the significance of that relationship was found with measures of correlation or with measures of group-differences.

different samples (e.g. males and females), each analysis is entered separately in the tables. Similarly, when a particular study yields useful information with more than one instrument, separate entries are made.

The symbol S+ means that smoking is positively associated with the personality trait listed at the top of the table and that the association is significant at the 0.05 level with a two-tailed test. Usually this means simply that smokers have more of the characteristic than nonsmokers, but not always. In some instances heavy smokers are compared with light smokers (e.g. Dubitzky and Schwartz, 1968); in others, moderate plus heavy smokers are compared with mild plus nonsmokers (e.g., Jacobs, Knapp, Anderson, Karush, Meissner, and Richman, 1965); in still others (e.g. Eysenck, Tarrant, Woolf, and England, 1960; Eysenck, 1963; Schubert, 1965) comparisons are made across groups (e.g. nonsmokers versus moderate versus heavy). In some studies different groups are compared regarding amount of smoking. Friedman and Rosenman (1959) studied the amount of smoking in each of two groups of subjects classified by personality "type." Lawton and Phillips (1956) compared neuropsychiatric patients and general medical surgical patients regarding amount of smoking. Raab and Krzywanek (1965) studied the amount of smoking in each of two groups classified in terms of emotional excitability. In all cases, however, the symbol S+ means that a significant positive association was found between smoking and the personality trait listed at the top of the table. Similarly, S— means that the association was significant and negative. When the association between smoking and personality does not reach the 0.05 level of significance with a two-tailed test, the symbol N.S. is entered in the table.

The meaning of S+ and S— is determined by the title at the top of the table, not by the title of the personality scale used. For example, whether a high score on a particular scale indicates high extraversion or high introversion, the symbol S+ means that smokers are significantly more extraverted than nonsmokers.

Some investigators reported results at the item level. When such results are incorporated in tables here, the word "items" follow the abbreviation for the test. Where a single item is used to test the association between personality and smoking, that item is reproduced in the legend of the table.

Extraversion

The information in Table 1, dealing with the association between smoking and extraversion, is based on twenty-five analyses found in

Table 1. Extraversion

Author(s)	Year	N	Sample Characteristics	Measurement Procedure	Result
Davis	1956	775	British males, age 16-54	S.Q.	Not Reported
McArthur et al.	1958	252	College males	SVIB	S+
Schubert	1959	226	College males and females	MMPI:Si	S+
Eysenck et al.	1960	2360	British males, age 40-70	S.Q.	S+
Eysenck	1963	3000	British males, age 45-64	S.Q.	S+
Straits and Sechrest	1963	125	College males	MMPI:Si	N.S.
Feather	1963	78	Australian college males	MPI	S+
Salber and Rochman	1964	131	High school senior males	MCI:items	S+
		153	High school senior females	MCI:items	S+
Schubert	1965	956	College males and females	MMPI:Si	S+
		314	College males and females	MMPI:si	S+
Cattell and Krug	1967	256	College males and females	16 PF:introversion	S+
Lane et al.	1966	675	Airmen	G-Z.:sociability	N.S.
Evans et al.	1967	1851	College males	MMPI:Si	S+
		1815	College females	MMPI:Si	S+
Smith	1967	512	Female nursing students	16 PF:introversion	S+
		700	Female nursing students	peer ratings	S+
		208	College males	peer ratings	S+
		121	College females	peer ratings	S+
Smith	1969a	188	High school males	peer ratings	S+
		198	High school females	peer ratings	S+
		80	Junior high school males	peer ratings	S+
		96	Junior high school females	peer ratings	S+
Smith	1969b	331	Puerto Rican high school females	peer ratings	S+
		568	Puerto Rican high school males	peer ratings	S+

fifteen reports. Of the twenty-five analyses reported in Table 2.1, twenty-two yielded significant associations between smoking and extraversion, and all twenty-two showed smokers to be more extraverted than nonsmokers. (Of the remaining three analyses, two failed to find a significant association and one did not report a test of significance.)

Significant association between smoking and extraversion has been found with various instruments (MCI, MMPI, MPI, 16 PF, special questionnaires, and peer ratings) and in various populations (United States adult males and females, United States high-school and junior-high-school males and females, British and Australian adult males, and Spanish-speaking high school males and females).

Anti-social tendencies

Table 2 presents 32 analyses from nineteen published reports dealing with the relations between smoking and what is called here "antisocial tendencies." This category includes measures of rebelliousness, belligerence, psychopathic deviance, defiance, misconduct, and disagreeableness. Of the thirty-two analyses, twenty-seven yielded significant relations; all twenty-seven indicated that smokers are more antisocial than nonsmokers.

As in the case of the data concerning extraversion, the data linking smoking and antisocial tendencies come from studies that vary widely in the instruments used (CPI, EPPS, G-Z, MCI, MMPI, NSA, special questionnaires, teacher ratings, and peer ratings) and in the populations studied (United States adult males and females, United States high-school and junior-high-school males and females, and Spanish-speaking high-school males and females.)

Response bias

Matarazzo and Saslow (1960) and Weatherley (1965) mention the possibility that the association between smoking and report of socially undesirable characteristics might be artifactual. Weatherley states: "It is possible that this kind of finding does not accurately reflect substantive differences between smokers and nonsmokers on the specific personality dimensions presumably measured, but rather is a product of a response-set artifact. Smokers may merely be relatively more willing than nonsmokers to acknowledge socially undesirable characteristics in themselves." Such an interpretation is consistent with the findings of Schubert (1965) and Evans et al. (1967) that smokers have significantly lower L scores on the MMPI than do nonsmokers.

The data on smoking and antisocial tendencies collected by non-questionnaire procedures is especially helpful in assessing the interpretation just mentioned. Stewart and Livson (1966) studied a sample of about 100 boys and girls who were annually evaluated by teachers, from kindergarten through ninth grade, regarding behavior in school, attitudes toward school, and conduct. These same students were rated annually (eighth through eleventh grades) on "resistance to authority . . . by three staff members who had observed the subjects in a variety of social situations." Subsequently, in their early thirties, these subjects were classified as either smokers or nonsmokers, and those two groups were then compared regarding scores on the earlier behavioral measures of "rebelliousness." Under these conditions of study, adult smokers were found to be significantly more "rebellious" as children, than were the adult nonsmokers.

Similarly, in a study of 1,029 adults and 568 preadults in which personality was assessed with peer ratings, Smith (1969a) found that smokers received significantly lower scores on each of six personality traits loading positively on a factor he calls "agreeableness" and received significantly higher scores on each of five traits loading negatively on that factor. The consistency of those results is unmistakable. In both the adult and the preadult samples each of the eleven traits differentiated between smokers and nonsmokers at or beyond the 0.001 level of significance. In a later study of 568 male and 331 female Spanish-speaking high-school students Smith (1969b) found further confirmation of these results. Of twenty-two analyses (males and females analyzed separately on each of eleven personality traits), all were in the direction of smokers' being more disagreeable than nonsmokers, and nineteen of those twenty-two were significant at or beyond the 0.05 level.

Internal-external control

Table 3 presents results of five analyses dealing with "Internal-External Control," defined by James et al. (1965) as a measure "of the extent to which a person perceives events as determined by factors intrinsic to himself or manipulable by himself versus the extent to which he views events as determined by fate, chance or the manipulations of others." Of these five analyses, four yielded significant associations (the fifth is almost significant), and all five showed smokers to be more externally oriented than nonsmokers; that is, smokers are more likely than nonsmokers to think that what happens to them is due more to chance than to their own efforts and skills.

Table 2. Antisocial tendencies

Author(s)	Year	N	Sample Characteristics	Measurement Procedure	Result
Lawton and Phillips	1956	63	General medical and surgical patients	SQ:grouchy, disagreeable	S+
Lilienfeld	1959	1806	Males and females, age 18-70+	NSA:items	S+
Schubert	1959	226	College males and females	MMPI:Pd	S+
Koponen	1960	1418	Adult males	EPPS:aggression	S+
Thomas	1960	657	Medical students (mostly males)	SQ:anger in response to stress	S+
Whiskin et al.	1962	402	Males and females, age 50-90	MMPI:Pd	N.S.
Straits and Sechrest	1963	125	College males	MMPI:Pd	S+
Salber and Rochman	1964	131	High school senior males	MCI:items	S+
		153	High school senior females	MCI:items	S+
Jacobs, Knapp, et al.	1965	97	Adult males	SQ:defiance	S+
		136	Adult males	SQ:defiance	N.S.
McDonald	1965	129	Unmarried first pregnancy females	MMPI:Pd	S+
Schubert	1965	956	College males and females	MMPI:Pd	S+
		314	College males and females	MMPI:Pd	N.S.
Weatherley	1965	182	Male college students	EPPS:aggression	N.S.
Jacobs, Anderson, et al.	1966	134	Adult males	SQ:defiance	S+
Lane et al.	1966	675	Airmen	G-Z:scales F & P °	S+
Stewart and Livson	1966	99	Males and females	Teacher Ratings	S+
		83	Young adult males	CPI & MMPI:Pd	S+
		82	Young adult females	CPI & MMPI:Pd	S+
Evans et al.	1967	1851	College males	MMPI:Pd	S+
		1815	College females	MMPI:Pd	S+
Smith	1967	762	College males and females	EPPS:aggression	N.S.†
		700	Nursing students	Peer ratings	S+

Author(s)	Year	N	Sample Characteristics	Measurement Procedure	Result
		208	College males	Peer ratings	S+
		121	College females	Peer ratings	S+
Smith	1969a	188	High school males	Peer ratings	S+
		198	High school females	Peer ratings	S+
		80	Junior high school males	Peer ratings	S+
		96	Junior high school females	Peer ratings	S+
Smith	1969b	331	Puerto Rican high school males	Peer ratings	S+
		568	Puerto Rican high school females	Peer ratings	S+

* Scales F and P are "Friendliness" and Personal Relations," respectively.
† One of four samples was significant; the other three were not.

Table 3. External control

Author(s)	Year	N	Sample Characteristics	Measurement Procedure	Result
Lilienfeld	1959	1806	Males and females, age 18-70+	NSA:item *	S+
Straits and Sechrest	1963	245	College males	JTIEC	S+
James et al.	1965	185	College males	JTIEC	S+
		272	College females	JTIEC	S+
Christiano et al.	unpublished		High school males and females	SQ:item ‡	N.S.†

* This item reads as follows: Do you feel you get more than your share of bad luck (Reviewer's comment: Lilienfeld's item does not precisely fit James' definition of Internal-External Control, but does relate to that concept; hence, results obtained with it are included in this table.)
† This t-value of 1.94 is just short of the 1.96 which is needed for p=0.05 with a two-tailed test. If significant, it would have been entered as S+.
‡ The item reads as follows: When a man is born, the success or failure he is going to have is already in the cards, and there is not much he can really do to change it.

Table 4. Impulsiveness

Author(s)	Year	N	Sample Characteristics	Measurement Procedure	Result
Lilienfeld	1959	1806	Males and females, age 18-70+	NSA:item *	S+
Whiskin et al.	1962	174	Males, age 50-90	MMPI:Gough's Impulsivity Scale	N.S.
		228	Females, age 50-90	MMPI:Gough's Impulsivity Scale	S+
Eysenck	1963	3000	British males, age 45-64	SQ	N.S.
Jacobs, Knapp, et al.	1965	97	Adult males	SQ:impetuousness	S+
		136	Adult males	SQ:impetuousness	S+
Schubert	1965	172	College males and females	SQ †	S+
Jacobs, Anderson, et al.	1966	134	Adult males	SQ:impetuousness	S+
Lane et al.	1966	675	Airmen	G-Z:restraint	S+
Dubitzky and Schwartz	1968	324	Adult males	MMPI:Block's Scale of Ego Control	N.S.

* This item reads: Do you often say things you later wish you had not said?
† Sanford, N., Webster, H., and Freedman, M.: "Impulse expression as a variable of personality." *Psychological Monograph,* 1957, 71, Whole No. 440.

Impulsiveness

Table 4 presents results of ten analyses dealing with "impulsiveness." Of these, seven showed significant association between smoking and impulsiveness; all seven indicated that smokers are more impulsive than nonsmokers. The study with the largest sample (3,000 British adult males) is one of the three studies (out of ten) that failed to show a significant relationship between impulsiveness and smoking (Eysenck, 1963). The study by Dubitzky and Schwartz (1968), which also failed to find a significant association, did not compare smokers and non-smokers; rather, it compared light and heavy smokers on a measure of "ego control" derived from the MMPI. The heavier smokers scored lower on this scale, but the difference reached only the 0.10 level of significance. Whiskin et al. (1962) failed to find a significant association between smoking and impulsiveness (measured with Gough's Impulsivity Scale) in their sample of 174 aged men (average age=70), but they did find a significant association in their sample of aged women. In addition to the study of aged females just mentioned, six other studies showed smokers to be more impulsive than nonsmokers. Three used a specially developed questionnaire called "Impetuousness" (Jacobs, Knapp, et al., 1965; Jacobs, Anderson, et al., 1966), one used a single item (Lilienfeld, 1959), one used a scale of "Impulse Expression" (Schubert, 1965), and one used the G-Z measure of "Restraint" (Lane et al., 1966).

Orality

Table 5 reports the results of four studies of the association between smoking and orality. In one, the Blacky Pictures were administered to seven heavy smokers and fifteen nonsmokers; the investigators report that smokers scored significantly higher than nonsmokers on "oral craving" and "playfulness" (Kimeldorf and Geiwitz, 1966). In the remaining three studies, all conducted in the same laboratory (Jacobs, Knapp, et al., 1965, Jacobs, Anderson, et al., 1966), orality was measured with a questionnaire containing items dealing with "nail biting, pencil chewing, beer drinking, excessive coffee intake or injestion of medicines" and other "non-nutritional oral intake activities." One of these three studies (N=97) found no significant association between orality and smoking, a second (N=134) found significantly more orality among smokers than among nonsmokers, and a third (N=136) found significantly more orality among heavy smokers than among nonsmokers.

Table 5. Orality

Author(s)	Year	N	Sample Characteristics	Measurement Procedure	Result
Jacobs, Knapp, et al.	1965	97	Adult males	SQ	N.S.
		136	Adult males	SQ	S+ [*]
Jacobs, Anderson, et al.	1966	134	Adult males	SQ	S+
Kimeldorf and Geiwitz	1966	22	College males	Blacky Test	S+

[*] The comparison of heavy smokers versus nonsmokers yields a t-value of 2.45. The comparison of moderate plus heavy versus mild plus nonsmokers yields a t-value of 1.50, which is not significant by the criterion employed here.

Table 6. Mental health

Author(s)	Year	N	Sample Characteristics	Measurement Procedure	Result
Lawton and Phillips	1956	85	Adult males	Groups compared re amount of smoking	S—
		63	Adult males	CMI:emotional disturbance	S—
Moodie	1957	156	Adult males	Nervousness; method not given	S—
Heath	1958	247	College males	Psychiatric rating of "personality integration"	N.S.
McArthur et al.	1958	252	College males	Physician's rating of "personality integration"	N.S.
				Physician's prediction of college adjustment	S—
Lilienfeld	1959	1806	Males and females, age 18-70+	NSA:neuroticism	S—
Schubert	1959	226	College males and females	MMPI:Ma	S—
				MMPI:Hs, D, Hy, Pa, Pt, Sc	S—
					N.S.
Eysenck et al.	1960	2360	British males, age 40-70	SQ:neuroticism	N.S.
Matarazzo and Saslow	1960	40	Psychiatric patients	TMAS	N.S.
				SPSI	N.S.
		114	Nursing students	TMAS	S—
				SPSI	S—

Author	Year	N	Sample	Measure	Result
		140 (Sexes combined)	College males, College females	TMAS	S—
				SPSI	N.S.
Thomas	1960	657	Medical students, mostly males	TMAS	N.S.
				SPSI	N.S.
				SQ:nervous tension [*]	N.S.
Ryle	1962	75	Males	CMI:neuroticism	S—
		85	Females	CMI:neuroticism	N.S.
Whiskin et al.	1962	402	Males & Females, age 50-90	MMPI & CMI	N.S.
Eysenck	1963	3000	British males, age 45-64	SQ:neuroticism	N.S.
Salber and Rochman	1964	131	High school senior males	MCI:emotional stability	N.S.
		153	High school senior females	MCI:emotional stability	N.S.
Gadourek	1965-1966	1382	Dutch adults	Interview: tensions, anxiety	N.S.
				SQ:emotional lability	S—
Jacobs, Knapp, et al.	1965	97	Adult males	SQ:emotional lability	N.S.
		136	Adult males	MMPI	N.S.
McDonald	1965	129	Unmarried 1st pregnancy females	SQ:emotional excitability	not reported
Raab and Krzywanek	1965	77	Males	MMPI:Ma	S—
Schubert	1965	314	College males and females	MMPI:Hs, D, Hy, Pa, Pt, Sc	N.S.
				MMPI:Ma	S—
		956	College males and females	MMPI:Hs, D, Hy, Pa, Pt, Sc	N.S.
Jacobs, Anderson, et al.	1966	134	Adult males	SQ:emotional lability	S—

Author	Year	N	Group	Measure	
Lane et al.	1966	675	Airmen	G-Z:emotional stability	S−
Cattell and Krug	1967	256	College males and females	16 PF:anxiety	N.S.
Evans, et al.	1967	1851	College males	MMPI:Hy, Sc, Ma	S−
		1815	College females	MMPI:Hy, Sc, Ma	S−
Smith	1967	512	Nursing students	16 PF:anxiety	N.S.
		700	Nursing students	Peer ratings: emotional	S−
		208	College males	Peer ratings: emotional	S−
		121	College females	Peer ratings: emotional	S−
Smith	1969a	188	High school males	Peer ratings: emotional	N.S.
		198	High school females	Peer ratings: emotional	N.S.
		80	Junior high school males	Peer ratings: emotional	N.S.
		96	Junior high school females	Peer ratings: emotional	S−
Smith	1969b	331	Puerto Rican high school males	Peer ratings: emotional	S−
		568	Puerto Rican high school females	Peer ratings: emotional	S−

* Differences between smokers and nonsmokers are tested separately for each of 25 items concerning habits of nervous tension. (No test is reported for the total scale of 25 items.) Only three items differentiate significantly; two are classified as S− and one as S+. Of the remaining 22 items, 15 are in the S− direction.

Mental health

Table 6 summarizes the data relating smoking to the admittedly broad and unwieldy concept of "mental health," referred to variously by different investigators as "neuroticism," "nervousness," "anxiety," "psychosomatic distress," "adjustment," "emotional stability," "emotional excitability," "emotional lability," and "emotionality." The results reported in Table 6 do not yield an internally consistent picture. This is almost certainly due, at least in part, to the great heterogeneity of material presented in the table. Slightly more than half the analyses show a significant association between smoking and some aspect of "mental health." In all instances where a significant association was found, the smokers had poorer mental-health scores than did the nonsmokers. Nevertheless, numerous studies failed to confirm this association, and in several instances such failures emerged in studies with large samples where significant associations *were* found between smoking and aspects of personality other than mental health.

Miscellaneous

The remaining findings, grouped in a miscellaneous category, will be mentioned briefly but will not be tabled. In one of the earliest studies reviewed (Vallance, 1940) nonsmokers were said to be "27.29% more suggestable than the smokers." However, the sample was small and the difference was not statistically significant.

Friedman and Rosenman (1959) found that eighty-three men characterized by a competitive, hard-driving style of life smoked significantly more than eighty-three men with a relaxed, easy-going life style.

Carney (1967) reports a significant positive association between smoking and achievement motivation, measured with the CPI.

McArthur et al. (1958) and Thomas (1960) studied differences between smokers and nonsmokers regarding Rorschach responses. McArthur et al. reported heavy smokers to have more "coarctated" (low color and human movement) responses, but Thomas failed to confirm this finding.

Three investigators have examined the relations between smoking and scores on the EPPS. Koponen (1960), who studied 1,418 males, reports that "the average U.S. male *smoker* scored significantly higher than the average U.S. *male* in his expressed needs for sex, aggression, achievement and dominance, and significantly below average in compliance, order, self depreciation and association" (italics added). (Although Koponen does not so state, it seems that he has used the terms "compliance," "self depreciation," and "association" to refer to the personality scales usually called "deference," "abasement," and "affiliation," respectively.)

Smith (1967) found that three of the EPPS scales ("order," "deference," and "heterosexuality") showed significant differences (with consistent signs) in two or more of four samples of college students (total N=762). Relative to nonsmokers, the smokers scored higher on the variable "heterosexuality" and scored lower on the variables "order" and "deference." These three differences agree with the results of Koponen. On the other hand, Weatherley (1965) failed to find significant differences between smokers and nonsmokers on any of the fifteen EPPS scales in his study of 182 male college students.

Jacobs, Knapp, et al. (1965) and Jacobs, Anderson, et al. (1966) studied differences between smokers and nonsmokers regarding "danger seeking" and "attitudes toward mother" in each of three samples of adult males (N=97, 136, 134). Two of these studies showed a trend indicating greater "danger seeking" among smokers than among non-smokers, but neither trend reached the 0.05 level of significance with a two-tailed test. In one of their studies (but not in the other two) they found that smokers were significantly more likely than nonsmokers to see their mothers as "controlling, cold, and harsh."

DISCUSSION

This paper set out to answer three questions, the first being, "What conclusions does this literature justify?" Anyone's answer to that question is obviously a matter of judgment, and different reviewers would assess the situation somewhat differently. This reviewer assesses it as follows.

Concerning "extraversion," twenty-two out of twenty-five analyses show smokers to be significantly more extraverted than nonsmokers; none shows a significant opposite finding. The twenty-two significant findings represent stûdies varying widely regarding instruments employed and populations studied; yet there is virtual unanimity of results.

Conclusion 1. Smokers are more extraverted than nonsmokers.

The results concerning "antisocial tendencies" also leave little room for doubt. Of thirty-two analyses, twenty-seven show smokers to be significantly more antisocial than nonsmokers; none shows smokers to be significantly less antisocial than nonsmokers. As with the studies of extraversion, the data linking smoking and antisocial tendencies come from studies varying widely regarding instruments used and populations studied.

Conclusion 2. Smokers have more antisocial tendencies than nonsmokers.

Concerning "internal-external control," the evidence is less solid but, nevertheless, reasonably convincing. All five studies of the relations between this concept and smoking indicate that smokers are more externally oriented than nonsmokers; that is, smokers are more likely than nonsmokers to think chance, fate, luck, and the like (rather than their own skill and effort) account for what happens to them. Four of these five results are significant, and the fifth is very nearly significant.

Conclusion 3. More information is needed to support what is now available, but it appears that smokers are more externally oriented than nonsmokers.

Concerning "impulsiveness," the evidence is again reasonably convincing but less solid than that for "extraversion" and "antisocial tendencies." Seven out of ten analyses show smokers to be significantly more impulsive than nonsmokers; none show a significant association in the opposite direction.

Conclusion 4. It appears that smokers are more impulsive than nonsmokers, but more information is needed to verify this finding.

Of four studies dealing with smoking and "orality," three yield positive associations that are statistically significant. However, of those three, one was based on a very small sample (N=22) and one achieved significance in one comparison but not in another (see legend of Table 5).

Conclusion 5. There is support for the hypothesis that smokers have stronger oral needs than nonsmokers, but more evidence is needed to confirm this hypothesis.

The data concerning smoking and "mental health" are highly conflicting. Numerous studies have shown that smokers have significantly poorer mental health than nonsmokers, but several well-designed studies that sought this relationship failed to find it. On the other hand, no studies have shown smokers to have significantly *better* mental health than nonsmokers.

Conclusion 6. Although the evidence suggests that smokers have poorer mental health than nonsmokers, more information is needed to confirm that suggestion, and additional work is needed to define more precisely the specific aspects of mental health on which smokers and nonsmokers differ.

Value of this literature

The second question this review promised to try to answer is: What value does this literature have? The questions of whether, and how, smokers differ from nonsmokers regarding personality are of interest for at least two reasons. First, the association between smoking and disease, although now widely accepted, is not uniformly interpreted. For example, Berkson (1958) and Fisher (1959), both statisticians, suggest that such genotypic factors as constitution and temperament might predispose some persons to develop lung cancer and also predispose them to become smokers. Whether or not that position has merit, the differential morbidity rates of smokers and nonsmokers will probably become more understandable as constitutional and psychosocial differences between these groups are further specified.

Second, little is currently known about the motivational factors underlying decisions whether or not to become a smoker; to continue or to quit; to reduce or not. Such knowledge is of considerable practical importance because the effectiveness of antismoking educational campaigns will probably improve monotonically with the accumulation of dependable and comprehensive information concerning the psychodynamics of smoking.

To optimize the beneficial effects of antismoking educational efforts, more must be learned about the psychodynamics of smoking, and such information should be sought with investigations differing widely in aims, assumptions, and methods. No one can say which approaches will, and which will not, succeed in generating pragmatically useful information.

Professors Hunt and Matarazzo, in the following chapter, assert that "the personality characteristics of smokers and nonsmokers have been well explored, and to no apparent advantage." Later they question whether the information resulting from such studies "is pertinent in any immediate sense to the problem of controlling smoking behavior." Lest the elegance of their success in being "both stimulating and contentious" obscure certain facts, let me assert, quite contentiously, that a thorough exploration of the personality characteristics of smokers and nonsmokers has *not* yet been accomplished; that what has been learned *is* of some apparent advantage; and that such information *is* pertinent to the problem of controlling smoking behavior.

As I see it, the literature reviewed in the present paper justifies only two positive conclusions: Smokers are more "extraverted" than non-smokers, and smokers are more "antisocial" than nonsmokers. Considerable evidence supports the belief that smokers also differ from non-smokers regarding internal-external orientation, impulsiveness, orality, and some aspects of mental health, but those matters remain uncertain, precisely *because* they have not been "well explored."

How advantageously such information (whether firm or tentative) can be used for the specific practical purpose of controlling smoking behavior remains to be seen; but in groping for an understanding of the *whys* of smoking, it would be folly not to accumulate information concerning sociological, psychological, and biological differences between smokers and nonsmokers.

The most certain cure for smoking is to stop it before it begins. To do that we must understand *why* people begin smoking in the first place. Adolescents and preadolescents are frequently exposed to information concerning the harmful effects of smoking; and at some level of awareness many of them must know that becoming a smoker is an irrational, self-defeating action. Yet each year a certain percentage in each age group decides to take that step. Why? Why some persons and not others? These are complex matters, but their elucidation is likely to come from a variety of types of investigations that approach the problem in quite different ways.

Research strategy

The third question addressed in this review was : What changes in research strategy might enhance the yield of future research on the relationship between smoking and personality? The paper by Coan (1967), in the book edited by Zagona, contains helpful advice, as do several other papers and discussions in that book.

My own work on the psychodynamics of smoking, supported primarily by the American Cancer Society, has built into it whatever ideas about strategy I have to share. I will therefore end this review by simply listing eight ways by which I hope to enhance the yield of my own work.

1. Measure all six categories of personality that the present literature shows to be promising: extraversion, antisocial tendencies, internal-external orientation, impulsiveness, orality, and mental health.
2. Where practicable, measure each area of personality with each of three methods of personality assessment: self-report questionnaires, peer ratings, and projective techniques.

3. Go beyond the domain of personality (to include attitudes, feeling, and beliefs about smoking) in the search for insight into the psychodynamics of smoking.
4. Study more subtle aspects of smoking behavior (such as depth of inhalation, vigor of smoking, style of smoking, and conditions under which the subject does and does not smoke) rather than simply the number of cigarettes the subject smokes per day or week.
5. Use the peer-rating method, as well as the self-report method, to study smoking behavior.
6. Conduct the study on a longitudinal basis, beginning at an early age.
7. Conduct the study in more than one culture—several, if resources permit.
8. Use multivariate statistical procedures (factor analysis, multiple regression, multiple discriminant analysis, and canonical correlation) to analyze the data collected.

Part Two
Learning Mechanisms and Smoking

Habit Mechanisms in Smoking

WILLIAM A. HUNT AND
JOSEPH D. MATARAZZO

APPROACHING the modification of smoking behavior through the application of principles derived from the experimental study of human and animal learning is by no means a novel procedure, particularly in view of the current popularity of classical and operant conditioning techniques in behavior modification and therapy. We feel, however, that our use of habit as a basic concept will offer something of a fresh approach, despite its time-worn usage in the common everyday vocabulary.

The presentation will begin with a definition of our use of the term, its differentiation from such terms as dependence and addiction, some further development of its characteristics and implications, its relation to the smoking behavior typologies of Tomkins and Horn, and a contrast of its potentialities with those of other approaches. Following this focus on the term, we will relate it to the learning literature in order to derive further explication of fruitful areas of research. While our primary focus is the modification of smoking behavior, we would like to believe that our approach has wider implications for the understanding of drug behavior in general. It is to be hoped that our paper will be both stimulating and contentious.

"HABIT"

Any justification of our use of the concept of habit should start with a definition. For a term as prominent in the popular vocabulary as habit, there is relatively little reference to it in the formal learning literature. This apparent neglect may reflect the fact that habit is, after all, merely a type of learned behavior and is adequately treated under other rubrics. A more likely reason may be that habit has been used to describe long-standing, well established behavior patterns, and learning researchers have been more interested in the acquisition than in the maintenance of behavior—as witness our relative ignorance of the phenomena of overlearning.

Since we are interested in behavior modification, we may well start with the definition offered by Wolpe and Lazarus (1967), "A habit is a consistent way of responding to defined stimulus characteristics." Berelson and Steiner (1964) are less terse: "As in common usage, this term refers to a connection between stimuli and/or responses that has become virtually automatic through experience, usually through repeated trials." To consistent responding automaticity has now been added; incidentally, it is often though not necessarily always, accompanied by diminished awareness. Dulaney (1962) has given a sophisticated treatment of some of these issues in discussing awareness and verbal conditioning. Since habit is learned behavior, Glaser (1969) deserves a hearing when he notes, "An adequately learned performance is characterized not only by the facility with which it occurs in different contexts but also in terms of its long-range properties; e.g., how well it is remembered, the extent to which it continues to be engaged in for relatively long periods of time, the degree to which it transfers to and facilitates new learning, and the extent to which it becomes increasingly independent from the supports required in earlier stages of competence." The salient addition here is the idea of increasing independence from the stimulus conditions responsible for the original learning, similar to Allport's (1961) concept of functional autonomy as "any acquired system of motivation in which the tensions involved are not of the same kind as the antecedent tensions from which the acquired system developed." In our terms this becomes a shift from primary to secondary reinforcement as the learned behavior continues. This observation is of particular importance for smoking behavior, where the traditional model has involved heavy reliance upon primary reinforcement and the attendant importance of conscious affect. We are not denying the importance of these in originating smoking behavior, we are merely stressing the importance of secondary reinforcement in maintaining the smoking behavior once it is established.

Our definition of habit, then, becomes *"a fixed behavior pattern overlearned to the point of becoming automatic and marked by decreasing awareness and increasing dependence on secondary, rather than primary, reinforcement."* For our purposes it stresses the importance of paying particular attention to the phenomena of overlearning in applying learning theory to smoking behavior, of being wary of the limitations of any affect model, and of realizing the importance of secondary as opposed to primary reinforcement. Since we are suggesting some relevance of habit to all types of drug behavior, it is pertinent, before expanding upon the above points, to contrast habit with such other terms as addiction and dependence.

We will make frequent mention of the term *awareness,* common in psychological usage though seldom defined, realizing the logical and methodological difficulties that attend its use. As Berelson and Steiner (1964) note, "the role of awareness is an unresolved and lively issue in the theoretical literature." As we use it, it may be interpreted in the subjective, phenomenological sense as a consciousness of what is going on; or in the objective, behavioral sense as the ability to make a verbal report upon a preceding or attendant stimulus situation. It is minimal or missing with the performance of repetitive, stereotyped behaviors and present with some intensity in the phenomenon of craving and with the withdrawal symptoms common to the addictive drugs.

The term *addiction* we would reserve for those situations marked by increased bodily tolerance, with the consequent need for an increased dosage, and by the prominence of withdrawal symptoms. The ultimate result of such an increasing spiral is the demand for dosage levels that cannot be tolerated by the body. Intense awareness would seem to be a prominent part of this experience.

Physical dependence is a related phenomenon in which the body develops a dependence upon a drug. As opposed to addiction, however, little tolerance develops, and there is no demand for an ever-increasing dosage. The result is a more or less stabilized, nonthreatening level of drug maintenance, the subject often being unaware of his physical dependence and withdrawal symptoms being minimal or missing. Actually, the relation between dependence and addiction is a cloudy area, and differentiation between them becomes difficult. At times one is tempted to remark that the difference in usage is at least in part dictated by the severity of the bodily reaction to the drug and by society's reaction to the induced behavior. Thus, these terms are used infrequently in relation to such a mild and socially accepted agent as tobacco, although scattered self-reports would indicate that in some cases a physical dependence accompanied by minimal withdrawal symptoms may develop with tobacco.

The difference between habit and physical dependence is complicated, not only by our relative ignorance of the psychopharmacology of the milder chemical agents, but also by the fact that the common objective criterion for both is the same—repeated usage. Where such repeated usage occurs and where physical dependence cannot be demonstrated, we would prefer to use the term habit or habituation.

The World Health Organization (1964) further complicates matters by speaking of psychic dependence as well as physical dependence, "psychic dependence" emphasizing dependence on the psychological accompaniments of drug usage not necessarily accompanied by physical dependence. This use of psychic dependence would seem to be a confusion of our terms "habit" and "awareness," with the added implication that the subjective experiences (i.e. consciousness per se) are the essential motivating agents, as opposed to some underlying physiological processes; such a position is no doubt dictated by reliance on an earlier, relatively unsophisticated phenomenological hedonism. More will be said subsequently of the dangers of such an existential hedonic model. At this point let the comment suffice that our use of habit plus awareness (a term that may be defined in ways acceptable to both subjective and objective interpretation) is a happier solution to the descriptive problem than relying on an outmoded model that flirts with the causal and dynamogenic properties of consciousness.

Much is assumed about conscious affect in smoking, alcoholism, and other drug behaviors; but the literature is lacking in carefully controlled introspective studies such as those of Mendelson and his associates in the field of alcohol (McNamee, Mello, and Mendelson, 1968). What has been collected is largely in the area of questionnaire studies, where the reporting is done on a retrospective basis, rather than being based on careful self-observation in actual stimulus situations. The senior author, veteran of many studies in the affective area, has long been suspicious of the casual reporting of hedonic tone. His suspicion traces back to an early study involving the affective values of colors, where it was obvious that after several presentations of a series of color stimuli, the observers were reporting affective values so rapidly that they could not have been based upon a genuine affective experience (Hunt and Flannery, 1938). The subjects' final judgmental reaction times approached their verbal reaction times, and it was obvious that they had learned a verbal response attached directly to the color and were now reporting it without any hedonic mediation. Both by treating variability in judgment as response error and by plotting reaction times, it was possible to produce typical learning curves. Perhaps most important were those occasional subjects who after achieving a stable set of responses suddenly realized that they were reporting a value for some color that did not represent their actual hedonic reaction to it. The reporting "habit" was thus persevering after its supposed hedonic base had radically altered. This circumstance is analogous to the situation in which smoking as a habit may occur, even though it is attended by extreme discomfort to the smoker (irritation of the nose and throat and the like).

In developing our concept of habit as a potentially enlightening approach to understanding the human use and misuse of drugs, we are not suggesting that the principles of learning are new and novel in the field; rather, we are calling for a renewed interest in their application and a more sophisticated use of the newer developments in the field of learning and of classical and operant conditioning in particular. Not only can learning theory bring much to our understanding of drug behavior, but further, the study of drug behavior as learned behavior or habit can do much to stimulate and enrich learning theory by pointing up overlooked and unsuspected gaps in learning theory and by highlighting new and suggestive interrelationships. Many of these have been bypassed previously on the grounds that there were not adequate analyses of complex human behavior—an excuse that appears much less telling in the light of contemporary developments in the field of operant conditioning and contingency management.

In differentiating habit from other learned behaviors by pointing out that it is marked by overlearning, therefore, we highlight the concern of learning theory with the *acquisition* of behavior to the relative neglect of its *maintenance,* although it seems that proportionately a greater part of man's adaptive activity consists of the emitting of already learned behaviors, rather than the acquiring of new ones. Standard texts usually mention the importance of overlearning and then dismiss it with the embarrassed comment that little is known about its phenomena. The longitudinal study necessitated by any investigation of extended temporal characteristics does, of course, make uncomfortable demands on laboratory procedures and resources, but long-established habit patterns, such as smoking, offer a ready-made and available approach to the problem. Through a study of smoking's resistance to extinction, to interference, and to substitution, much can be uncovered about overlearning and about the maintenance of fixed, stable patterns of behavior.

That habits are overlearned can hardly be denied, but we have also called attention to two other characteristics, or perhaps *suggested* two other characteristics. These are diminished awareness and increased control by secondary cues and secondary reinforcements as a temporal function of habitual behaviors. Here the ground is far from solid, but the hypotheses seem both reasonable and stimulating.

Not much can be said about awareness, since not much is known. With all its phenomenological implications, it can hardly be expected to play a prominent role in a field dominated by animal experimentation, although the application of operant principles in the area of verbal conditioning has resulted in some attention. Interestingly enough, as behavior modification turns its attention to the problems of covert conditioning, many of the problems of an older, subjectively oriented psychology are reappearing in a new objective guise. In any case, it seems fair to say that where awareness has been considered, it has seemed to bear a close relation to the learning process, a relation that in general is facilitory (as in Matarazzo, Saslow, and Pareis, 1960).

Awareness also seems a more prominent aspect of the acquisition of behavior than of its maintenance. One may well ask about its relation to overlearning if it is decreased in the repetitive, stereotyped behaviors we have called habits. How does awareness relate to stimulus differentiation, contingency management, and covert conditioning? And what are its implications for the hedonic model so commonly used in the discussion of smoking, drinking, and eating behavior? If people smoke for pleasure, how can smoking be explained when smokers are barely aware of doing it? Or, in Olds' terms (Olds and Milner, 1954), does one self-stimulate if one does not know one is doing it? Or, in terms of a humorous rallying cry frequently heard in our habit laboratory, "Let's take the habit out of our vices and put the pleasure back in."

We are not suggesting an existential psychology nor leading a revolt against the behavioristic tradition of the last forty years in American psychology. We are merely noting that awareness seems an interesting phenomenon. It might be profitable to sort behaviors on the basis of whether or not they are attended by awareness, and to what degree. Such a classification might lead to new insights about behavior, particularly in that area that we have called habit and that seems so prominent in smoking. Eriksen (1962b) has given a detailed discussion of some of the problems involved and has pointed out that "A broad-scale attack on the problem of awareness should include experimental studies not only of how overlearned perceptual-motor responses become automatic, but also should orient itself toward investigating ways and techniques by which behavior that has become automatic is brought back into awareness."

We are not denying the importance of affect or of primary reinforcers as instigators of behavior, but we are challenging their continuing effectiveness in maintaining those repetitive behaviors we have called habits. In defining a primary reinforcer as a stimulus whose reinforcing properties do not depend upon a history of conditioning, and conditioned or secondary reinforcers as ones established by conditioning, we are saying that as a behavior pattern develops into a habit, secondary conditioning to incidental stimuli may in time result in the production of a series of stimulus cues far removed from the primary satisfactions responsible for the original establishment of the response in question. Such secondary stimuli may ultimately produce a response under circumstances where the consequences are no longer congruent with the original motivations, or they may even become aversive and directly oppose them, as in smoking despite a sore throat and the like, where the behavior results in actual pain and discomfort to the smoker.

We might speak of the gradual ascendance of secondary cues, of anticipatory responses, of mediational mechanisms, and of cognitive complications until a behavioral independence of the original primary reinforcement is achieved. Schacter (1968) finds a similar situation in obesity, where he notes: "These persistent findings that the obese are relatively insensitive to variations in the physiological correlates of food deprivation but highly sensitive to environmental, food-related cues is, perhaps, one key to understanding the notorious, long-run ineffectiveness of virtually all attempts to treat obesity."

Such habitual, relatively affectless behavior has been recognized among tobacco users. Both Tomkins (1966) and Horn (1969) classify this as "habitual" smoking and include it among their types of smokers. Horn, indeed, describes it much in our terms: "This kind of smoker is no longer getting much satisfaction from his cigarettes. He just lights them frequently without even realizing he is doing so. He may find it easy to quit if he can break the habit pattern he has built up." Horn later relates such habitual behavior to diminished awareness in our terms by noting, "The key to success is becoming aware of each cigarette you smoke. You can do this by asking, 'Do I really want this cigarette?' You may be surprised at how often you decide that you do not."

In their unusually comprehensive study, "The Natural History of Cigarette Smoking," Mausner and Platt (1968) refer to some smoking as habitual and add, "It may well be that smoking represents an example of Allport's functional autonomy; that the smoking which began as a gesture of role definition turns into either a purely habitual response, a response based solely on social stimulation, or a response supported by its pleasurable or tension reducing characteristics."

We have, then, no fundamental disagreement with Horn, Tomkins, or Mausner and Platt. Our difference lies in the importance we attach to habit. With them it would seem to be a minor category of behavior; they attach their major interest to affect and see smoking as an attempt to gain positive affect or to avoid negative affect. Mausner and Platt add the importance of social stimulation. We admit the importance of the affect model in understanding the acquisition of behavior, but we feel it to be of less importance in understanding the maintenance of behavior. Put simply, we admit that people learn to smoke because it relaxes them, stimulates them, eases social tension, and the like, but we are proposing that the reasons they continue smoking may become quite different and that a pattern of habitual response may be established that has little relation to the original satisfactions experienced. Much of the supporting data for the affect model as used by Horn and Tomkins has come from questionnaire or interview data, where the respondents may be suspected of having answered retrospectively, on the basis of the original satisfactions initially derived when they began smoking. Thus, an individual who in reality is a "habitual" smoker may answer that he smokes because it gives him a pleasant sense of relaxation, even though he is no longer aware of this satisfaction when smoking.

Mausner and Platt (1968) seem to have run into a similar problem in comparing their results from different data sources. "Much of the qualitative material from the respondents in our studies of college students deals with the properties of the cigarette as a pacifier. However, for the two groups for whom we obtained scores on the expanded Horn-Waingrow test, the scores on negative affect reduction were relatively low. In addition, the number of individual instances of smoking in which the respondents in the diary study reported the reduction of negative affect was extremely low. Yet when asked to rate themselves during the interview on a scale of negative affect reduction, many respondents rated themselves well above the midpoint. The inconsistencies among these various data may be due to the fact that most of the cigarettes smoked by our respondents do not actually reduce negative affect. However, where the cigarette does act to reduce an externally caused tension, the impact on the smoker is very great; such impact would undoubtedly affect the smoker's perception of his smoking quite deeply." Or one might suggest, as we have, that there are habits of reporting as well as habits of smoking and that such habits may produce distorted reports.

In closing our discussion of the characteristics of habit, we would like to offer three plausible suggestions concerning this class of behaviors:

1. Habit is larger and of greater importance than previously assumed. We have discussed this point in relation to the Horn and Tomkins model of smoking behavior; we can only emphasize again that the behavioral sciences, in their interest in the *acquisition* of behavior, have largely overlooked the problems inherent in the *maintenance* of behavior, and that fully as much time is spent in emitting older, already learned responses as in learning new ones. Not for nothing has man been called a creature of habit.

2. Habit represents the common, ultimate resolution of many behavior patterns originally instigated by primary reinforcement. One might almost speak of a flight from affect or view the chaining mechanisms of secondary conditioning as affect reducing, diluting, and the like. The blandness of habit is one of its major characteristics.

3. The maintenance of habit in the drug area is largely a matter of learning principles rather than of physical dependence or addiction.

Let it be clear that we are not suggesting all repetitive behaviors be classed as habits, nor all drug behaviors. Primary reinforcement with pronounced awareness of gratification is typical of the more powerful drugs, such as the hallucinogens and opiates. One can hardly call the withdrawal effects attendant upon heroin usage secondary stimuli and assume that their relief would not be accompanied by acute awareness of their departure.

In proposing habitual behavior as an important aspect of drug usage, we would stress its relative importance in connection with the milder drugs and deemphasize its importance with the severe ones. Thus, if drug usage is scaled from such mild practices as coffee drinking and smoking up through alcohol and marihuana to the more severe reactions produced by the hallucinogens, psychedelics, and opiates, habitual behavior as we have defined it would be expected to decrease. As we might paraphrase it, the *more* the repetitive behavior involves a pronounced physiological reaction and the possible development of physical dependence, the *less* it will resemble habit and the more it will involve awareness and primary gratification.

We must also, of course, admit that even such commonly habitual behaviors as smoking, tying shoelaces, and the like, are sometimes attended by primary reinforcement and by acute awareness. The problem reaches beyond the simple intensity of reaction and involves the complications introduced by environmental stimuli, dependent on such intricate factors as ease of access to the drug, ease of ingestion, social ritual attendant upon ingestion, frustration, and so on. It has been said that man's crowning glory is his ability to learn, with the resulting potential for flexibility in his behavior; but it also furnishes a crowning frustration for the scientist attempting to understand him.

Before we end our discussion of habit, mention should be made of the importance of habitual behaviors as "something to do." For the heroin addict, his addiction offers him a way of life. Problems of role, identification, life purpose, career, and so on, are pushed aside by his addiction, and the satisfaction of his need for drugs becomes his major purpose, to which his entire life is dedicated and the demands of which offer him little uncommitted time or choice of activity. In a small way habits also serve a function in answering man's need for activity. They are the available behaviors ready to be utilized when tension builds up a stimulus potential beyond the capability of the ongoing activity to absorb, and their emission need not disrupt the major behavior in which the person is engaged at the moment. This is particularly true of those habits, such as smoking, that involve a great deal of manipulatory activity. At a higher level they offer a minor activity (accompanied by the dignity of purposive behavior) that can be used to fill an empty space in time. Thus, smoking a cigarette while waiting for a friend, not only permits activity, but also seems a more logical, purposeful, and dignified activity than pacing back and forth or standing in one place tapping one's foot or twirling one's hat.

Lest our stress on the concept of habit seem unduly limiting, let us hasten to point out that habits are, after all, learned behaviors and that anything we find out about them will enrich our understanding of the learning process. Broadly speaking, our approach is a "learning" approach, and we have used the concept of habit to suggest certain parameters of seeming importance to habitual behavior that certainly have implications for learning in general, but that have been relatively neglected in the study of learning: overlearning, awareness, and secondary conditioning. The study of smoking behavior along these parameters should contribute further to knowledge of the field.

After all, concepts are not absolutes. They are cognitive tools, functional in nature, to be evaluated by a careful blending of Occam's razor and Kohler's principle of scientific fertility. It is to the point to quote the wise words of Gordon Allport (1968): "We do not solve our problems; we only grow tired of them. New labels, we think, identify new problems. We grow weary of suggestibility and so investigate persuasability; personality and culture give way to systems theory

. . . problem solving dissolves into programming; pleasure and pain become positive and negative reinforcement; maladjustment becomes alienation; volition gives way to decision-making; no longer does one possess character, one has ego-strength. The average life of popular concepts is, I estimate, about two decades. After that, they begin to taste as flat as yesterday's beer." But a stimulating concept can live a lot in twenty years and can make its own particular and valuable, though possibly evanescent, contribution.

We will conclude our discussion of habit per se by reviewing some of the implications of the parameters mentioned above, the problems they pose, and the approaches they suggest. Following this, there will be a section discussing the alternative strategies available, such as an approach to the modification of smoking behavior through the study of the pharmacology of tobacco, the personality of the smoker, or the cultural factors in society that sanction and encourage it. The final section will relate smoking behavior to learning in general and will attempt to derive some suggestions from the current literature for its control.

It is pertinent at this point to discuss further some implications of our position for the control of smoking behavior, beginning with overlearning. It must be remembered at all times that the habitual behaviors here dealt with are overlearned in a tremendously more stringent sense than those produced in the laboratory. We are not dealing with a response reproduced one or two hundred trials beyond criterion. Assuming the puff to be the crucial unit reinforced or reinforcing in smoking, there may be ten puffs per cigarette, twenty cigarettes per pack, two packs per day for a heavy smoker, and 365 days in a year, making a total of 146,000 reinforcements (a correction of 1/1,460th of this may be added to take adequate statistical account of leap year). And the subject may have been smoking for twenty years! Granted the puff has been selected arbitrarily as a unit and that not all responses may have been reinforced positively, we are nevertheless faced with overlearning to an extent not hitherto produced in a learning laboratory, with the possible exception of Skinner's pigeons. One must conclude that in dealing with smoking behavior, we cannot study within the laboratory the development of habits subject to that much reinforcement, but must rather accept the already established habitual behavior and study its alteration or removal through such phenomena as extinction, interference, substitution, and the like. We can study under controlled conditions the acquisition of a behavior, and we can study the alteration of already acquired behaviors; but the longitudinal study of the development of a behavior into a habit through continuing overlearning or reinforcement would appear to be a task beyond our laboratory means or at least our present inclination.

Although the intricacies of modern learning models may not offer much specific aid in interpretation, there is ample evidence that overlearning does strengthen response and that old behaviors apparently long forgotten can reappear, sometimes at awkward moments. Jost's Law that, other things being equal, the older of two learned responses has precedence over the newer, however superseded this formulation may be by modern work on the dissipation of inhibition and the removal of interference; Pavlov's old "inhibition of an inhibition"; and the appearance of regressive behavior under stress—all illustrate that out of sight is not out of mind, and that response potential can linger on long after the behavior in question disappears from our actual performing repertoire.

Yet this fact is neglected in smoking "therapies," most of which are short-term, a few weeks at best; and the criterion of success is abstention or the disappearance of smoking. If, at the conclusion of the course or treatment, the smoker is still smoking, the treatment is assumed to have failed; if he has quit, it is successful. Little attention is paid to partial success as might be demonstrated in reduced smoking rate or in success after continued treatment. When the abstainees are followed over an interim of time, the majority of them are found ultimately to resume smoking. If abstention is viewed as a learned behavior, the data on follow-up look very like an extinction curve.

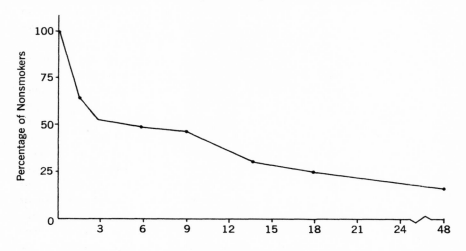

Figure 1. Abstemious Behavior as a Function of Time After Successful Therapy

Figure 1 presents graphed follow-up data from seventeen treatment studies that we considered valid and reliable. The beginning point of 100 per cent is based on those subjects who were not smoking at the end of treatment. Each subsequent point represents the average percentage of originally successful abstainers who were still abstaining after that interval of time. The data at the six-months point are roughly in agreement with the latest report of Lichtenstein and Keutzer (1969), and the one-year and two-year points roughly coincide with the figures reported for a civil-commitment program for drug addicts as reported by Kramer, Bass, and Berecochea (1968). The result is a typical "forgetting" or extinction curve. Adding data from studies we considered unreliable merely increases the distribution around each point but does not change the shape of the curve. Certainly some sort of learning or "unlearning" seems involved here, with implications for any treatment program.

It seems obvious that some sort of booster shot or retreading is necessary to support and sustain the abstinence behavior subsequent to its acquisition. To base the criterion of successful treatment on the disappearance of symptomatology at the end of therapy can be as disastrous here as it was with some of our wartime venereal programs. Since the curve is negatively decelerated with a rapid decline at first, it may be assumed that such added support should come fairly shortly after the original success. Provision for individual differences in rates of progress should also be made, rather than adoption of a fixed period of treatment. On the research side not only is better follow-up data needed, but the length of abstinence must also be related to measures of habit strength before and during the treatment program.

As shown subsequently, altering behavior is more than simple habit manipulation through reinforcement. Some type of attitudinal acceptance or rejection mechanism resembling encoding seems to be present. In this regard, it should be pointed out that the universal use of complete abstinence as sole criterion of success in habit modification, as is the custom throughout all areas of drug usage, involves possible secondary losses. Such an all-or-none criterion deprives the subject of the reinforcement value of partial success and unnecessarily damns him as a lost soul after one slip either of conscious indulgence or unconscious habit. After years of heavy cigar smoking, the senior author now regards himself as a nonsmoker, yet he occasionally does indulge, perhaps on an average of once every six weeks. The reasons are immaterial and will be considered later; the important point is that such incidents are always greeted by his colleagues with, "So you can't give it up," "Once a smoker, always a smoker," "Well, you're back on the habit"—remarks not calculated to reinforce a pattern of abstinence. Moreover, a certain anxiety and self-doubt usually intrude themselves into his thinking at such times, and it is necessary for him to remind himself that without errors there can be no learning curve.

In discussing the importance of secondary conditioning in smoking behavior, we have suggested that as an acquired response develops into an overlearned habit, there may be a gradual ascendance of secondary cues (through anticipatory responses, mediational mechanisms, cognitive complications, and the like) until a behavioral independence of the original primary reinforcement is achieved. No neat learning or response model exists by which to chart this transition, except possibly the Dollard and Miller position (1950) that postulates "thoughts" as mediating links in the stimulus chain, but over time and with repetition such secondary cues or stimuli might well develop a response eliciting power challenging or superseding the original physiological needs and satisfactions. A further discussion of the part that verbal operants might play in such mediation may be found in Verplanck (1962) and indeed in the entire symposium edited by Eriksen (1962a) in which it appears along with the previously mentioned papers by Eriksen and Dulaney.

If we hold to our definition of habit as a fixed behavior pattern overlearned to the point of becoming automatic and marked by decreasing awareness and increasing dependence on secondary rather than primary reinforcement, it would seem reasonable to assume that its importance in understanding drug usage would diminish with progress from those drugs with milder, less disturbing effects upon the organism's metabolism, such as caffeine and nicotine, through alcohol to the more dramatic hallucinogens, amphetamines, and hard drugs, such as cocaine and morphine. One would expect the more pronounced effects of the stronger drugs to produce a sharper stimulus definition and more reliance upon primary reinforcement mechanisms with a narrower range of usage behaviors.

To continue at a hypothetical level, might not one expect more variability and flexibility of behavior to be associated with smoking than with "shooting" STP or heroin? Smoking behavior should be easier to place under voluntary control but perhaps more difficult to keep in complete abstention. The availability of secondary cues of an environmental nature might produce a greater temptation, while at the same time the milder and often secondary reinforcements could more easily be overcome. In terms of any treatment program, one might expect more frequent slips or relapses in smoking, but with each relapse asserting less prejudice upon the final outcome of abstention than in the case of the "harder" drugs.

It certainly might be supposed that in treatment programs involving tobacco the use of substitute drugs would be less efficacious, the major results coming from an attack on retraining habitual behaviors. Evidence in favor of such a view is forthcoming on review of the use of such drugs as lobeline in breaking the smoking habit and comparison of their relative inefficiency with the use of methadone in controlling heroin usage. What success has been achieved with lobeline seems to come when it is used as a supportive adjunct in behavior training programs or when it is supplemented with attitudinal supports or exercises. The contrast with methadone is very clear.

In fact, it might reasonably be asked whether the effects achieved with nicotine substitutes are attributable to the drug per se or to its placebo effect. Placebo effects are too well known and the use of placebos is too firmly entrenched in our therapeutic practice to need discussion here, but it should be pointed out that placebos need not be inert drugs, and that any drug even while exercising a desired and specific effect upon behavior also has a placebo overlay. Our current experiences with hallucinogens has pointed up the fact that what one gets from a drug is in part determined by what one brings to it and expects of it. Any nicotine substitute, then, would have an expected efficacy, determined by the actual value of the drug in relieving any physical need for nicotine *plus* the effects anticipated by the subject.

The relationship of learning to awareness and the relative lack of awareness in much habitual behavior suggest that the controlled introduction of awareness in the retraining program might be helpful. As Estes (1967) notes in discussing verbal conditioning, "Although awareness of the constituent relationships on the part of the subjects would not be a necessary condition for this learning, it could be expected to be a correlated variable since the conditions which give rise to awareness are in general the same as those which tend to lead subjects to attend to stimulus-outcome relationships and thus to be in a position to learn them."

The relationship between awareness and stimulus discrimination cannot hope to be a favored problem in a learning generation committed both to animal studies, where we have dubious criteria for its measurement, and to human studies conducted under a rigid objective philosophy, where phenomenology is ruled out by ideological fiat. Nevertheless, this facilitative relationship, largely overlooked in practice but seemingly commonly believed in, could bear investigation. In the habitual behavior called smoking there are many unpleasant concomitants of the response of which the smoker seems unaware at the moment, or at best is only vaguely aware, so that the full negative reinforcement value of such unpleasant experiences seems lost. The deliberate introduction of awareness under such circumstances might help in breaking the habit, or at least in providing sufficient negative reinforcement to diminish the response potential. It is our belief, for instance, that much of the success in the use of satiation in eliminating behaviors comes not alone from satiation per se, nor from the aversive context that is created, but from the intense awareness accompanying the forced experience in such settings. When the individual is smoking under an arbitrary schedule governed by external factors, his adherence to the schedule demands voluntary action, and awareness seems to accompany this. We might summarize by suggesting that whenever a human being is aware of what he is doing and of the consequences of his action, stimulus discrimination is facilitated.

We have mentioned the fact that the senior author, while a nonsmoker to all intents and purposes, does still smoke an occasional cigar. He will not deny temptations occur, but most of these smoking incidents are voluntary and purposive, carried out deliberately under conditions selected to provide negative reinforcement and therefore to bolster the general pattern of abstention rather than to weaken it. Society has so stressed the immorality and catastrophic nature of any recidivistic behavior that we have completely overlooked the fact that controlled experience of forbidden fruit under conditions encouraging gastric distress can lead to mature progression rather than immature regression. Such techniques are found in modern behavior-modification therapies, but here the awareness is apt to be an incidental correlate of the strength of the aversive stimulus rather than a deliberately manipulated variable.

This is, of course, what was meant earlier with the mention of taking the habit out of our behavior and putting the pleasure back in, except that in abstention the goal may be said to be removing the behavior itself by putting the pain back in. In any case, the time may not be ripe (except among the existentialists) for suggesting the controlled manipulation of subjective experience in the facilitation of the learning process, but it does have the economic advantage of being cheaper than the modern psychologist's use of candies as a reinforcing agent with children. Actually, this is taking place in behavior modification therapies today when covert stimuli—or "coverants," as Homme (1965) would say—are used; it is amusing to see how the term "covert stimulus" can apparently make "ideation" and "imagery" respectable operant phenomena.

Someone once said of Titchener that he was so busy discussing experience that he had no time for it. This failing of Titchener's has been true of the ideological hedonist throughout history. He has been so busy manipulating the abstract concept that he has tended to neglect the concrete reality. We have already cautioned against an easy overreliance on the affect model in explaining smoking behavior, pointing out that some reporting discrepancies in previous studies may be due to retrospective rather than to introspective reporting. For many reasons we suggest that more and more careful phenomenological investigation into the nature of the smoking experience is indicated. Such research could consist of free experiential reporting of an introspective variety, or it might be accomplished more objectively, through a stylized interview or even with the use of a checklist or questionnaire, provided proper phrasing of the questions focuses attention on valid reporting of the immediate experience.

ALTERNATIVES

Having made a case for the study of habit mechanisms as an approach to mastering the control of smoking behavior, let us defend this approach by considering some of the alternatives. No attempt will be made to supply a comprehensive survey of the field, such as already exists in the two symposia edited by Zagona (1967) and by Borgatta and Evans (1968). If these are a bit weak in their representation of current behavior-modification techniques, the remedy exists in Bernstein (1969, 1970) or Keutzer et al. (1968). Smith (1967, 1970) has presented a summary in the area of personality. A possibly prejudiced position in favor of learning approaches is explained by the primary interest in the most efficient and immediate way of controlling smoking, and not in a complete understanding of the factors governing its genesis and existence. Thus, study of the cultural aspects of smoking has shown its beginning among adolescents to be a matter both of rebellion and of the attempt at adult identification. In many aspects it serves the purpose of a primitive puberty rite. This finding is of interest and value in understanding and even ultimately controlling the behavior, but it does not have the heuristic value of immediate interference of an aversive conditioning technique.

In comparing the potential value of various approaches to the control of smoking behavior, we will draw an analogy with the field of alcoholism, not only for its illustrative value, but also to encourage consideration of the many commonalities throughout the continuum of drug usage. Habits are not confined to tobacco. The early history of the study of alcoholism was dominated by an interest in its pharmacological and metabolic aspects, perhaps following the medical model of the first quarter of the century. Much has been contributed and is being contributed—such as Nichols and Hsiao's (1967) recent claim for a genetically based common susceptibility to both morphine and alcohol in rats—but alcoholism still remains. With the rise of dynamic psychiatry insight was achieved into the famous 3 Ds of alcoholism—dependence, denial, and depression—but the problem still exists. The cultural approach typical of sociology followed and again has contributed much to our understanding, particularly in terms of demographic data. The Plaut (1967) report of the National Commission represents this influence when it calls for a cultural acceptance of the use of alcohol with the establishment of and training for youth in reasonable and acceptable drinking patterns. Finally—and I would like to call this period "psychological"—we are beginning to apply learning principles in treatment, although at present these are largely limited to the behavior-therapy techniques of desensitization and aversive conditioning. We have taken liberties with history in this thumbnail sketch, but two things are clear, and they are as typical of smoking as of drinking: one, we have progressed in our current use of drugs way beyond our satisfactory pharmacological and psychopharmacological knowledge of them; and, two, we are dealing with a multivariate problem.

On the pharmacological side relatively little is known about nicotine. Its immediate effect on the human system seems to be in terms of a short period of stimulation, followed by a more lasting depressive effect. There is scattered evidence of possible physical dependence, or at the least some general metabolic adjustment to its continued use. Individual differences and interaction with other drugs, such as alcohol, used in association with it are largely unexplored areas. The delivery of nicotine in some other fashion than smoking and the use of substitute drugs seem to have little effect on the behavior. The direct use of behavior modification techniques currently seems more efficacious.

Perhaps because of the superabundance of personality measures and measuring techniques and the relative ease of running significance tests upon differences in group means, plus the ubiquity of simple correlational methods, the personality characteristics of smokers and nonsmokers have been well explored, and to no apparent advantage (Veldman and Bown, 1969). As Coan (1967) notes: "Common failings in personality research stem from fixation on haphazardly chosen concepts, preoccupation with particular forms of measurement, and overdependence on available instruments." Where group differences have been found, their statistical significance is inflated by large samples, and the overlapping in the groups renders individual prediction of little value. Smith (1967) comments, "Examination of current literature concerning personality differences of smokers and nonsmokers indicates that accuracy of classification typically ranges from 50% (chance accuracy) to about 60% (.50 SD separation). Such accuracy offers only modest support for the hypothesis that smokers and nonsmokers differ regarding certain constitutional variables." Smith proposes a multiple discriminant analysis employing a composite score, and he raises his accuracy of discrimination between smokers and nonsmokers to 68 per cent and between nonsmokers and heavy smokers to 76 per cent. It can still be asked whether the resulting information is pertinent in any immediate sense to the problem of controlling smoking behavior. It is interesting to know that male smokers are more heterosexual, more extraverted, and less deferent than nonsmokers; but proposing a program of preventive emasculation, thus reducing heterosexuality, and producing an interaction resulting in less extraversion, with presumably greater deference, is hardly a practical solution to the problem of the abolition of smoking. We must hasten to add that the proposal is ours and not Smith's.

The same pragmatic criticism can be raised concerning the sociological approach and much of the demographic and cultural data it is giving us. It is good data, and ultimately it will fill in the complete picture needed for a perfect understanding, but much of it has little implication or promise for a crash program of smoking control. Thus, when Straits (1967) finds that successful quitters tend to have nonsmoking wives, while people who try to quit and fail tend to have wives who smoke, he is telling us something about the importance of social supports. In terms of our habit analysis, the smoking wife provides an added set of environmental cues for smoking and a greater probability of recidivistic behavior, but to suggest that if you wish to stop smoking and your wife smokes, you had better divorce her would be completely impractical. Much better for both of you to try aversive conditioning.

SMOKING AND LEARNING

And now we come to learning. Admittedly we have been somewhat cavalier in our treatment of other approaches, but our motivation has been one of immediate expediency rather than ultimate evaluation. Certainly any comprehensive preventive health program will necessitate a thorough knowledge of the pharmacological, personality, and cultural factors conducive to the initiation of smoking; and more knowledge of the communication process, and of the part that threat plays in it, will be necessary if we are to support our program with a campaign of public education. If we can find some way of attacking the behavior directly, however, through the interference techniques of behavior modification, we can diminish the threat immediately and gain time for the research necessary in evolving the broader program.

We have noted that we are dealing with a multivariate problem, one that has many and varied etiological factors, all interacting with one another. Multivariate analysis is a statistical method for evaluating the influence of the factors involved in such complex situations, but unfortunately no simple technique of multivariate therapeutic action exists for their control. Fortunately, despite the many different reasons (metabolic, personality, and cultural) that lead people to smoke, there is one common, universal element—the behavior itself. All smokers smoke. If some simple, direct means of attacking this behavior can be found, then it can be controlled, regardless of the complexity of its genesis. This is the promise of behavior modification.

The problem, of course, is not as simple as here implied. The transposition of conditioning procedures from the animal laboratory to the human organism existing in a social environment is beset with complications. One of them, to which too little attention has been given, is the apparent existence of two kinds of learning—or perhaps we should say two kinds of performance or two kinds of behavioral control. One is the familiar, classical type of acquisition, with behavior developing gradually over time as a function of reinforcement. This is represented by conditioning or learning as studied in our learning laboratories. The other is an immediate acquisition or suppression as a function of decision processes or attitude. A person may learn (in the classical sense) to smoke or to stop smoking, but he also may *decide* to smoke or to stop smoking, and do so.

One of the most vivid (and amusing) examples comes in a case history recently reported by Nolan (1968). His wife desired to stop smoking but was unable to and asked for help from her husband, a psychologist. Aware of the importance of supportive environmental cues, Mrs. Nolan's smoking was prohibited unless she smoked in a designated "smoking chair" so placed that she could not conveniently watch television or carry on a conversation. No one was permitted to approach or to speak to her, and she was denied reading materials.

Under the conditions, which she faithfully maintained, her rate dropped to twelve cigarettes per day, less than half her normal consumption. However, her smoking rate stabilized at this figure. Further improvement was obtained subsequently by moving the chair to an isolated location in the cellar of the house. Thereupon her rate dropped to five cigarettes a day. At this point she ceased keeping a formal record of her smoking, and the daily rate advanced to seven, apparently because of the aversive implications of the recording task. This "monitoring" effect has recently been commented on by McFall (1969). It is interesting to note, however, that the reinforcement provided by the act of smoking per se, without the added reinforcement from the usual environmental satisfactions accompanying it, was insufficient to maintain her previous rate.

Up to this point the ground is familiar. Unfortunately an unforeseen development occurred, and after two weeks of consuming seven cigarettes per day, she said that "she was disgusted with her inability to quit smoking and that she was disappointed with the self-control program," whereupon the following day she stopped smoking completely, and at the time of Nolan's reporting she had not smoked for six months. Apparently standard conditioning techniques weakened the habit behavior to the point where it could be "voluntarily" controlled.

This transformation from standard stimulus control to some kind of broader, hierarchically organized behavior of an "attitudinal" nature or "set" is, of course, a common phenomenon. It is not clear whether it represents a simplification of behavioral control through some type of hierarchical organization or, as Mandler (1967) might say, is an encoding process whereby some transformative set is superimposed on incoming information, since little is known about the development of such control mechanisms.

One of us recently had an interesting example of the development of such an attitude or set in his six-year-old daughter. It is a family custom at times to serve wine with dinner. If the child requested to taste the wine, she was permitted a "sip." Sometimes she was offered a taste without asking. In all cases the behavior was the same. Following the tasting, she would grimace and make some derogatory comment of rejection, but she would continue to "taste" on the infrequent occasions when wine was on the table. After some two years of such behavior, when offered a trial sip one evening at dinner, she suddenly said, "No thank you, I do not drink wine." From a simple trial-and-error behavior she had suddenly shifted to a generalized attitude of rejection.

As in Mrs. Nolan's case, there is an interaction between such mechanisms of control. Some people can and do stop smoking "voluntarily." Others can be taught by behavior-modification procedures. For still others, conditioning techniques seem necessary for a preliminary weakening of the response strength before voluntary control can be instituted. Such an interaction offers a fascinating area for investigation and represents the type of problem (under the rubric of "generalization"?) that intrudes itself when interest is shifted from animals to humans.

It is obvious that, in speaking of behavior modification, we are relying largely upon the classical use of conditioning techniques. One of the prevalent objections to the clinical use of conditioning techniques in behavior therapy is that they furnish at best a symptomatic treatment; and since they are not directed at the root of the patient's problem, they are transitory in nature and symptom substitution is inevitable. The neurotic relieved of one manifestation of his basic anxiety will find another outlet for it. Actually, such recent studies as that of Gordon Paul (1968) have failed to reveal evidence of such symptom substitution over periods as long as two years. The danger of the occurrence seems to have been vastly overrated.

Our clinical experience over the years leads us to advance two further arguments against the assumed dangers of symptom substitution. The symptom is not an isolated behavior maintained in a dynamic vacuum; as part of the patient's behavioral repertoire, it is a reality with which he must interact and to which he must now adapt, adding to the difficulties he encounters and exacerbating his problem of adjustment. As the late Carney Landis once quipped, "Any man who has hallucinations and doesn't develop delusions is crazy." The anxiety neurotic who develops tachicardia has acquired a further cause for hypochondriacal anxiety. Lader and Sartorius (1968) have recently discussed this circumstance in relation to increased anxiety level in hysterics following symptomatology. The development of a pronounced tic or of such gastric symptoms as flatulence does nothing to alleviate difficulties of social interaction. As a rule, the removal of such symptomatic behavior does much to relieve the patient's difficulties, sometimes to the point at which he can either handle his basic problem or at least make progress toward its control.

Finally, symptoms as well as smoking behavior may become habits that persevere well beyond any utility to the adjustmental situation that originally produced them. In such cases the symptomatic behavior may linger on after the basic anxiety has departed. The patient's remaining problem then is the symptomatic behavior per se, and its removal clears up the remaining difficulty. In such a case there is no reason for symptom substitution.

In the case of smoking, moreover, where the behavior is a definite health hazard, most reasonable behaviors, such as chewing gum, that might be substituted for smoking can certainly be considered a lesser evil. While there are reports of increased smoking or coffee drinking following abstention from alcohol, we know of no reports where cessation of smoking was followed by an increased consumption of alcohol. Such incidents may have occurred, but we are not aware of their presence in the literature. Increases in body weight following the cessation of smoking have been reported (Brozek and Keys, 1957), but the phenomenon presumably is as much a function of metabolism as it is of increased intake or between-meals nibbling. Actually, the fear of such weight increase is often quoted as a deterrent to stopping smoking, and diet control is built into many smoking-control programs.

In suggesting that there may be two different mechanisms controlling smoking (and any similar habit), we are complicating what may well be, and in fact is usually assumed to be, simply a matter of the relative response weighting involving various contingencies. As Resnick (1968a) notes in discussing satiation as a means of controlling smoking, it may be that "satiation provides sufficient weakening of the response so that when the program ends, numerous aversive contingencies (danger of cancer, cost, etc.) which previously were relatively impotent compared to the overlearned response can now operate to continue the response in its weakened state. These aversive contingencies continually counteract the effects of potentially new and attractive reinforcements." He propounds a standard learning-theory interpretation.

In suggesting two elements of the problem—one a decision-making process, resulting in some encoding mechanism or attitudinal set, and the other the usual association process governed by the contingencies involved (or, if you will, by the relative stimulus and/or response weights existing)—there are four phenomena that encourage us:

1. The change in behavior (abstention or ceasing to smoke) may be sudden and not gradual as would be assumed were it solely a function of a building up of imbalance among competing response systems.

2. Related to the above, the shift may be complete. There is no vacillation (or oscillation), no wavering. The response may disappear completely for a long period of time.

3. It occurs when the strength of the habit still seems considerable by any measure available before the change, as in shifting from two packs of cigarettes per day to none at all.

4. The change may persist apparently independently of the prevailing reinforcement values, as in the case of the affective judgment and some instances of smoking behavior.

Two immediate objections arise: the phenomena above can also be explained on the grounds of competing habit strengths; and we are coming dangerously close to reinstating the forbidden but not forgotten problems of volition and will.

To the first criticism we can only answer: true, competing habit strengths could cover the salient points we have mentioned without the introduction of a second concept, but we doubt that such an interpretation does the job as well. In the first place, there seems to be too much lag in the system for it to be a unitary process. The response potential of the behavior does not appear to be as sensitive to changes in current reinforcement values as might be expected. Related to this fact are the cases of perseveration of behavior, where the independence of immediate reinforcement goes well beyond "lag" and approaches functional autonomy. Finally, a competing-habit-strength interpretation would seem to demand more sudden and more intense build-ups of reinforcement than could be handled by even a system of amplifiers such as Estes posits.

To the claim that we are flirting with the concept of volition and will we can only answer that the flirtation is not of our doing. The phenomena are there. We would rather avoid the issues involved, but we will accept the risk rather than brush the behavioral phenomena under the rug.

The interactions between the decision-made set or attitude and the contingency-based habitual behavior are worthy of further study. At one extreme are the people who show no difficulty in dropping a habit pattern once they decide to, despite its apparent strength. At the other extreme lie those who, irrespective of their desire to quit, are unable to do so. Little attention has been paid to them, perhaps because they represent the common therapeutic "failure" and hence are a source of embarrassment. It would be interesting to continue behavior training with them beyond the course of the usual program (which is quite limited in time) to see whether, with added learning, the behavior can eventually be brought under control. In between are those individuals, like Mrs. Nolan, who can decide to quit and do so after some contingency management has weakened the habit.

As yet unanswered is the question of what happens when the techniques of behavior modification are applied to someone who does not wish to stop smoking. This course raises knotty problems of dissimulation and the invasion of privacy, but the health hazard involved in smoking would seem to justify its exploration. Such experimentation would also contribute further to answering the question of the universal potency of conditioning techniques in modifying behavior, as well as shedding light on the possibility of some double aspect of habit control as we have suggested.

It would be tempting to try some integration of this two-process hypothesis with conventional learning theory, but we have neither the expertise nor the data to support such an interpretation. At the level of simple analogy, in Estes' terms we are suggesting something like an automatic tuning mechanism for scanning that would set the organism in a preordained direction and limit the range of stimuli or responses scanned. In Hullian or Spencian terms, it would take out of the system some aspects of motivation in any dynamic sense and put them back in structurally in terms of some hierarchically organized set or encoding mechanism. These suggestions are not to be taken too seriously. In any case, our comments here in no way alter the case for habit as a special sort of behavior as set forth at the beginning of this paper.

In essence we have adopted what might be called a naturalistic stance, describing an observed behavior, habit, which we feel has certain definable characteristics, with practical implications for the control of smoking behavior. Our conception of habit, then, is an experiential one and is not derived analytically from any fixed theoretical system. Whether it can be fitted into one of the existing systems and whether the attempt to do so would be valuable must be answered by someone more knowledgeable in the field of learning.

There are exciting times ahead. American behaviorism is shedding its early parochialism, as any movement must that from its very beginnings has committed itself to applying the knowledge of the experimental laboratory to the worldly problems of man. In this broadening of horizons behavior therapy has played an important part. But the days of simple conditioning and counterconditioning are over. Neal Miller's (1969) recent work on the specificity of the autonomic nervous system is going to force a reexamination of anxiety and of its role in psychosomatic medicine. The shift from external stimulus control to covert control with the use of subjective, covert, ideational stimuli in desensitization techniques and aversive conditioning, marked by Homme's (1965) use of the term "coverants," takes us inside the black box with a vengeance (or should we say, inside its shadow), as does the Eriksen symposium mentioned above. No longer can we escape responsibility by some vague reference to mediational processes; we now have techniques for investigating them.

It may even be that the black box will turn out to be Pandora's box, as I am sure it does in Skinner's nightmares, and that more has been unleashed than can be controlled. Certainly modern behavior therapy is moving toward increasing sophistication, as witness Carlin and Armstrong's (1968) recent warning on the interpretation of aversive conditioning: "all behavior change occurring in conditioning therapies should not be assumed a function of conditioning." And again, "cognitive consistency within belief systems and expectations may be a powerful factor in all behavior change." We hope this conference, by creating an interface where the "pure" and the "applied" can meet, may contribute something to our mechanisms of control, either to restore the lid to Pandora's box or to so regiment and train its troubling creatures through operant techniques that they become our slaves rather than we theirs; and in time we may even explore the box more deeply and find therein the hope that was left behind when Pandora's curiosity released man's ills upon a troubled world.

Comments on Paper by Hunt and Matarazzo

CHARLES B. FERSTER

THE IMPORTANT dimension of behavior emphasized by the preceding discussion of habits is its maintenance and persistence rather than the acquisition of performance. Such a discussion also emphasizes the frequency of the habitual act as an important property. The general problem for the modification of certain habits is that of self-control: there is a performance whose reinforcement is immediate and effective, but which also has delayed aversive consequences. The immediate positive reinforcement of the behavior leads to a persistent activity, whereas the long-term aversive consequences of the activity lead to the disposition to control the activity by reducing its frequency.

Self-control refers to performances that alter the conditions of a person's life so as to reduce the frequency of the habitual performance and hence reduce the long-term aversive consequences that result from these behaviors. The long-term aversive consequence is the reinforcer that maintains the self-control behavior. Self-control activity is reinforced because it reduces the aversive consequence resulting from the behavior to be controlled. The frequency of the self-control performance is due to termination or reduction (negative reinforcement) of the long-term aversive effects. The development of self-control behaviors would not be a problem unless the performance to be controlled were not reinforced immediately, while the aversive consequences occur considerably later.

When Hunt and Matarazzo speak of internalization of self-control, they refer to the many self-control performances—some verbal, some overt, and other covert—that are a firm part of the repertoire because they bridge the temporal gap between the performance and its long-term aversive consequences. Practically, the problem is how to reduce the frequency of the performance by manipulating all the variables of which the performance is a function. Before these variables can be manipulated, however, they have to be identified. Every behavioral process we know of in psychology is relevant.

The repertoire of taking and eating food is a useful example of the self-control needed to alter an effective and strongly reinforced performance. In the control of overeating the performance of putting food in the mouth is reinforced by the chewing and swallowing that follows. Sometimes eating is reinforced because it is prepotent over other activities that are aversive. The long-term aversive consequences of overeating include health problems and the social consequences of excess weight. The variables of which the eating behavior is a function are the individual's body weight and the time since his last meal; the presence or absence of circumstances normally surrounding the individual's eating; the kind of food that is available; the amount of performance required to obtain each kind of food; and the other kinds of performances, incompatible or prepotent over eating.

Drinking alcohol is another example of a behavior whose immediate reinforcement and delayed aversive consequences require self-control. The performance—drinking alcohol—is reinforced by a variety of consequences, including those behaviors that can occur only in the drugged state. Some of these are the social behaviors facilitated by alcohol, such as less inhibited conversation. Others are the social customs, such as participation in the conversations at the bar or the cocktail environment. The drugged state also removes aversive stimuli by interfering with their control over the individual's behavior. The aversive consequences of drinking may include long-term health deterioration, interference with normal eating patterns, a hangover, delerium tremens, interference with normal work activity, economic loss, deterioration in interpersonal relations, and unintended social effects on others caused by inappropriate behavior while under the influence of alcohol. The frequency of drinking may be reduced by avoiding places where alcohol is served, strengthening social behaviors that may be prepotent over those made possible by alcohol, eliminating aversive situations, and solving difficult problems that are the aversive stimuli attenuated by alcohol. Self-control as an actual performance that reduces the frequency of a habit is most clearly seen in a simple interchange between host and guest described by Skinner (1953). The host increases the frequency of drinking as a means of stimulating the party by serving salted peanuts, while the guest, in order to decrease the frequency of drinking, has several glasses of water just before entering the party.

The child who, facing the expensive bric-a-brac, puts his hands behind his back shows the self-control performance plainly. The past aversive consequences of parental punishment reinforce (negatively by removal) an actual performance. The effective maintenance of the performance requires an aversive event, present at the time the child is inclined to reach for the bric-a-brac, which will reinforce the incompatible performance. Hunt and Matarazzo's example of Mrs. Nolan illustrates the reinforcement of a specific performance that in turn altered the habit. While punishment and other aversive stimuli sometimes appear to subtract from a positively reinforced performance, the process is more likely to occur as the reinforcement of an incompatible behavior that in turn reduces the frequency of the habit.

The view of self-control as a performance that in turn controls the habit suggests that attention must be paid to its maintenance—its durability and frequency. Even after an individual acquires a self-control performance, its frequency can vary over a wide range. The usefulness of a self-control behavior in influencing a habit depends on its sufficiently frequent occurrence. Thus the development of self-control is a continuous and gradual phenomenon, rather than an all-or-none phenomenon, despite apparent instances where it appears to be acquired suddenly.

Because self-control comes from specific operant behaviors reinforced by avoiding aversive stimuli, their reinforcement is difficult because most of the aversive consequences of the habit are considerably delayed. Therefore there is no immediate reduction in aversive stimulation when the self-control performance reduces the frequency of the habitual act. Some way is needed to bridge the gap between the performance and its consequences so that there is a conditioned aversive stimulus, deriving its aversiveness from the ultimate consequences of the habit. Such a conditioned aversive stimulus can provide a reinforcer that can follow the self-control behavior immediately and thus effectively increase its frequency and maintain it.

The general analysis of self-control as a behavioral phenomenon provides a framework for organizing some of the common observations that can be made about smoking. Smoking is a very specific series of acts producing the final consequence of smoke in contact with the mucosa of the mouth and lungs. We need to find (a) the reinforcers maintaining smoking; (b) the short-term and long-term aversive consequences of smoking; (c) a way to bridge the temporal gap between the performance and its aversive effect; and (d) the performances, reinforced by terminating aversive consequences of smoking, that will reduce the frequency of smoking by reinforcing an incompatible behavior or by altering some of the reinforcers maintaining smoking. A critical step in the analysis is the discovery and amplification of the actual aversive consequences of smoking.

THE REINFORCERS MAINTAINING SMOKING

The most obvious consequence of inhaling cigarette smoke is its absorption into the mucosa of the lungs and mouth. The mechanism appears to be similar to that of drug addiction, where the absence of the physiological effect of the drug creates an aversive stimulus that only the drug can terminate. I do not know whether anyone has actually measured the conditioned and unconditioned reflexes involved in the aversiveness of withdrawal, but the situation appears to be clear behaviorally. Smoking is negatively reinforced by altering aversive physiologic states. Although the physiologic effects of smoking are undoubtedly conditioned and controlled by stimuli characteristically surrounding smoking, there are many other secondary consequences of smoking, independent of primary physiologic changes, which also reinforce. As Hunt and Matarazzo point out, the act of smoking interacts in very complex ways with many other repertoires; reinforcers other than smoke in the mouth maintain smoking. This interaction needs to be analyzed before an understanding can be reached of the events reinforcing smoking.

Non-metabolic simple effects of smoking

Smoking is also reinforced because it is a regular simple repeatable way of manipulating the environment—like doodling; nail chewing; tics; a hand gesture; scratching the body; grooming of the nails, hair or skin; or rubbing the chin or stroking a beard. It is probably not useful to think of these behaviors as reinforced by conditioned or secondary reinforcers because this view implies that their reinforcing effect is derived from a more primary behavior. For most purposes it is clear that the simple direct consequences of these acts sustain them—the pattern of the doodlers' drawing, the change in the condition of the fingernail, and the tactile effect of rubbing the skin or pulling the hair. These may not be powerful reinforcers, but in the absence of a strong competing behavior they seem capable of sustaining much behavior. Doodling, for example, is much more likely to occur at a conference that does not sustain the interest of the participants and where most of the possible items in the individual's repertoire cannot be emitted. It is the bored boy, during the long hot summer, who will spend thirty minutes running a stick over a picket fence; such behavior, having such a high frequency under these conditions, will be unlikely to occur at all when it is competing with major items in the boy's repertoire.

All the elements of the chain of performances that comprise smoking have these similar elements. There is the taking of a cigarette out of the pack and a ritual of tapping and manipulating it. There is the striking of a flame and the manipulation of match or lighter, also frequently with a ritual. There is the immediate, direct stimulation of smoke in the mouth, functionally similar to chewing a candy, biting the cheeks or lips, or picking the teeth. The pattern of smoke coming out of the mouth is one direct consequence of smoking that probably reinforces it. There is the change in the length of the cigarette. The color of the lighted end, which changes in a fine-grain relation to the performance of sucking air through the cigarette, is also a consequence of smoking. The ash that forms on the end of the cigarette requires further behavior and is another of its reactive features. Many smokers have elaborate rituals surrounding the disposal of the cigarette ash. Finally, the cigarette in the hand is an object whose manipulation can be directly reinforcing just, as a person may manipulate a coin, "play with a knife" at the dinner table, or handle a pencil during a conference. The effective reinforcement of these performances by their simple consequences is undoubtedly related to other events and circumstances. It does not seem profitable, however, to describe the relationship as conditioned or secondary reinforcement. Such a relationship implies that one stimulus derives its reinforcing properties because it is in a chain to the next one.

Smoking as a performance that avoids aversive social patterns

Smoking a cigarette may have some of the significance of "speaking to break a silence." The absence of conversation, or of some other performance to fill the gap, is often an aversive situation that reinforces compulsive talking. Some people use silence as a technique of social control. Speaking increases in frequency because it terminates the silence (negative reinforcement). A pause in the conversation is functionally shorter if one person is lighting or puffing on a cigarette. The process is present in exaggerated form when the elaborate rituals of pipe smoking are involved. There is probably some truth to the cultural stereotype of the pipe smoker as a taciturn, slow-speaking person. Smoking a pipe and speaking tend to be incompatible.

THE LONG-TERM AVERSIVE CONSEQUENCES OF SMOKING

The health damage caused by smoking appears to be its main long-term aversive consequence. The gap from the day-to-day smoking activity and its aversive consequences seems so remote that few smokers are controlled by it. Most people lack direct experience with cancer and heart disease that can provide the experiences from which day-to-day behavior about the ultimate aversive consequences can be generated. It is said that physicians who frequently see the lungs of smokers and who are frequently in contact with the relationship between cancer and heart disease and smoking are more likely to give up smoking because of its probable effect on producing these diseases. But for the average person these consequences seem rather too remote to be effective negative reinforcers. The possible use of these long-term aversive stimuli occurring in the immediate vicinity of the smoking performance depends upon a fairly elaborate repertoire, mostly verbal. This repertoire needs to occur with a sufficiently high frequency and with a sufficiently adequate form to be effective in the face of a strong inclination to smoke. In general the two repertoires are incompatible. These factors will be discussed with the dynamic problems in using aversive consequences of smoking as reinforcers.

THE SHORT-TERM AVERSIVE CONSEQUENCES

One of the aversive effects is the dirt that results from the ashes and the difficulty of maintaining ash trays and disposing of butts. Some smokers handle the ashes very efficiently, but others find themselves in conflict when they are in places where there is no ash tray when they need to dispose of an ash or cigarette end. Further, habitual smoking produces considerable irritation of the mouth, tongue, throat, and bronchi. These and other effects of smoking are referred to by some smokers as cigarette hangover, which occurs the morning after a party, as a result of the large number of cigarettes smoked the night before. Other smokers have continuous unpleasant symptoms resulting from smoking. The inability to be without cigarettes, except for brief periods, causes many smokers difficulty. Frequently important activity needs to be interrupted in order to go out and purchase cigarettes. Many smokers feel a general cultural disapproval from their inability to control their smoking behavior. The addictive aspects of smoking represent a lack of control that is socially disapproved and internalized by most people. For some individuals the cost of smoking may be one of its aversive consequences.

DYNAMIC PROBLEMS IN USING THE AVERSIVE CONSEQUENCES
OF SMOKING TO REINFORCE SELF-CONTROL PERFORMANCES

Such, then, are the potential consequences of smoking that may serve as reinforcers for behaviors that in turn will reduce the frequency of smoking. But these events are not static phenomena that can automatically be effective for reinforcing self-control. These potential reinforcers will be effective only under certain conditions. The possibility of applying these ultimate aversive consequences to reinforcing self-control behaviors is a delicate problem that requires careful adjustment of all the components of the individual's repertoire. Since most of the potential aversive stimuli are displaced in time from the smoking behavior, it follows that the major means of bringing them to bear and bridging the temporal gap is verbal behaviors under control of the short-range or long-range aversive consequences of smoking. Before the behaviors can even develop, there is a problem, first, whether the person can observe the existence of these aversive consequences and, second, whether or not the repertoires of describing them exist in any substantial form. The self-control performances need to have sufficient fluency and durability to occur in competition with a strong inclination to smoke. The long-range aversive consequences of smoking may be potential reinforcers in the case of most smokers, but their effective use depends on the person's ability to observe the aversive consequences of smoking, the ability to speak about them in a sufficiently fluent form to allow them to be applied, and a sufficient frequency and durability of the self-control behavior to persist in the face of a strong tendency to smoke.

The use of the aversive consequences of smoking as reinforcers for self-control behavior requires a delicate balance between the removal of the aversive stimuli by self-control behavior that reduces the frequency of smoking and the occurrence of a mechanism, such as denial or suppression, in which the aversive stimuli reinforce behaviors that are incompatible with observing the aversive stimuli. An imbalance between an effective current level of self-control and a full development of the aversive consequences of smoking will lead to a continuation of smoking without thought or talk about the long-range or short-range aversive consequences. It would seem that the development of a verbal repertoire about the ultimate aversive consequences of smoking would have to be very carefully paced with the person's ability to control smoking in some way. This writer's experience with teaching weight control indicates that the ability to think or talk about the long-term consequences of being overweight depended upon the subject's having some successful experience in controlling his eating patterns. This was accomplished in the weight-control experiment (Ferster, Nurnberger, and Levitt, 1962) when the subjects altered their eating patterns by restricting all food intake to meals but still had not reduced their weight or their food intake. Thus it was possible to achieve some self-control with minimum development of the long-range aversive consequences and without any loss in weight or reduction of food intake. This small amount of self-control, reinforced by the reduction of the aversive stimuli associated with being overweight, provided a base for the next steps—additional verbal behaviors about the aversive consequences of being overweight that could reinforce new self-control behaviors. There was repeated evidence of active denial of the aversive consequences of being overweight before the subjects had achieved any control over their eating patterns. It was possible for the subjects to speak fluently, realistically, and in detail about their overweight only after they had already achieved some control.

THE SITUATION WHERE SMOKING OCCURS

An important determinant of the frequency of smoking and of procedures for controlling it is the wide range of circumstances under which a person smokes. The Nolan case illustrates self-control performance which reduced the overall tendency to smoke by restricting the circumstances in which smoking occurs. The frequency of smoking was therefore reduced on other occasions. Such a procedure had the obvious advantage of producing long periods of abstinence, which in turn reduced the addictive and withdrawal problems. Limiting the circumstances under which a habit may be reinforced is one of the main avenues by which performances of various kinds can be controlled. In the control of eating this is accomplished by limiting eating to certain times, to certain distinctive places, and to specific foods.

It is important not to confuse the occasion when smoking occurs with secondary reinforcement. The occasion in which smoking occurs is a situation in which a performance is reinforced, in contrast to another situation in which it is not. As a result, the one occasion controls high frequency of a performance and the other a low frequency. Most people who have stopped smoking can vividly recount many stories in which an old acquaintance or a party increased the frequency of smoking to the point where smoking became prepotent over self-control. Because these situations had not been encountered since smoking had stopped, there had been no opportunity to reduce the tendency to smoke on these occasions. It seems that the disposition to smoke has to be reduced on each and every occasion the person is likely to encounter.

EMOTION AND STRESS

"Emotional variables" is a term referring to the kind of experiences or procedures that increase or decrease the generic classes of behavior. Thus, when someone is angry, there is a noticeably high frequency of performances reinforced by the harm he produces on other persons. The changes in hormones or physiological conditions that might accompany these changes in behavior are corollaries of the emotional behavior. Frequently the most apparent behaviors observed when someone is "under emotion" are not necessarily the most significant. For example, if someone is biting his nails in an obviously emotional state, it is more significant that there is a low frequency of all other items in his repertoire that would normally be present at that time. With the increase in emotional symptoms there is frequently a major cessation in most of the ongoing repertoire the person might engage in. With such a temporary decrease in the frequency in most of the items in a person's repertoire, the relative importance of even the minor reinforcers increases enormously. Thus the relative position of smoking items of the repertoire are depressed. Smoking becomes something to do in the entire repertoire is increased considerably when other major when no other behavior is appropriate.

It is also possible that smoking may in some cases be one item of a general class of aggressive behaviors that occurs because it produces injury. The line of reasoning is speculative, but the parallels to clinical theory and the consistency ·with a behavioral analysis of the phenomenon suggest that it is substantial enough to be considered. The standard clinical expression that "depression is anger turned inward" illustrates a phenomenon that may also be described behaviorally. Casual observation of people under stress will, I think, generally indicate a much higher frequency of smoking when they are angry than at other times.

Similar forms of self-punishment may be observed when someone strikes his own head or a table, kicks a piece of furniture, destroys one of his own possessions, digs his nails into his palm until it hurts, or clenches his fist and jaw to the point of discomfort. In all these cases the significant fact is that a performance is taking place that is inflicting pain. These behaviors belong to a class of performances whose frequency increases in anger, and their occurrence, which is inappropriate to the condition that generated them, is probably the result of the severe punishment that occurs as a result of aggressive acts toward many people. Smoking a cigarette may have the same relationship to the emotional state as "kicking the cat" or screaming at a child.

INTERACTION BETWEEN SMOKING AND THE INDIVIDUAL'S ENTIRE REPERTOIRE

In the discussion of emotion I have already mentioned that a decrease in the frequency of any segment of the individual's repertoire may increase the frequency of smoking. Smoking interacts with broad aspects of the individual's repertoire in many other similar ways. First, smoking is incompatible with many activities. For example, most movies and theater performances require that a smoker abstain for two hours or more. It would be virtually impossible for the same individual to refrain from smoking in other circumstances. The theater and its social sanctions result in a very strongly controlled performance that is prepotent over smoking. A common device for those who try to stop smoking is to keep busy with as many activities as possible that are prepotent over smoking. This suggests that there is a general personality factor in which the overall state of the individual's repertoire is a significant element that partly determines the persistence, addictiveness, or habitualness of smoking. The problem is like that of the autistic child, characterized by a very minimal social and intellectual repertoire. In such children simple, primitive consequences of behavior support enormous amounts of activity, essentially by default. Such children will sit for hours throwing sand, touching a spot, walking back and forth, repeating simple sounds over and over, or engaging in other kinds of rituals. Simple reinforcers, such as the direct effect of the behaviors, sustain them in the face of any other stronger competing behavior. Lindsley's observations (1959, 1963) in his experiments with psychotic subjects who were pressing a bar on schedules of reinforcement (provided by cigarettes and candy) is relevant to the same point. He found that actively hallucinating schizophrenic patients carried on the "crazy behavior" only during the pause after each reinforcement in the key-pressing behavior generated by the fixed-ratio schedule. Pressing the key under the control of its reinforcer was prepotent over these psychotic symptoms.

Part of the answer to the control of smoking may lie in an assessment of the individual's basic repertoire that allows the minor and major reinforcements of smoking to produce a performance that is prepotent over so many elements of the person's life. While it is true that smoking may be compatible with many other kinds of activities because it can occur concurrently, there is still the problem of why the other activities are so insufficiently maintained as to allow room for another concurrent behavior.

SUMMARY

The development of self-control depends on the opportunity for the aversive consequences of the habit to reinforce actual behaviors. The child about to reach for the bric-a-brac generates conditioned aversive stimuli that come from his history of punishment when he played with similar objects in the past. Withdrawing his hands and putting them behind his back is reinforced because it terminates or reduces the conditioned aversive stimuli and it constitutes an actual behavior that in turn decreases the frequency of the punishment and hence is self-controlled. The child who is about to giggle in class and who has been punished for such behavior in the past puts his hand over his mouth, bites his lip, looks the other way, or inflicts pain on his body so as to produce a reaction incompatible with laughing. All of these actual behaviors terminate a conditioned aversive stimulus because they reduce the frequency of potentially punishable behavior. These types of self-control occur readily in the course of normal development because the aversive consequences follow actual behavior closely.

To control smoking it is necessary to examine all the reinforcers that sustain the performance and search for all the behavioral processes that can either reduce the frequency of smoking by reinforcing an incompatible behavior or alter the environment if the normal reinforcer does not occur.

An analysis has been made of the many different consequences that sustain the frequency of smoking. It is not necessary to decide whether these are conditioned or primary reinforcers. In all probability they derive their reinforcing properties from some preceding experiences, but their practical control does not appear to depend upon these in every case. The problem is more empirical because the discovery of a reinforcer comes from observing the frequency of a performance when its consequences are changed. Thus, if the tactile manipulation of the cigarette is an important reinforcer for smoking, then altering the smoking situation so that the individual is unable to touch the cigarette with his hands should produce a decrease in the frequency of smoking, all other things being equal.

The development of self-control in behavior depends on identifying the actual aversive consequences of smoking and constructing a verbal repertoire that can be brought to bear fluently and immediately.

A behavioral analysis of smoking suggests the distinction between a strong habit and addiction. A habit can be described as a performance having an unusually high frequency and prepotent over most items in the individual's repertoire. "Addiction" refers to an aversive physiological state that appears during abstinence and whose termination reinforces the smoking.

The development of self-control was posed as a dynamic problem, in which the frequency of the various relevant performances need to be adjusted to each other. This view suggests the observation of the maintenance of behavior over a long period of time rather than the learning or acquisition of new forms. The basic problem is that of increasing the frequency of some performances so that they are sufficiently stable to maintain self-control behaviors and be prepotent over the smoking behavior. Thus the issue is not the presence or absence of a particular kind of behavior but whether it has a sufficiently high frequency to compete with or alter the smoking behavior significantly. A successful program of self-control in smoking would necessarily involve very careful pacing of the development of self-control with the conditions with which it can be reinforced successfully. A procedure to use the long-term aversive consequences of smoking needs to be carefully paced with the development of actual self-control, so that self-controlled behaviors are reinforced rather than denied or repressed. A program for self-control should not force the person into a degree of coercion, deprivation, or abstinence that exceeds the self-control repertoire he has developed at the particular stage of the program.

General Discussion

BORGATTA pointed out the difficulty of defining the "field" within which people operate. It consists of many complex aversive and attractive factors, both direct and, in the social sense, indirect—as in the case of the individual's identity, his self-evaluation, and the responses that other social beings make to him. While he did like the idea that not all rewards and punishments are sensual in nature, he questioned whether the knowledge and understanding of the determining factors in behavior as given in the Hunt-Matarazzo paper was complete enough to render application profitable.

LOGAN objected strongly to the statement that there were two kinds of learning in the sense used by Hunt and Matarazzo, pointing out that Hull's "pure stimulus act" and Miller and Dollard's "cue producing response" refer to behavior that produces stimuli that in turn control behavior. The difference is not in kind of learning, but in type of controlling stimulus. One is external and impinges upon the organism. The other consists of those feedback stimuli one gets from one's own behavior. Some of our behaviors have no other function than to produce stimuli to control subsequent behavior.

TOMKINS interjected his feeling that Hunt and Matarazzo were making the point that the difference was essentially a quantitative one, that the consequences of a particular kind of self-statement or self-feeling were disproportionate to what one would have expected on a purely quantitative reinforcement basis.

BORGATTA pointed out the difference between manipulating the system in which the person lies and dealing with the problem of the variables in the system. In some conditioning experiments external limitations are imposed on the system; here the control is direct. In other situations the control may be indirect through the individual's self-motivation. Conceptually at least, these different levels of complexity must be handled. Furthermore, in smoking more is involved than a singly determined system. There is a multiple determined system; and when an input is made, a multiple set of consequences is likely to ensue.

PREMACK came in at this time to comment that two points seemed at issue. In the first place, every act inevitably has an intrinsic consequence (and possibly an extrinsic consequence as well). In general, control of the act is easier through the extrinsic, because it is more easily grasped. Thus, in the case of controlling x by y, the extrinsic factor may be more convenient, but the intrinsic factors may complicate the problem.

Secondly, the extrinsic-intrinsic differentiation is not the whole story. One has to ask whether in imputing to the individual the ability to deny or to permit himself to smoke, a belief or value system is not forced on this person. This is where x is manipulating x, as in self-control. One must ask: What are belief systems? What are values? Can they be operationalized? What role do they play in self-control?

At this point JARVIK intervened to say that he thought the importance of nicotine in maintaining smoking behavior was being overlooked. HILL commented that in many cases where behavior seems to be self-maintained without reinforcement, the problem actually may be an inability to identify the reinforcer rather than the absence of one. PREMACK agreed, saying that in the adult and veteran smoker the extrinsic consequences are not the main factors in maintaining the behavior. The extrinsic factors refer to the control exercised by the external world on a response that is maintained on a base level by intrinsic factors. Here the heavier weight will have to be assigned to the intrinsic factors.

The discussion then turned to the complexities and importance of external factors, with BORGATTA stressing the necessity of differentiating between habit acquisition and habit extinction. He pointed out the complexity and variability of social situational factors and the need for introducing them into analysis of behavior; but he ended by conceding that, despite the importance of external stimulus control, it would be impossible to ignore the baseline JARVIK, HILL, and PREMACK had been mentioning. PREMACK, in turn, added the caution that stimulus control is by no means confined to cases in which the act is being maintained by an intrinsic consequence, but that it has been maintained by extrinsic consequences.

TOMKINS concluded the discussion by stressing the fact that his model of smoking behavior did deal with habit and that one of his categories is the "habitual" smoker. There was no intention of treating such behavior as trivial. He had two major objections, however, to the Hunt-Matarazzo paper. One was the definition of habit, and the second concerned the questioning of the validity of introspective evidence— or rather, the retrospective reporting of introspective evidence.

He pointed out the terminological ambiguity of "habit" and stated that there are two aspects of habit as overlearned behavior. All habits, he assumed, have some storage site in the nervous system, whence they can be retrieved. What is retrieved can by-pass consciousness— largely as a computer program by-passes consciousness—and still control target organs. The organs move in accordance with the program, as is the case when someone is driving a car while having a conversation with a passenger. This is the sense in which he interpreted the Hunt-Matarazzo usage. But habitual behavior can be conscious, as when one is asked one's name and responds. This, too, is habit, but it occurs with full consciousness. When habits work reasonably well in a fairly constant environment, that program is going to by-pass consciousness and free it for new learning. It is not necessary to learn something more thoroughly when it works well as it stands. But the moment the environment makes new demands on old habits, to restrict habit to a behavioral program that by-passes consciousness is to impoverish the organism and make it impossible to meet the new demands.

On the question of the validity of the retrospective reporting of introspective data, he pointed out that one cannot take literally any kind of evidence, including the introspective report, but neither should one decide in advance that it has no validity. That view is equally naïve. The critical question about introspective evidence is not whether or not it is valid, but whether or not it has any predictive power. He had found that the answers people give to the question as to the kinds of occasions under which they smoke are lawfully related to what they will say and what they will do in terms of renunciation and the consequences of renunciation. The data hang together. If they did not, he would be more suspicious about the validity of what people say about the occasions on which they smoke and the reasons they give for doing so.

As to a hedonic model of smoking, while his language sounds like an affect theory of smoking, his model is by no means limited to the specification of affects, and it is not completely accurate to call it an affect model. American psychology in the last sixty years has been deluded into thinking that a human being can be understood in terms of some small part of the total system.

The meeting had been told that the only thing that matters about a person is his behavior, or his cognition and expectations, or his drives, or his affects. The simple and obvious fact of the matter is that a human being acts, he thinks, he feels, he has drives; and to exclude any of these from the systematic study of the human being is to ask for trouble.

Mechanisms of Self-Control

DAVID PREMACK

THERE is a strong reluctance to discuss observations from the laboratory in the same breath with those from everyday life. This compartmentalization may represent an intelligent policy for many purposes, protecting data from anecdote and theory from common sense. But on other occasions it can impose an anomalous barrier between sets of information that would otherwise profitably influence one another.

A case in point is the recent mass of unsuccessful attempts to train people to stop smoking. A variety of behavior modification techniques reflecting diverse theories have been unable to produce more than a temporary reduction in smoking (Bernstein, 1969; Keutzer, et al., 1968). On the other hand, the government reports that millions have quit smoking voluntarily; HEW estimates put this number at about twenty-one million (Horn, 1969). These observations have been perfectly sheltered from one another. Recent reviews of the behavior-modification work, though exhaustive in their coverage of that work, make no mention whatever of the contrasting achievements from outside the laboratory (Bernstein, 1969; Keutzer, et al., 1968). In terms of an analogy from another field, it is as though laboratories were uniformly unable to perfect an internal combustion engine—and in the meticulous write-up of their failure neglected to mention the twenty million cars driving by outside.

But the paradox between the failure inside and success outside the laboratory is important for more than a striking example of compartmentalization. How is the paradox to be resolved? Why are millions able to do by themselves outside the laboratory what apparently they cannot be trained to do inside the laboratory? The answer to that question contains, I believe, important suggestions as to how people actually control themselves, in contrast to the kinds of control mechanisms with which they are endowed by current behavior theory. The typical laboratory reaction to the failure is, of course, quite different: nothing is needed beyond the usual tightening up: greater ingenuity and better controls. But this is a reasonable reaction only if one looks exclusively at the laboratory data. If one attends to both sets of observations, different conclusions are in order, the most important of which, I think, are as follows.

First, the failure of behavior modification to produce a lasting cessation of smoking is not, as some suggest, a disconfirmation of behavior theory. Rather, it is substantially predictable from behavior theory that if one were allowed only the kinds of mechanisms that behavior theory allows, it would not be possible to produce a lasting cessation of smoking by people living in an open society. This view states that current behavior theory is not so much false or incorrect as it is radically incomplete. Second, the success of people outside the laboratory comes not from a more ingenious use of those mechanisms that have not worked in the laboratory, but from the use of mechanisms different from those behavior theory talks about. Third, these "different" mechanisms are of the highest importance to society, for it is to them —and not the mechanisms of behavior theory—that society owes its existence.

The paper is organized as follows. First, to understand the failure of laboratory procedures to control smoking, I consider possible causes of smoking and the practice each would implicate as a control for smoking. Each case raises the same question: is there any evidence that masses of people actually engage in these practices? Second, a process of elimination suggests that punishment or some other aversive procedure would be the most effective approach against smoking; in fact, punishment is the procedure adopted by virtually all behavior modification; but punishment does not work, and it is necessary to show why. Third, as a prelude to a theory of self-control, I ask whether the medical evidence on lung cancer causes people to quit smoking or whether this evidence is less cause than catalyst. Fourth, several versions of an informal theory of self-control are examined. I conclude by indicating why society, unlike an institutionalized population, may require not only control of one individual by another, but also self-control.

POSSIBLE CAUSES AND IMPLICATED CONTROLS FOR SMOKING

In general, responses are maintained by either their intrinsic or their extrinsic consequences or both. In the case of smoking, examples of intrinsic consequences are the stimulation resulting from the inhalation and exhalation of smoke, as well as the increased heart rate produced by nicotine. Extrinsic consequences, on the other hand, can include indefinitely many possibilities; some frequently suggested examples are social anxiety, which smoking may reduce; or attention, which smoking may increase. In addition, a response can be maintained jointly by both kinds of factors—at one level by the intrinsic consequences, at a still higher level by the addition of appropriate extrinsic consequences. These factors limit the ways in which a response can be eliminated.

For example, an attack on intrinsic consequences might include a cigarette with reduced nicotine content, which may maintain a lower base level of smoking than an ordinary one. But if so, tne problem would still remain of inducing people to smoke such cigarettes. And this problem would confront any attempt to reduce the base level of smoking through attenuating the intrinsic factors that maintain smoking.

An attack on the extrinsic consequences might include reducing social anxiety; or arrangements might be made to eliminate the attention smoking receives, or to give some other response—a socially desirable one—more attention than smoking receives. For example, if smoking were caused by social anxiety, it could be reduced by so-called de-sensitization—that is, by progressively reducing the anxiety a person experiences in social situations. The success of desensitization in other areas (Wolpe, 1958) suggests that it might succeed in this area too, if in fact smoking were caused by social anxiety. However, nothing compels the view that the millions who have quit were primarily social smokers who somehow desensitized themselves (or, alternatively, learned to stay out of social situations); whereas those who have not been "cured," either by themselves or in the laboratory, were not social smokers and thus could not be aided by desensitization. To begin with, there is no evidence that people desensitize themselves. More important, many of those who quit were not primarily "social smokers" but were more nearly "solitary smokers"—people who indulged heavily in the early hours of the morning, when alone with a book or a manuscript.

An alternative view is that people smoke because they are rewarded for doing so—by attention, for example, or by a gratifying self-image. It is not difficult to generate this hypothesis: in some parts of the country one need do no more than drive his son to school. There, on the street corners, near the school, short skirts and long cigarettes rehearse awkward gestures that plead for eyewitness. If no one looked at these young people, it seems certain that some percentage of them would quit smoking. But the hypothesis is less reasonable if it is extended to the adult sector of the population. Few adults smoke to illuminate the image of, say, Humphrey Bogart, and it is they, not the young, who account for the millions who have quit.

Attention and a gratifying self-image do not exhaust the possibilities of reward. Smoking rarely occurs alone; more often it is accompanied by or itself accompanies drinking, snacking, talking, reading, watching TV, or simply thinking. Even though these events are not contingent upon smoking, they might still be considered to reinforce smoking (Skinner, 1948). To determine whether they do would require comparing a base frequency of smoking with frequencies obtained after the suspect events had been first eliminated and then restored. If smoking were rewarded by these events, their elimination would reduce, and subsequent interposition restore, the frequency of smoking. Unfortunately it does not seem likely that such data will be obtained in the near future; fortunately they are not really needed. Although these measurements alone could tell whether smoking were reinforced by drinking and the like, that question need not be answered in order to decide how people actually quit smoking.

There appear to be no reports of people turning off the TV, putting aside reading materials, pushing back the snacks and then, abstaining from speech and even thought, smoking until the room is hazy. Yet this is precisely what extinction would require. That is, if smoking were rewarded by certain of its co-occurrents, extinction would require that smoking occur in the absence of these co-occurrents. Alternatively smoking might be reduced by latent extinction; if the stimuli that normally followed smoking, which were themseves followed by snacking, drinking, and so on, no longer led to snacking and the like, smoking could be extinguished without actually having to occur. But this would require a major rearrangement of one's life, and there is no evidence that such changes have ever taken place, especially on the scale that would be required to account for the millions who have quit. In brief, I do not question the efficacy of the extinction paradigms—that has been shown in the laboratory—but whether in fact they have any currency outside of the laboratory.

Moreover, even if smoking were a behavior that was first rewarded and then extinguished, there would still be a failure to reproduce much of the data reported by HEW. At least some of the estimated twenty-one million have quit smoking, not merely cut down, and extinction is better suited to reducing a behavior than to eliminating it. That is, extinction carries a response to its prereinforcement level which is almost always greater than zero, if only because of the difficulty of initiating reinforcement in responses whose base frequency is zero. Finally, it is a mistake, albeit a common one, to assume that because two events occur together in time, one must be reinforcing the other one. Some theories appear to lead to this view, but on the few occasions when this implication was tested, the theories were not supported (Premack, 1963). Co-occurrence is a necessary, not a sufficient, condition for reinforcement.

The folklore, if not the literature, of smoking contains accounts of outcomes that can only be called paradoxical. If in a choice between cigarettes with and without nicotine, people chose the latter and in this way smoked less, this would be a paradoxical outcome and would require special explanation. Similarly, if in a choice between smoking that in one case leads to no extrinsic consequence and in another case to electric shock, people chose the latter, thereby smoking less than normal, this too would be decidedly paradoxical. The standard outcome is for choice and base rates to be proportional (Greeno, 1968; Premack, 1965), and any actually obtained outcomes to the contrary would require special explanation (perhaps along the lines of the mechanism for self-control that will be proposed here). The point is that "paradoxical outcomes" cannot be offered as a procedure for quitting smoking; if they occur at all, they must be a source of puzzlement until a theory is provided that can account for them and can show how they can be reliably produced.

RELIANCE OF BEHAVIOR MODIFICATION ON
AVERSIVE CONTROL

Almost all forms of behavior modification use an aversive procedure, either simply associating smoking with an aversive event or, as in punishment, making the aversive event contingent upon smoking. The smoker may be assailed with stale smoke or electric shock each time he smokes, or he may be shown a film on lung cancer while he is smoking, or he may be instructed to hold his breath for an uncomfortable duration each time he thinks of smoking. If desensitization, extinction, rewarding another response at a still higher rate, or attenuating intrinsic factors prove to be ineffective, then aversive procedures emerge as the only alternative. Moreover, punishment is an effective way of eliminating behavior, and smoking is not impervious to it. For example, when electric shock was made contingent upon smoking, or upon opening a box containing cigarettes, the suppression that followed was typical of response suppression generally (Powell and Azrin, 1968). Then why does punishment fail to control smoking?

Punishment fails to eliminate smoking for the same reason it would fail to eliminate any other response to which it was given the same relation: it is possible to smoke outside the training situation without being punished. This problem has already been encountered in a somewhat different form in the reduction of smoking that might be achieved through reducing the nicotine content of cigarettes. Both the nicotine and electric-shock procedures will reduce smoking, but the problem is then to induce people to confine their smoking to the circumstance in which these factors apply. Most people cannot be induced to smoke only when smoking produces electric shock. In certain basic essentials the situation is like that of a rat that has two activity wheels available for exercise, one of which produces electric shock. At first the rat may fail to discriminate the wheels and not run at all, or the suppression in the punished wheel will transfer in part to the unpunished one, but the transfer will be temporary. The magnitude of the transfer can be enhanced by increasing the similarity between the wheels, but this device cannot be relied upon to eliminate running in the rat. On the other hand, if when the rat ceased to run, the disposition to run were itself to decay, then any procedure capable of producing even temporary abstinence might also be capable of producing permanent abstinence. There is, however, no evidence that the disposition to run decays during periods in which running does not occur. Nor is there any evidence of a similar process in smoking; on the contrary, many people quit for weeks or even months, only to resume with a vengeance.

In summary, if a response with a base level greater than zero cannot be punished in all of the situations in which it can occur, it cannot be eliminated by punishment. This view is predictable from behavior theory. It is within the range of demonstration in the animal laboratory and, it would seem, is well on its way to being demonstrated with human subjects. But now the fact arises that, although in the present circumstance behavior theory has no way in which to eradicate smoking, an estimated twenty-one million people have quit smoking.

FEAR OF CANCER AN INSUFFICIENT
CONDITION

As a first step toward clearing the way for a theory of self-control, what may seem the simplest alternative explanation must be considered: people quit smoking because of the threat of lung cancer. This alternative cannot be eliminated on the grounds that the effective dissemination of the evidence linking cigarette smoking to lung cancer has had no relation to the data. Furthermore, the medical information has at least some of the qualities of an effective deterrent—high aversiveness—plus a special quality lacking in traditional punishment and accounting for its ineffectiveness in the present case. People cannot escape the dread of cancer merely by changing the room in which they smoke—as they can so easily escape the electric shock that may be contingent upon smoking in the laboratory merely by smoking at home. Then why doubt that the fear of lung cancer directly caused millions of people to quit smoking?

There appear to be a great many individuals who do not dispute the medical evidence, who unquestionably fear lung cancer, and who smoke nevertheless. But do they really believe? This is not apt to be a profitable line of inquiry; we may have no more reason to doubt their statement of belief in this case than in any other. Moreover, it has been shown possible experimentally to increase a person's belief that smoking causes cancer without affecting either the amount the person smokes or the likelihood that he will quit (Lichtenstein, Keutzer, and Himes, 1969). The concordance between belief and behavior is not that simple.

The fear of cancer may start out as a sufficient condition and then extinguish. Even the individual who is so unfortunate as ultimately to incur lung cancer will have smoked many times without experiencing negative feedback—a condition that makes for extinction in normal circumstances. Additionally, if a person reaches middle age without having been afflicted, he may consider his odds to have improved. If each time the person smokes, the medical evidence took the form of a "little heart attack" or some other negative feedback, the deterrent would be more effective. Finally, we may even wish to invoke the seemingly uncanny ability of people to defend a sense of immortality against all merely probabilistic threat.

The fear of cancer is not a cause but a catalyst, setting in motion in some people a process that leads ultimately to the termination of smoking. If the medical evidence is assigned this role, it accounts, first, for the obvious conjunction between the statistics on quitting and the dissemination of the medical information; and, second, for the otherwise puzzling inefficacy of the medical evidence in those cases where the evidence is not disputed. The task now is to make clear the causal process catalyzed by the cancer evidence. The character of this process is directly suggested by the case histories of people who have quit smoking. I will describe three such cases, deliberately in a quasi-anecdotal manner, so as to retain their intuitive flavor, that may help the reader to recognize similar processes in himself and predispose him both to join in the attempt to elucidate the process and to judge the accuracy of the elucidation proposed here.

Use of humiliation in self-control

A forty-year-old male smoked two packages a day for twenty years before quitting abruptly and completely; he has not smoked in seven years. Despite the lengthy period of abstinence, he is not able to discuss the topic dispassionately. "It is humiliating to be duped by those goddamn cigarette companies. They know their product causes cancer, but they do absolutely nothing to prevent it. Instead they spend millions on advertising, to keep all the old suckers smoking and to start as many new suckers as possible. Can you see those bastards down there sitting around a pool—Virginia, Kentucky—counting the loot, patting one another's back, laughing it up and not a one of them smoking? You're right, absolutely, the blacks are the ones you see smoking down there." This tirade could be enriched along numerous lines, but the speaker's attitude has already been adequately conveyed. If this person were to contemplate the possibility of smoking, he may be apt to hear not so much the clinical warning, "You may get cancer," as a sniggering invitation in a Southern accent calling to him across the splashing of a pool, "Smoke, suckah, and make me rich!"

A second case involves a thirty-year-old physician who had smoked approximately a package a day for over ten years and who quit only recently. His case is of too recent vintage to be regarded as true quitting, but it is interesting nonetheless for the suggestion it contains as to how the outside world may influence quitting. Again the provocation or catalyst was cancer, this time communicated by a TV short prepared by the American Cancer Society. The film shows a father and son strolling through the woods, the son imitating the father in ways that are either innocuous or socially desirable until, at the end, the father takes out a cigarette and prepares to smoke. The viewer is then asked, in effect, is this what you are teaching your child? The physician reported that as he watched the film for the second time, he suddenly recognized himself as just such a father; he was leading his son to smoke despite his intimate knowledge of the cellular irritation that accompanies each inhalation on those "vile things." With this realization he abruptly stopped smoking.

The third and last case also involves a father, in this instance one who had smoked heavily for twenty years and then quit with characteristic abruptness—forty cigarettes one day, none the next—approximately eight years ago. This man dates his quitting from a day on which he had gone to pick up his children at the city library. A thunderstorm greeted him as he arrived there; and at the same time a search of his pockets disclosed a familiar problem: he was out of cigarettes. Glancing back at the library, he caught a glimpse of his children stepping out in the rain, but he continued around the corner, certain that he could find a parking space, rush in, buy the cigarettes and be back before the children got seriously wet. The view of himself as a father who would "actually leave the kids in the rain while he ran after cigarettes" was—I think the word is appropriate—humiliating, and he quit smoking—an accomplishment for which he had been prepared (softened up)—by the cancer statistics but which they could not accomplish alone.

Rather than multiply case histories, I think from these few cases the critical features may be abstracted that are common not only to them, but to the vast majority of the rest of the case histories. Each person has a set of attitudes or beliefs that entail a conduct that is acceptable to him. In old-fashioned language these are called moral or ethical standards. In each of the examples the person realized that smoking involved him in behavior incompatible with the conduct required by his ethical standards. The person in the first example found that in smoking he became a member of the class of people who contribute to sinister companies (companies knowingly marketing a product causing a nearly incurable disease). In the second case smoking placed the father among those who set an extremely dangerous example for their children. And in the last case rain conspired with an empty cigarette package to show a father that his addiction had reached the point where he put his own pleasure above the welfare of his children. Duped by a malevolent company; setting one's child a dangerous example; setting a self-destructive pleasure above the well-being of his children: each of these describes a class. For many people the discovery of membership in such a class is a humiliating shock.

INTERNAL CONTINGENCY

The discovery of membership in an ethically repugnant class could act to affect behavior in several ways. The discovery alone cannot be the whole story. It is, so to speak, only knowledge, a cognitive-emotional state of affairs, and a mechanism must be devised that will enable this knowledge to affect behavior. In one alternative the humiliation attendant upon the discovery would act like any other aversive event—with, however, some considerable potential advantages over the standard aversive events of the laboratory. All laboratory cases involve *external* contingencies: a conditional relation between an antecedent consisting of a response by the subject and a consequence consisting of an event in the world *external* to the subject. In classical examples, if a subject presses a lever, a food pellet is released or an electric shock is turned on or off. The antecedent is instanced by the subject, the consequence by the world outside him. The weakness of this kind of control mechanism has already been demonstrated for worlds containing more than one room.

If not only the antecedent but also the consequence is put inside the subject, what might be called an internal contingency obtains, a seemingly far more powerful mechanism of control. The power would come from the fact that the person is then his own source of food pellets or, in this case, electric shock and would be so no matter which room of the world he chanced to be in. At least it would be so if the moral standards were constant and did not fluctuate notably from room to room. Even though this view is not strictly true, the approximation may hold sufficiently to give the internal contingency its special power.

Some of the awkwardness of this machinery can be alleviated simply by invoking standard anticipatory mechanisms. To suffer humiliation, the person would not actually have to smoke but would merely have to contemplate smoking. The contingency would then be wholly internal—that is, the antecedent would no longer be smoking but the thought of smoking, and the consequence would be the equally internal humiliation. Now one could be guilty by intention alone, and the control mechanism would seem to have achieved not only power but elegance as well.

In summary, for an individual to discover that he is a member of a strongly interdicted class can be acutely humiliating. Each time the person engages in behavior that made him a member of the class—

smokes or contemplates smoking—he reexperiences the humiliation. If humiliation acts like aversive shock it suppresses or, if the magnitude effect is proper, even totally eliminates smoking. But an internal contingency, though possibly a necessary condition for quitting smoking, is not a sufficient one; and other factors must be considered, not the least of which is smoking itself, an act conditioned to virtually every time and place in the individual's environment.

SELF-INSTRUCTION: THE OPERATIONAL CONSEQUENCE OF A DECISION

The process that eventuates in an internal contingency will also give rise to a decision to quit smoking. Whatever else a decision may be, its prime operational consequence is self-instruction. Having decided to quit smoking, the individual will henceforth have a tendency to say to himself, "I'm done with that business, I'm through with smoking," and the like. A person who has made a decision may be likened to two people—one an agent or potential locus of behavior, the other a speaker who at critical times offers the agent advice, "Don't do that," or "Do do that." Indeed, in a rich man decisions might be expected to take this form explicitly: a lackey trailing the potentate about, reminding him at critical moments of the decision he has made, "No, sire, do not do that; you asked me to call to your attention," and so forth. The poor man must substitute his own inner voice for that of the lackey; and if it is less certain, is also less cumbersome.

Far from being idle, self-instruction can serve to restore thought to behavior sequences that, as a result of frequent occurrence, have become automatic or thoughtless. Thus, although smoking is conditioned to virtually everything, thinking about smoking is probably conditioned to very little; in the inveterate smoker thinking about smoking is a rare event. But if the thought of smoking can be intruded at critical points, the act of smoking can either be stopped before it starts or aborted at some early point in the sequence. Disruption of this kind depends upon self-instruction's becoming conditioned to the same external events that hitherto have controlled the act of smoking

Given an internal contingency and the decision to quit, thoughtless or automatic smoking can be reduced in several ways. To begin with, the decision to quit will tend to result in the cigarettes being thrown away. Although it is possible to buy more in an unthinking way, this action is less likely than the resumption of automatic smoking in the event the pack is not discarded. In addition, the self-instruction has some probability of being evoked by the same events that previously evoked smoking. That is, if the thought of smoking strongly evokes instruction against smoking, events similar to the thought—for example, opening the pack or watching others smoke—should also have some tendency to evoke the same self-instruction. If the stimuli that previously evoked smoking now evoke the thought of smoking, or the negative instruction itself, the individual should be well on his way to becoming a quitter.

One point that cannot be stressed too keenly is that a decision to quit is not the equivalent of extinction, any more than a decision to start a new behavior is the equivalent of conditioning. A decision is not a magical event that can abolish all the control that months or years of learning have established. Decisions per se have no effect upon the degree to which the external world does or does not control a response, and thus they are no substitute for learning. As was stressed, they can play a unique role in modifying established behavior patterns. In view of the self-instruction they entail, which may be supposed to work essentially like any other instruction, they can intrude thought between motor links of smoothly flowing behavior sequences and thus disrupt the sequences. Moreover, the self-instruction should be conditionable to the same stimuli that previously evoked the to-be-eliminated response. In short, decisions do not act magically but by disruption, through the restoration of cognitive elements and ultimately through the counterconditioning of negative self-instruction.

This treatment may be seen to reject two traditional views of decision-making and conditioning. First is the view that either cognitive mechanisms or conditioning is the true process, the other being false or trivial, as the case may be, the judgment varying with the expert. Second is the view that dispute between these processes is impossible because there is only one process, described in different languages— philosophical monism. In the present account conditioning and decision-making differ in process not merely in language, but this leads not to the question of which is correct, but rather to questions of how the two processes may relate to or affect one another.

IDEAL LINKAGE BETWEEN THE EMOTIONAL
AND DECISIONAL PROCESSES

At some point the reader may have wondered why internal punishment is unable to do the job alone. It might be supposed that the internal punishment would suppress smoking beyond any need for extinction or counterconditioning. Though a behavior sequence may be strongly conditioned, nevertheless, if a highly aversive event is made contingent upon the sequence, punishment alone should suppress the behavior, with no requirement from additional mechanisms. Is the humiliation inadequately aversive to cope with a response whose base rate is as great as that of smoking? To my knowledge there is no way of estimating that aversiveness, but the problem is less one of magnitude than one of stability or invariance of the aversiveness. That is, the internal contingency is, I suspect, a fragile process that, if it is to make a contribution, must do so early or be destroyed by overuse.

The process is not well understood, but the emotion that accompanies a discovery tends to be strongest on the first occasion and to weaken progressively thereafter. A joke, for example, is scarcely funny the second time, less still the tenth time. Similarly, the repeated contemplation of behavior that, if carried out, would place one in an offensive class may be expected to lose its original emotional character. Before long the individual will be able to view his possible villainy with clinical dispassion; and if he then had no means of suppressing temptation but emotion, he would be unable to control himself. In view of this possibility, it is questionable whether a serious parallel can be genuinely accepted between the role of humiliation in an internal contingency and that of electric shock in an external contingency. Electric shock can retain its physical intensity from trial to trial, but humiliation and emotional processes generally appear to lack this capacity.

But the emotional and decisional processes are not incompatible. The point may be to combine them in a way that would maximize their efficiency. There is a simple and rather surprising way in which the two mechanisms can be linked together for maximal effectiveness.

If the decisional process is instigated both early and successfully, it will serve to keep the emotional process at nearly full strength. That is, if the self-instruction is successful, the humiliation cannot be habituated by repeated activation, for the individual has no occasion either to contemplate or to return to the offensive class. Thus an important by-product of an early and successful decisional process will be the preservation of the emotional component. But by preserving the emotional component, the decisional process will at the same time assure its own preservation. So long as the emotional process is viable, remaining as the potential source of a highly aversive condition, the decisional process may be likened to the instrumental response in an avoidance-learning situation. The success of the decisional process prevents the occurrence of the aversive event, and as the laboratory has demonstrated, responses leading to the successful avoidance of aversive events can be maintained at good strength indefinitely.

What is anomalous and interesting about the linkage between these two mechanisms is that a response is maintained by an event that it is itself responsible for maintaining. Normally the instrumental event avoids the occurrence of the electric shock, but the intensity of the shock does not itself change over trials. In this situation, however, each time the decisional process fails, the shock occurring on the next trial will be a little weaker. And each failure will make the next failure more likely, for the probability of an avoidance response is an increasing function of the intensity of the aversive event. Thus the ultimate contribution to the individual of a successful linkage between the emotional and decisional processes is highly dependent upon *initial* success. If the decisional process is not successful from the start, the emotion will dry up, and the individual will lose both mechanisms: humiliation as a form of internal punishment and humiliation as the aversive event, the avoidance of which would maintain the decisional process.

THREE VULNERABILITIES IN THE INTERNAL MECHANISM

It is assumed that each individual has a set of beliefs—a conscience. How these beliefs are inculcated is a question of the highest interest, though not one that will be dealt with here. Instead, beliefs will be treated as primitive and their consequences will be considered. The conscience has the effect of prohibiting many acts and countenancing others; but it cannot be assumed that everything an individual does is in perfect accord with his conscience. We may foresee discord on three grounds.

First, there is what amounts to ignorance of the law. For example, the person who is strongly opposed to setting children dangerous examples must still discover that smoking in the presence of children is a possible member of this class, and to do so he must even entertain certain views about imitation and the like. That is, we cannot assume an automatic process sweeping through the mind, setting up hypothetical conditional relations, testing out the possible ethical consequences of each and every act. If I smoke, I may "get cancer; a bad cough; foul breath; burned shirt fronts; stained fingers"; but never, "set children a dangerous example." That is, there is no guarantee that the search will terminate effectively, in a consequence of sufficient emotional voltage to be an important potential source of internal punishment. People doubtless engage every day in acts that are incompatible with their conscience for no other reason than that of ignorance. The injunction against setting children bad examples was obviously not implanted in the context of smoking, but more probably in a context such as "don't tip your chair back or ride your bike in the street, and things like that, because if you do it, Timmy will do it, and if he does it, he'll get hurt." There is no reference to smoking in this example, and while this fact raises the interesting question of how information is stored in the conscience, I think it most reasonable to guess that it is stored in the form in which it was first learned. There is, therefore, some cognitive distance that will have to be traveled in order to relate smoking in front of one's children to an injunction based upon not riding one's bike in the presence of a smaller brother; and I see nothing that guarantees that that distance will be traveled in each and every case.

Ignorance of the law would not apply to the sexual taboos, since these acts—masturbation, adultery, incest—are prohibited as such. One does not have to travel uncertainly through the middle-class conscience, setting up hypothetical relations to see if by chance these acts can be linked up to unforeseen prohibited consequences. The acts are directly prohibited by name. Nevertheless these acts are widely engaged in, I assume, by people whose consciences prohibit them, and we must appeal to some factor other than ignorance of the law to account for these discords between behavior and belief.

We have already seen one such factor in the attentional rivalry between control by the external world and the usurpation of that control by the reemergence of thought and the negative self-instruction. The individual may be entirely clear that he rejects the act and yet, through a lapse in attention, awaken to find himself in the midst of the act. This would be a doubtful excuse for, say, stealing, since to offer it as such would be to admit that stealing was widely conditioned to one's environment and that one did a great deal of it; but it is a reasonable explanation of backsliding in an ex-smoker. This factor also points to the advantage of prevention over treatment. If smoking can be prevented in the first place, the internal mechanisms will not have to compete with established external controls.

A third factor needs to be considered, however. Despite full knowledge and excellent attention, the individual may still succumb to temptation. Picture the lackey at the foot of a bed, bemoaning the action of his patron: "But, Sire, you have promised yourself to give up this sort of thing!" Here there is no deficiency in either the decisional or attentional processes; the only deficiency is in the internal punishment, which is insufficient to supress the ongoing act. We may expect the adverse emotion to return in a few minutes, but for the moment it is supplanted by a different emotion. The question is essentially parametric: is the strength of the punishment sufficient to suppress the behavior in question? We know that in all cases it is not. Recall the teenage youth who in the first summer of his maturity will repeatedly relinquish the handle of the lawn mower only to substitute for it, behind the locked bathroom door, another hard object.

In brief, the internal machinery is vulnerable at three points. Even though an individual may have a well-formed conscience, an act may not come to be recognized as a member of a prohibited class. Even if it is recognized, the attempt to establish new discriminative control of a competing event may be overcome by the existing control of the old event. Even if the act is both recognized and attended to, it may prove to be stronger than the aversive emotion that is available to suppress it. Thus, at forty-five an individual may suddenly become a model husband for no reason other than that the emotional voltage is now able to cope with the weakened challenges. Similarly, people who have been unable to quit smoking at one age may suddenly prove able to at a later age.

RECAPITULATION

It is assumed that the individual has a conscience—a set of beliefs that prohibit certain acts—and further, that the discovery that one is engaged in behavior that makes one a member of a prohibited class can be acutely humiliating. It is assumed that the discovery can give rise to an internal contingency, a conditional relation between the contemplation of the act in question and a reactivation of the original humiliation. The discovery may also give rise to a decision to desist from the act, the main consequence or form of which is negative self-instruction. I envisioned a possibly ideal linkage between the decisional and emotional devices, one in which an early successful decisional process would preserve the humiliation against the habituation of heavy use, and in so doing would assure its own continuation in a manner analogous to that of an avoidance response.

The advantages of a conscience are straightforward. If one lived in a world with only one room or, like a child, in a world over all of whose rooms hovered a godlike presence, there might be little need for a conscience. The external contingency might then be a sufficient mechanism of control. With the whole show in one room, it should be easy enough for society to assure that to everything that (it considers) should be controlled an external contingency will apply. The laboratory rat and the institutionalized person tend to live in one-room worlds, though even there the approximation is imperfect, for the problem arises occasionally whether the contingency that applies in the test box is not violated in the home cage. Although the child does not live in one room, society solves this problem by moving with the child, accompanying him from room to room, assuring that critical contingencies do not break down in any of the rooms. If all control were restricted to the external contingency, there are only three forms society could take: a one-room world; a world of many rooms but with supervision in each of them; or partial supervision of its many rooms, along with the hope that the learning parameters will keep things from collapsing in any one room before they can be reestablished in some other room. The hope here is that there will be great transfer from room to room and that the extinction rates will be adequately countered by those for reacquisition. Needless to say, there will be an appeal to intermittent reinforcement schedules and the increased resistance to extinction that they engender.

But it would seem that no more complex example is needed than that given by smoking to observe that, whether or not society *could* survive with no control mechanism other than that of the external contingency, it apparently regards this approach as risky and has chosen not to try it. That is, if attempts are made to control smoking with only the external contingency—say, punishing it in one room—they are unsuccessful, presumably because in this case the hope for an accommodating transfer from one room to the others and a favorable reconditioning rate relative to that for extinction is not realized. Apparently the person distinguishes between the lab or clinic in which smoking is punished and the living room in which it is not, much as a rat might discriminate between safe and not-safe periods in a differential-punishment routine. But many people have quit smoking. Since the attempts to do this with the external contingency are largely unsuccessful, and the people who have succeeded give no sign of having done so by external contingencies, it seems proper to conclude that society does not rely exclusively on the external contingency and that people are equipped with other mechanisms—mechanisms of self-control. These internal controls, however, are merely another kind of mechanism; they are not infallible.

Comments on Paper by Premack
WINFRED F. HILL

DR. PREMACK has done an excellent job of explaining why the disappointing results of so many attempts to modify smoking behavior are predictable from learning principles. The studies that Dr. Bernstein summarized for us seem typically to follow the pattern Premack would predict—often an initial reduction in smoking, but then a relapse, either as the contingencies are withdrawn or as the subject forms discriminations among the various rooms in his environment.

Having fulfilled his first goal of relating predictions from the lab to data from everyday life, Premack then goes on to another syncretism, this time between behavior theory and ego psychology. The most potent factor in overcoming smoking, he suggests, is the humiliation of recognizing what kind of person one is as a smoker—a sucker for exploiters, a heartless parent, or (if one has previously tried to quit and failed) a weakling without self-control. We might paraphrase his thesis as, "A discrepancy between the perceived self and the ego ideal serves as an aversive stimulus which reduces the rate of the smoking operant." If this phraseology has the same jarring sound as a mixed metaphor, I think Dr. Premack and I agree that this is more an advantage than otherwise.

Dr. Ferster referred to the various approaches a discussant can use. Since I do not have either of his advantages—experience as a behavior therapist or a personal history of smoking and quitting—I am forced to address myself solely to Premack's position. I want to do so under two headings. The first is the practical matter of how people can be helped to give up smoking, the topic that justifies our being here today. The other is the theoretical matter of the implications of Dr. Premack's paper for behavior theory; and I have the impression that the American Cancer Society will not mind an excursion into that issue.

Regarding the practical issue, the first question is why the experience Premack calls humiliation should be so effective a punisher. Why can a person who is not deterred from smoking by fear of disease and death be deterred by this recognition of a self-ideal discrepancy? Part of the answer is a mixture of probability and delay: "If I smoke, I may get cancer later, and I will definitely be a contemptible person right now." However, this answer only raises more questions. On the one hand, fear of electric shock can suppress behavior even when the shock is both delayed and uncertain; why, then, does fear of cancer not act in this same way? Admittedly the time span is a long one, but humans are well provided with verbal mediators for bridging the gap. On the other hand, there is no reason why a single experience such as Premack describes must have humiliating consequences; the person might rationalize that the incident is so atypical and he is generally such a strong-willed person or such a devoted parent that his minor slips can easily be overlooked.

Since fear requires learning and humiliation calls for even greater learning, there is room for a detailed exploration of individual differences in responsiveness to these two kinds of aversive stimulation. Dr. Smith has provided us with some information about personality differences between smokers and nonsmokers. He tells us that comparable information is not available about differences between current smokers and former smokers who have quit, but it would not be surprising if the pattern were similar. If that is indeed the case, then the people most likely to give up smoking would be those who are more introverted and more prosocial. These are just the people whom we might expect to be especially concerned about their ego ideals, and hence especially susceptible to the sort of humiliation described in Premack's anecdotes. Admittedly this is a tenuous argument. However, I think we have reached the point in our investigations of smoking where we can stop asking about either the mechanisms of smoking or the personalities of smokers and start asking about the interactions of these two kinds of variables.

Just as Hunt and Matarazzo earlier distinguished decision from habit, Premack notes three ways in which a decision to stop smoking may be obstructed by the snares of habit. Again the need for more specificity in our attacks on smoking becomes clear. If a person's habits of information-seeking are such that he never discovers the discrepancy between his ideals and his behavior, and hence never makes the decision to stop smoking in the first place, the answer lies in education (or propaganda, depending on whether it is labeled by the American Cancer Society or the tobacco companies). If smoking is attached to so many cues that a person who has decided to stop smoking nevertheless finds himself automatically lighting up, we need the whole armamentarium of tricks that behavior-modification therapists have worked out. The person can get rid of all his cigarettes. He can make bets with his friends that he will quit, so that if they offer him a cigarette, they will do it with an "I-win" leer that will serve as a reminder. He can identify the stimuli that most often give rise to smoking, so as to attach new responses to them. Finally, if overwhelming temptation is the problem, various gratifications as substitutes for smoking may help. Perhaps there are hard-core addicts whom nothing will help, but if they can be identified, their failures can be kept from discouraging other smokers.

Probably one reason attempts to modify smoking behavior have not been more successful is that they have not recognized how many different approaches are useful for some people some of the time and then concentrated on making the appropriate specific linkages. This suggestion is scarcely original, and it applies just as well to any aspect of education or of psychotherapy. With smoking, however, the goal is so specific and at least relatively reliable to measure that the problem of finding out what works best when and for whom should be easier to solve than when the goal is "better general adjustment" or "a fuller understanding of society."

Turning now to the theoretical implications of Dr. Premack's talk, I am struck by the extent to which internal stimuli, responses, and reinforcers dominate the analysis. Let me summarize his analysis as I think I understand it. An external stimulus that has in the past been followed by smoking arouses the thought of smoking, which arouses the thought that one has resolved to stop smoking. At that point the person may either stick to his resolution and not smoke or go ahead and light up anyway. If it is the latter, his behavior is then punished by another thought, that such behavior is unworthy of him, which produces a punishing feeling of humiliation. Several people, including Hunt and Matarazzo, have commented with amusement on the contrast between the behavioristic language and the mentalistic content of such analyses as this. I share their amusement, yet I think if we come to laugh, we should remain to pray. To the extent that Premack or any of the rest of us is successful in analyzing thoughts and feelings according to the same laws as overt responses and in generating useful predictions from the analysis, he deserves not our ridicule, but our respect and gratitude.

I was particularly interested in Premack's notion that situations cannot continue indefinitely to arouse humiliation. If, therefore, humiliation is to continue to be an effective deterrent for someone, it must be not humiliation itself, but the anticipation of possible humiliation that carries the burden. Something akin to Solomon and Wynne's (1954) anxiety conservation is protecting the capacity to experience humiliation under certain conditions from extinction. However, the situation that Premack has described has not only all the problems of the standard avoidance situation, which have proved enough to tax some of the best intellects in psychology, but the additional problems of how the tendency to be humiliated under certain conditions was originally learned and how resistant it is to extinction. Again individual differences are brought in, but now in an attempt to explain them rather than to use them as explanations. These problems will have to be solved before Premack's model can be considered at all complete. Fortunately they do not all have to be solved before practical use can be made of the model. If it can be determined how effective humiliation is as a form of aversive control for whom, and if there is enough ingenuity to make use of that knowledge, Premack's formulation will have contributed amply to the purposes for which this conference was sponsored.

General Discussion

WHEN Premack raised doubts concerning the extinction process as a technique for abolishing smoking behavior, TOMKINS mentioned the apparently successful use of satiation is some recently reported work. PREMACK replied that he had done quite a bit of work using habituation but had usually found considerable recovery. He has not been able to find in the laboratory a behavior analogous to smoking that can be eliminated permanently through a satiation procedure. It is conceivable that using satiation might result in a low probability for a behavior, and this probability in turn might make it possible to operate effectively upon the behavior through counterconditioning and other procedures, thus exploiting its low probability; but he doubted the efficacy of satiation by itself. However, since the system is multivaried, it will have to be acted upon in many ways, so that any procedure that would assign it a low probability would help to bring in a competing response.

Later PREMACK, JARVIK, GREEN, TOMKINS, KORNETSKY, and SPENCE became involved in discussing the role of fear of cancer in controlling smoking, SPENCE pointing out that there are two factors governing an individual's fear of cancer: one based on his knowledge of the objective probabilities based upon statistical data, the other on his subjective estimate of whether *he* will contract cancer.

As Premack discussed the decision-making aspect of stopping smoking, BORGATTA complained that he was talking about decision-making in the concept of "big" decisions and that in one sense one could say that a person makes a decision any time he is conscious about something. PREMACK admitted that he was dealing only with "big" decisions, which he described as having the prime operational consequences of self-instruction; and, despite further provocation by BALTER and TOMKINS, he refused to be drawn into a discussion of decision-making in general.

In responding to Hill's discussion of his paper, PREMACK commented on the irony of saying that external contingencies alone would not do the job of controlling smoking but that undoubtedly they were among the main mechanisms by which the internal controls were inculcated. Reward and punishment can be used not only to modify the frequency of arbitrary responses, but also to build in systems, be they "language" or "conscience," that confer greater power of behavioral control than can exist without these systems.

KNAPP commented that the simple problem of trying to influence people to abandon an apparently simple act (smoking) forces the investigator into a comprehensive psychology and reveals how often theoretical, experimental, and therapeutic approaches have used over-simplified models. The similarity of much of our knowledge of smoking is in sharp contrast with the quite different theoretical frameworks within which it can be understood.

He has interviewed about 150 smokers to get histories of how they started, the problems that resulted when they quit, and the circumstances of any backsliding. Innumerable factors seem to be involved; for instance, not only the fear of death, but also increased motivation for living. The adolescent seems much more caught up in external cuing, whereas the older adult is more apt to show signs of physiological dependence. He has also been studying the relation of the acute withdrawal phase to acute depression, suggesting that antidepressants might be helpful in treatments of this phase.

MATARAZZO stressed the fact that the cessation model emerging from Premack's treatment was not necessarily based upon humiliation but had wider implications.

BORGOTTA mentioned the existence of a long research tradition in sociology involving the internalization of norms, beginning with James Mark Baldwin and running through Charles Horton Cooley, George Herbert Mead, and others. They would not use humiliation, however, and he was not optimistic about a model that does. Before good models can be attained, more accurate specification is needed of all the variables involved. The present tendency is to take a piece here and a piece there and to articulate them and then derive certain consequences, but most of the specific mechanisms involved are omitted. It will be necessary to specify the criteria that must be predicted and then to predict these criteria before a level of understanding can be achieved. TOMKINS commented that no science, no matter how highly developed, has aimed at prediction in nature, but only at prediction under controlled conditions—quite a different proposition. BORGATTA demurred but progressed to a final criticism of the reliance that had been placed on case histories, which are open to the unreliability of varying interpretation.

The Smoking Habit[1]

FRANK A. LOGAN

NOBODY ever quits smoking—except perhaps in Mark Twain's sense of having done so hundreds of times—simply because habits are permanent. The "ex"-smoker may for a while "cut down to zero" and may even continue at that frequency for the rest of his life, but he is irrevocably different from the never-smoker. One of the most obvious ways to prove the difference is to let both smoke a few cigarettes: the latter *may* treat it as a lark, while the former *may* resume habitual smoking. And there are more subtle behavioral differences between the two, such as their emotional reactions to the smoking behavior of others. The principle that habits (as I shall develop the term) are permanent has important practical implications if one wants to control any behavior, such as smoking. Most obviously, preventing the habit from being formed in the first place is the only way permanently to

1. This paper does not provide scholarly references to the relevant literature, nor acknowledgment of its theoretical background. It is most dependent on the ideas of Clark L. Hull, Kenneth W. Spence, and Neal E. Miller, but a complete genealogy would be both prohibitive and distracting. Responsibility, of course, is mine.

eliminate it. And less obviously, smokers should be accepted for what they are.

These are several of the implications that can be drawn from the experimental psychology of animal learning and motivation. This field is less than a half-century old and is self-conscious of its infancy. Yet its subject matter concerns the most fundamental principles of learned behavior. This is not to deny the importance of "characteristically human" psychology. People talk—and in doing so, generate a variety of complexities unknown elsewhere in the animal kingdom. But people cannot escape their animal heritage and the behavioral principles that have evolved with them. These are not always palatable; indeed, sometimes they are painful; but they are also inescapable. The purpose of this paper is to explore some of the statements about the smoking behavior of people that a behavior theory based largely on the running behavior of rats and the pecking behavior of pigeons can say.

A DEFINITION OF THE SMOKING HABIT

Learning is a hypothetical process inferred from objectively measurable changes in behavior that result from practice and that cannot be ascribed to such temporary processes as fatigue. Although learning is therefore not directly observable, there are increasingly good reasons to believe that it reflects basic neurophysiological and/or biochemical changes in the organism. Following the Hull-Spence tradition the outcomes of these still hypothetical changes may be called habits.

Learning combines with motivation to determine performance. The principal basis for distinguishing between factors that affect learning and those that affect motivation is their relative permanence. Motivation can be changed rapidly in either direction, whereas learning requires the gradual accumulation of a persisting process. The distinctions and interrelationships between these constructs have not yet been unequivocably determined by experimental analysis, but they must be recognized if the present theoretical approach is to be understood. Most specifically, the smoking habit does not alone imply smoking behavior; that habit must be motivated to appear in performance. However, since the term is so well ingrained in the vernacular, the smoking "habit" will be used to refer to the actual practice of regular smoking. These distinctions have at least the following implication: breaking the smoking habit means removing the motivation to smoke.

Habit is an acquired association of a response with a stimulus. For present purposes it is not necessary to deny the existence of other kinds of associative processes, such as exist among stimuli. Nor is there any need to deny that learning about stimuli and learning how to make responses are important effects of experience. Indeed, it is evident that "pure stimulus learning" and "pure response learning" are important precursors of associative learning. But the habit construct under discussion here is conceived as a bond, connection, or association between a stimulus and a response. To make a stimulus-response approach effective in naturalistic contexts requires considerable enrichment (or, in Neal Miller's terms, liberalization) of the basic concepts of stimulus and response.

The smoking response

Technically smoking is a behavior chain. That is to say, smoking comprises a sequences of activities beginning with the reaching for a cigarette, then lighting it, and then engaging in periodic inhaling and exhaling of its smoke. There is no rigorous formula for breaking up the continual flow of behavior into discrete units called responses. Nevertheless, it is conventional to treat a behavior chain as a single response once it becomes fully integrated in the sense that later members of the chain are elicited by feedback from earlier members without external stimulus support. Accordingly smoking will be considered as a unitary response objectively identifiable by some component of the chain, such as lighting a cigarette.

There are both qualitative and quantitative variations in the ways these activities involved in smoking are performed, and for some purposes these may be significant. Specifically, for example, the person who draws heavily on a cigarette that he holds tightly in his partly clenched fist may be revealing a substantially different form of behavior from the person who holds a cigarette at his fingertips and takes occasional light puffs. These features of the smoking response are themselves learned and hence comprise one aspect of the smoking habit. In effect, learning to smoke equally involves learning how to smoke. Nevertheless, such differences in topography probably reflect personality factors and, without discounting their probable importance, they will here be ignored. "Smoking" will mean manipulating a lighted cigarette so that it is occasionally brought to the lips. The length of the cigarette, filters, fingers, puff rate, and depth of inhalation are interesting but tangential to the present theme. Any sequence of events that deliberately puts cigarette smoke directly into the lungs is an instance of the integrated act of smoking.

The smoking stimuli

The identification of the events that can be effective stimuli is functional: any descriptive property of an environment that can be shown capable of controlling the behavior of the organism in question may be treated as a stimulus. It is thus not necessary that stimuli can be directly pointed out. Fully to define the smoking habit requires the recognition of several important classes of stimuli in this sense. One such class is feedback. Feedback may be interoceptive: cues emanating internally from behavior, both muscular and glandular, that provide direct information about the state of the organism. Feedback may also be exteroceptive: cues emanating from the environment in response to behavior that also provide information. The smoking response may become associated with feedback stimuli; in effect, other responses may, through their response-produced stimuli, evoke the smoking response. For example, smoking may first become associated with feelings of anxiety after which any stimulus situation that produces anxiety will tend also to elicit the smoking response.

Stimuli also include the notion of the stimulus trace: stimulus events initiate a temporally decaying process that persists for some period of time and that is somewhat distinctive at each instant. Events, therefore, need not be physically present in order to control behavior. Of special interest in the context of smoking is the concept of the trace of feedback stimuli. If a response recurs during the decaying trace of the stimuli produced by a previous occurrence, a response can become associated with itself. Specifically, once one reaches a frequency of smoking in which the next cigarette is being smoked while the trace of the preceding cigarette is still present, the response can become self-perpetuating. Smoking elicits smoking elicits smoking. . . .

Other events must be recognized as potential stimuli. These include decreases in stimulus energy as well as increases, since terminations or reductions are effective in gaining control over behavior. Relationships among stimuli may themselves be treated as stimuli capable of controlling behavior. The general context in which behavior occurs is also part of the total stimulus complex, so that simply being in a particular environment may importantly affect the rate of responding. In short, the present conception of the stimulus is considerably larger than simply the lights, sounds, and touches typically studied in the laboratory.

Smoking behavior

By and large, smoking is an operant response—one that is freely available to the organism, as is typically true of smoking (unless one has run out of cigarettes). Smoking may not be permitted in some contexts, but it is still available and is suppressed by the aversive consequences when the stimulus "No smoking" is in effect. The most general measure of an operant response is its overall rate of occurrence; in this case, for example, the number of cigarettes smoked per day.

The experimental analysis of operant conditioning has established the close dependence of the rate of a freely available response on the schedule of reinforcement. Four basic schedules—fixed and variable interval and fixed and variable ratio—together with a myriad of more complex combinations of these, have been studied extensively. While a number of suggestive inferences may be drawn from this literature, there is one reason why this experimental background cannot yet provide a complete description of smoking behavior.

Operant conditioning is typically studied in a rigidly controlled environment in which few stimuli are available. In such a context the observed response is sometimes thought of as emitted by the organism, since there is no obvious stimulus with which it is associated. This is, of course, a reasonable strategy, since it enables one to determine the pure effects of a reinforcement schedule uncontaminated by extraneous influences. In contrast, however, the everyday environment of smokers presents a continual flux of stimulus events that may come to elicit smoking. Let us first disregard this difficulty to illustrate the way the rate of smoking might be controlled as a simple free operant.

First, let me assume that there is some reinforcement for the act of smoking produced by the biological reactions to the nicotine content of a cigarette. I will subsequently discuss the intrinsic and extrinsic sources of motivation/reward for smoking; suffice it here to elaborate the assumption that the reinforcing value of a cigarette is in part dependent upon the time since the preceding cigarette. While chain-smoking is a familiar phenomenon, the typical smoker finds such behavior not only unsatisfying but actually aversive.

These assumptions produce what in the laboratory is called a differential reinforcement of low-rate schedule. That is to say, responding too rapidly leads to less reward, no reward, or possibly even punishment; maximal reward requires a pause ˙after each response. Such a schedule generates a low steady rate of responding in which the organism occasionally responds too quickly to receive reward but also rarely waits much longer than the required interval. Hence, if it is assumed that a cigarette is reinforcing only if say a half-hour has elapsed since the last cigarette, a person would gradually come under control of that schedule. He need not be consciously aware of the contingencies, but he will gradually come to reach for a cigarette about every half-hour.

There is every reason to believe that these underlying principles of operant conditioning are involved in the smoking habit. As noted above, for example, if smoking is also punished in certain environments, the rate of responding would be expected to become appropriately differentiated. But the fact that the human environment contains a variety of changing stimulus events, coupled with the basic principle of stimulus-response associative learning, suggests that smoking is more than a simple free operant emitted at a rate determined solely by its schedule of reinforcement.

The smoking habit

The smoking habit is actually a constellation of habits in which the smoking response has become associated with a large number of stimuli. Such associations are formed simply as a result of practice. That is to say, each time a person smokes a cigarette, there is a resulting increase in the habit strength of the elements of the existing stimulus complex to elicit the smoking response. The tendency to smoke in particular situations therefore depends on the frequency with which smoking has occurred in that context in the past. As such, any individual's smoking habit depends upon his unique past experiences. However, there also appear to be large areas of communality in this regard. Arising in the morning, finishing a meal, leaving a theater, and a variety of similar contexts are ones in which most smokers have learned to smoke.

Less conspicuous stimuli that need to be included in the smoking habit involve primarily internal feedback stimuli. Being in doubt about one's next move, being anxious about an impending event, being worried, being in a quandary, or any of a variety of emotional states may become associated with smoking. And since a cigarette is always smoked at some time after the last one, the decaying traces of that event will come along to elicit smoking when other events in the environment have not precluded their occurrence.

Summary

Smoking is a chain of behavior that may be conceptualized as an integrated act. It is typically a freely available operant response, and as such its rate of occurrence depends in part on the schedule of reinforcement. It also becomes associated with environmental events present when it occurs, and these also come to control its occurrence. The smoking habit is the convergence of these determinants on a single response. But the principles governing its occurrence are not unique, they are those that apply to any learned response.

ON LEARNING THE SMOKING HABIT (AND THE NOT-SMOKING HABIT)

It has already been noted that habits are acquired simply as a result of practice. Any person who begins to smoke will, to some extent and progressively, develop habit associations of the smoking response with stimuli. This is true even of a person who does not intend or desire to develop the habit. At the present time one can only speculate upon the original reasons for making this response. Sometimes exploratory curiosity motives are involved; smoking may be engaged in to obtain peer approval or to avoid peer disapproval; smoking may represent a rebellion against the restrictions imposed by the environment; and smoking may simply be a premature way to try to be grown up. Whatever the reasons—and they are undoubtedly numerous, complex, and individual—it is important that they be discovered.

The importance of doing so has already been indicated: habits are permanent. Learned behavior can subsequently be modified by the superimposition of stronger habits, but the underlying process is irreversible. Extinguished habits are subject to spontaneous recovery, disinhibition, and rapid relearning. In the case of undesirable responses, the value ratio of prevention to cure is vastly greater than an ounce to a pound.

Knowledge of the motives for beginning to smoke might enable one to reduce the extent to which smoking is a really effective way to deal with those motives. In most of the above speculations, for example, the motive for smoking involves the conflict contained in the situation that youth are restrained from smoking while adults can and do smoke. It could thus be concluded that smoking would be less frequent among young people (and later, when they are adults) if the existing prohibitions against the behavior were completely removed. (For that matter, all age restrictions on behavior are questionable, since our present laws do not recognize a minor as personally responsible for his acts.) Were there no restrictions whatsoever, smoking would not be a success-ful rebellion against control, it would not be grown-up, and one's peers would therefore probably be less interested in the behavior. It might even become childish. In general, one way to eliminate a response is to remove the reward for it.

This approach, however, is probably not desirable if used alone. As I will argue, drives have to be satisfied. However, it is also possible that one could direct the reduction of the motives that originate the smoking response in alternative and more acceptable ways. Toward this end, I would like to entertain the concept of "neutral control." Existing techniques vis-à-vis smoking involve aversive control: punish-ment or threat of punishment for engaging in the behavior. Positive control may sometimes be tried, as when a parent offers a child money for not smoking. Neutral control does not involve the use of any explicit rewards or punishments.

This is not to deny the importance of motivation in behavior. Rather, it is to suggest that there are often various ways in which a drive can be satisfied, and particular ways to reduce a drive can be taught simply by insuring that the desired responses repeatedly occur and that the undesirable responses do not occur. Let me give an example in a completely unrelated context: toilet training. Certainly the need to eliminate gives rise to a compelling psychological drive, which is reduced when the act occurs; motivation and reward are therefore clearly involved. But for that purpose, it makes little difference where the act is performed. A child may be trained to use the toilet by positive control: the parent applauds appropriate behavior as a source of additional reward. More commonly the parent uses aversive control: mistakes are punished. By neutral control I mean the use of no extra rewards or punishments; instead, the parent simply insures for a period of time that elimination takes place more or less regularly in the bathroom, and those habits will be acquired. The child learns to use the toilet, not because it is particularly good to do so or particularly bad not to do so, but simply because that is the way it is done.

I believe that this concept can be used effectively in the social control of behavior in general. In the present context, if one first determines the motives that underly the onset of smoking, one can arrange to have those drives satisfied in alternative ways. Of course, doing so would require that society face squarely the needs that are engendered in youth. But if it did so realistically, it could decrease the number of adults who smoke, not because they have been rewarded for refraining, not because they are afraid of the consequences, but simply because they never smoked. I personally believe that no other approach offers as much promise for controlling the smoking habit.

THE MOTIVATION OF THE SMOKING HABIT

All behavior is motivated. The source of motivation may be obscure both to the individual involved and to independent observers, but the mere fact that a response persistently occurs establishes the presence of some source of relevant motivation. For its part, motivation has two aspects: drive and incentive. Drive motivation is conceptualized as related to the needs and desires of the organism, being primary when these are unlearned—as in the case of hunger, thirst, and sex—and secondary when they are acquired, as in the case of learned fears. Incentive motivation is conceptualized as reflecting an expectation of reward or punishment for making a particular response based upon past experience of these consequences. Both sources of motivation are necessary to activate habits. Loosely, for a response to occur, one must want something and also expect to get it.

If one adopts the drive-reduction hypothesis about the nature of rewards, at least in its weaker form that any event that occasions a decrease in a drive can serve as a reward, then the distinction between drive and incentive is relatively unimportant in identifying sources of motivation for a response. Hence, if one says that the youth's motivation for smoking is peer approval, one is simultaneously saying that he has the drive motivation to obtain approval and that he has learned that smoking is one way to obtain it. But understanding the distinction is still important, because controlling behavior through the control of motivation has different consequences depending on whether drive, incentive, or both are involved.

Intrinsic motivation to smoke

Some responses by their very nature directly reduce a drive: eating reduces hunger, drinking reduces thirst, copulating reduces the sex drive. Such consummatory responses may normally be thought of as intrinsically motivated by the drives they reduce. But drives can motivate responses other than consummatory ones, as is the case when a person works for money; furthermore, consummatory responses can be motivated by other drives, as when a child eats to get himself excused from the dinner table. Hence the present concept refers to a relationship among the drive, the response, and the reward. If the response naturally reduces a prevalent drive, that drive is said to be intrinsic for that response.

Steady smoking produces a physiological need that gives rise to a psychological drive to smoke. It is a kind of positive feedback situation in which the response produces events that, in turn, tend to lead to more of the same response. It is true that the withdrawal symptoms from nicotine are relatively mild compared with some other addicting drugs, and it is also true that they may be attenuated to some extent by compensatory drugs, but they are nevertheless real. Smoking may therefore become intrinsically motivated by a drive arising from bodily reactions to nicotine and then deprivation of it. This is the essence of a habit-forming drug.

This source of motivation can be readily eliminated by breaking the positive feedback loop. If a person does not smoke for a while, the physiological reactions at first increase, but then decrease and eventually disappear altogether. Thus the intrinsic motivation for the performance of the smoking habit is eliminated, and response tendency is correspondingly reduced.

The typical approach to accomplishing this break in the positive feedback loop is the "sink or swim" technique: the individual decides to quit and sometimes makes this decision public, so as to enable social pressures to bolster his personal resolve. Not infrequently, however, he swims for only a limited period of time and then sinks again into the smoking "habit," perhaps with increased feelings of weakness or inadequacy. If, alternatively, he defines the goal as cutting down to zero, a more gradual shaping process may ease the strain produced by the intrinsic motivation to smoke.

Shaping can be accomplished by reducing the number of cigarettes smoked, gradually approaching the target number of zero. However, an alternative and possibly better approach, at least initially, is not to reduce the number of cigarettes but rather to reduce to one or two the number of puffs per cigarette. Somewhat surprisingly, people following this approach may not increase the number of cigarettes lit per day, even though they have reduced their nicotine intake to a tenth or less of its previous level by restricting their puffing behavior.

The reason can be found in the principles of classical conditioning. Physiological reactions elicited as unconditioned responses to nicotine may be thought of as learnable responses. That is to say, they may become associated with stimuli initially incapable of eliciting them simply by being paired with those stimuli in a classical conditioning paradigm. One set of stimuli regularly preceding and accompanying these physiological reactions are the feedback stimuli from the responses of reaching for, lighting, and holding a cigarette. These stimuli can eventually produce these reactions almost as effectively as nicotine itself. This is one psychological basis of the "placebo effect."

Accordingly, smoking a cigarette but taking only one or two puffs can, at least for a while, be as rewarding—in the sence of reducing the intrinsic motivation—as would taking twenty or more puffs, but the positive feedback is progressively being reduced because of the smaller amount of nicotine absorbed. Furthermore, cutting down in the presence of available cigarettes more faithfully reproduces the originally effective stimuli and hence fosters persistence of the reduced (zero) rate. In time the person can begin to reduce the number of cigarettes and get to zero quickly and painlessly. He can, that is, provided the only source of motivation is intrinsic.

Extrinsic motivation to smoke

Organisms perform responses that do not intrinsically reduce a prevailing drive but that lead to such drive reduction as a result of environmental circumstances. A hungry rat, for example, will press a bar to obtain food even though there is nothing inherent in bar-pressing that reduces hunger. So too, smoking may be (and must inevitably initially have been) motivated by some drive or drives extrinsic to the act itself.

The importance of recognizing this fact is that, if an organism is denied the performance of a motivated response and is not provided with an alternative response for the satisfaction of that drive, he is left in a state of tension, conflict, and often misery. The result may be the development of behaviors that are more detrimental to his individual well-being or to society than the response that he was denied. Suppose, for example, that an adolescent begins to smoke in rebellion against his parents and the establishment; denied that response, he may satisfy this natural aspect of growing up by turning to more dangerous drugs or to more damaging forms of overt aggression. Another example is the adult who smokes as a source of relaxation from the anxieties and tensions of his life; denied that response, he may excessively increase his alcohol consumption or else endure developing physical symptoms such as ulcers. The implication is that one should never deny himself or be denied a response without, at the same time, attending to the drives motivating that response.

As indicated earlier and generally recognized, individuals are not always aware of their motives. The often heard expression, "I smoke, but I really don't want to," is a nonsequitur; behavior is always motivated. If the motivation to smoke is intrinsic, then it can be harmlessly eliminated. If, however, the motivation is extrinsic, care is necessary. The person, in shaping the elimination of intrinsic motivation to smoke, might profitably ask himself each time, "Do I really want this cigarette?" If he keeps responding affirmatively, that is good evidence that some source of extrinsic motivation is also involved, and he might then be well advised to continue uninhibited smoking until his circumstances change or until he better understands his own motives and can deal with them in preferred ways.

Summary

The occurrence of behavior implies drive motivation. Initially smoking must be motivated extrinsically; youth learn to smoke to be accepted, to rebel, to reduce their feelings of inferiority, from curiosity, or the like. Society should not condemn youths' smoking without providing them with other satisfactory ways to deal with these inevitable drives. In time smoking generates its own intrinsic motivation, which may make it functionally autonomous even after the initiating drives are no longer present. In such cases smoking can be safely eliminated by breaking the positive feedback generating this motivation. However, smoking may continue to be motivated in part by extrinsic sources of drive, and these should be recognized and dealt with before smoking is eliminated.

THE PERSISTENCE OF THE SMOKING HABIT

From the claim that habits are permanent it might be concluded that there is nothing more to say about the persistence of the smoking "habit." But if overt behavior is examined, the question may arise why smoking persists in the person who admits he gets little or no pleasure from the act and is fully aware of its possible harmful effects. Habits have to be motivated to be performed, yet some responses persist even after there is little or no apparent reinforcement and/or there is punishment.

The persistence of behavior has long been of special interest to the student of learning, to some extent because of its clear practical significance: desirable responses often seem transitory, while undesirable responses often seem to persist indefinitely. Conceptually more important, however, is the typical finding that persistence is not perfectly related to other measures of learning. Indeed, there is often an inverse relationship that I would dub the "law of the cursedness of habits": the worse the conditions for learning, the more persistent the habit!

Partial reinforcement and punishment

There are several experimental demonstrations of this law involving persistence; let me mention only two. The first is the familiar partial reinforcement effect: responses persist longer the lower the frequency of reward they have encountered. This is important in the context of smoking because it is rarely the case that every cigarette "satisfies." Indeed, heavy cigarette smokers may enjoy only a very few of the cigarettes they smoke; but this fact, rather than encouraging them to quit, leads inexorably to a persistent high rate of responding.

The second factor is punishment. There is ample experimental evidence for the familiar principle of punishment: responses followed by aversive consequences tend to occur less frequently. But there is also experimental evidence that, if those aversive consequences are ineffective in completely eliminating the response, then punishment actually "fixates" the response, resulting in an increase in its persistence. To some extent this factor is inherent in smoking, since one's first cigarettes are likely to burn and to produce coughing and even nausea. But in that same light must be considered the parent who admonishes his child not to smoke but nevertheless tolerates the usage, or the increasing publicity that "cigarette smoking may be hazardous to your health." These and similar aversive control techniques may be ineffective in eliminating the response of many smokers and potential smokers and hence may .result in more strongly fixating the habit than would be the case if the behavior had simply been ignored.

Other factors could be used further to illustrate these problems concerning the persistence of behavior. For example, small rewards lead to greater persistence than large rewards; and few people would smoke if they really had to walk a mile for every cigarette. Responses learned in the face of obstacles are especially persistent; and the young person rarely finds smoking easily accessible. In short, the prevailing conditions for learning to smoke could hardly be better designed to insure that, if smoking is once acquired, it will be extremely persistent even in the face of low rewards and punishment.

Eliminating undesirable responses

Nevertheless, undesirable responses can be eliminated. Apart from the possibility of removing the stimuli that enable a response to occur, there are three basic techniques: extinction, punishment, and counter-conditioning. Extinction of an operant response refers to removal of the reward for its occurrence, as a result of which the rate of responding decreases. In the case of smoking, this method would require making that response ineffective with respect to the intrinsic and extrinsic sources of motivation. The by-product of this technique, however, is that the drives are left unsatisfied and may come to motivate even less-desirable behavior.

Punishment of an operant refers to the application of an aversive event consequent upon making the response, as a result of which the rate of responding is suppressed. If suppression is not complete, however, fixation may occur; in any event, punishment produces conflict. That is to say, simultaneous tendencies to approach and to avoid the response are generated by its reward and punishment, leaving the person constantly struggling in the conflict between these opposing tendencies. Punishment is therefore likely to lead to undesirable by-products unless rewards for the response are simultaneously removed.

There are more specific rules for the effective use of punishment. The first is that the proper punisher is one that elicits responses incompatible with the punished response; in the case of smoking, one would need an event that elicits rejecting cigarettes. Punishment should be applied immediately following a response; in the case of smoking, the threat of lung cancer is quite remote. And punishment should be applied in the presence of the stimuli eliciting the response; in the case of smoking, aversive events should occur in the very context of smoking. In general the effectiveness of punishment depends importantly on what punisher is employed and when and where it is applied.

In view of the by-products of extinction and punishment, counterconditioning is usually the most promising technique for eliminating undesirable responses. The technique of counterconditioning is to establish stronger tendencies for competing responses that are incompatible with the response in question. This requires insuring the practice of such incompatible responses under conditions in which they are more rewarding than the response being eliminated. Insofar as oral satisfaction is one basis for the smoking habit, chewing gum or sucking mints may be effective counterconditioning techniques, and they could be even more effective if other effects of nicotine were available in such forms.

Summary

Habits are permanent, but behavior is modifiable. Responses tend to be more resistant to modification the worse the conditions for their acquisition, including small and infrequent rewards and ineffective punishment. Nevertheless, responses can be extinguished by removal of reward, they can be suppressed by appropriate punishment, and they can be supplanted by competing responses that have been counter-conditioned to the controlling stimuli. Some combination of these procedures that insures the satisfaction of the motivating conditions is likely to be most effective and least fraught with undesirable by-products.

The smoking "habit" refers to the overt practice of smoking cigarettes with some regularity. As such, it reflects the presence of two underlying processes: the smoking habit proper and motivation to smoke.

The smoking habit is a constellation of conditions that have acquired control over the integrated act of smoking. In part, control is exerted by the temporal schedule of reinforcement; in part, by a variety of environmental and feedback stimuli that have become associated with smoking as a result of that response occurring in their presence. Motivation to smoke is in part intrinsic: the psychological drive based on the need for nicotine engendered by the drug. There may also be extrinsic sources of motivation such as rebellion in youths and anxiety in adults. Rate of smoking depends jointly on habit and motivation; increasing with larger numbers and frequency of controlling events and stronger motivation.

The smoking habit is acquired as a direct result of smoking. The usual conditions of learning to smoke—especially small and infrequent rewards and ineffective punishment—are precisely ones that foster persistence of the smoking "habit." Behavior modification is still possible in the habitual smoker, but it requires sensitive understanding of the underlying mechanisms. Prevention is the only sure cure.

Comments on Paper by Logan
JANET TAYLOR SPENCE

PROFESSOR Logan has given an excellent theoretical account of the factors underlying the acquisition and maintenance of smoking behavior. Here I have chosen to restrict myself to comments on only several of the many points raised in this paper and to develop their implications for techniques designed to modify smoking behavior. I will do so within the context of several assumptions.

First, it seems reasonable to assume that few of the participants in this conference are concerned with smoking behavior and the possible habit mechanisms underlying it primarily because of intellectual curiosity. Our dominant concern is rather with the development of programs and techniques that will persuade individuals never to start to smoke or, if they already do so, to reduce their rate of consumption, preferably down to zero.

Smoking has a number of undesirable aspects: it is among other things smelly, messy, a fire hazard, and expensive. I will assume however —and this may be somewhat idiosyncratic—that these disadvantages, though genuine, are of only incidental importance here. Ideally the goal is to persuade people not to smoke at all. But I, at least, would be willing to settle, if necessary, for a lesser goal: arranging for conditions that would prevent the inhalation into the lungs of the noxious pharmacological products of burning tobacco. The former will guarantee the latter, of course, but the converse is not necessarily true.

As Professor Logan correctly reminds us, on a behavioral level smoking is a chain of responses. One can conveniently use as a unit of description the smoking of one cigarette (referring, for convenience, to the most frequently used tobacco product): pulling it out of a pack, lighting it, taking puffs, and in most instances eventually extinguishing it. The response chain, as is commonly realized, is not highly rigid: within a given individual any given sequence can, for example, be interrupted, changed, or modified, by external stimuli, and it can be resumed at any point. Further, individual smokers often show considerable variability in their smoking behavior, their smoking pattern changing in response to circumstances—such as puffing in leisurely fashion while contentedly reading the Sunday paper and drinking an after-breakfast cup of coffee, versus a rapid, intense set of smoking behaviors while under emotional stress. Constant repetition of this general class of behavior chains leads, all agree, to the formation of a "habit." In fact, as Professors Hunt and Matarazzo have pointed out, the behavior may become so highly practiced as to become automatic; the veteran smoker may find himself smoking a cigarette without having made any conscious decision to do so or having had any prior awareness of executing earlier portions of the chain.

While these characteristics of the response chain have some practical significance in themselves, the nature of smoking behavior becomes important to consider, in my opinion, only when one simultaneously takes into account the stimulus conditions, both interoceptive and exteroceptive, that elicit the behavior. Further, reference to the strength of the habit is to the strength of the stimulus patterns in *eliciting* the response chain that is crucial, not to the degree of learning underlying the smooth sequence of motor behaviors called smoking.

These eliciting conditions, as the earlier papers have emphasized, are numerous even within the same smoker. On a theoretical level, this heterogeneity in conditions suggests in turn that a variety of drive and reinforcement conditions may and typically do operate to maintain smoking behavior. One may smoke, for example, while waiting for meals in order to distract oneself from hunger pangs; one may light a cigarette to give oneself time to think of an answer to a difficult question or to have something to do with one's hands when talking to strangers. The situations that lead one to "light up" are endless—and so are the rewards. Interestingly, it is probably the individual trying to *stop* smoking who is most aware of the variety of internal and external stimulus situations that elicit a desire to smoke and the variety of ways in which he has used smoking as a coping device.

But even for the smoker trying to quit identification of the triggering stimuli and the reinforcers for smoking is likely to be incomplete or even inaccurate. Particularly difficult for the smoker to determine is the role of nicotine: the extent to which, in initiating the response chain on any given occasion, he is responding in whole or in part to a complex set of physiological cues associated with "nicotine deprivation" or the extent to which the reinforcing consequences of smoking a particular cigarette is related to physiological reactions to nicotine ingestion. (The role of nicotine is, of course, unclear not only to a smoker in considering his own smoking behavior, but on a more general and objective level, to scientists working in the field. The evidence does suggest, however, that in many smokers nicotine plays some role in the maintenance of smoking behavior.) For any given individual on any given occasion, then, the motivational-incentive conditions for smoking may, in Professor Logan's terminology, be purely intrinsic, purely extrinsic, or a mixture of both. This complex state of affairs in and of itself makes extinction of smoking behavior difficult. When one attempts to extinguish the behavior while leaving underlying motivations intact and without providing any substitute satisfactions, the challenge becomes greater. Logan suggests, in fact, that when extrinsically motivated smoking is involved, it is not merely difficult, but perhaps even undesirable, to persuade an individual to stop smoking unless alternate sources of drive reduction can be arranged.

The procedures developed to date, including behavior-modification techniques, have been at best only modestly successful in assisting individuals to reduce or eliminate their cigarette consumption for protracted periods of time. Perhaps one of the factors contributing to the lack of success of many techniques is their failure to take into account the kinds of complexities just outlined; in other words, a treatment of smoking as if it were a single response or response chain, elicited by a rather simple, consistent set of stimuli, with uniform motivational underpinnings (if, indeed, one bothers to be concerned with the latter at all) is inadequate. But if the attempt *were* made to take all these factors into account, the diagnostic problem would be formidable: it would be necessary to identify for each individual smoker all the stimulus patterns that regularly elicit smoking behavior and then to attempt to infer the underlying motivation and the presumed reinforcers. Having done this, the researchers' ingenuity would then be tested by attempts to devise adequate substitute behaviors that could be counterconditioned to each set of eliciting conditions—or at least that it is *hoped* would be amenable to countercondition.

Professor Premack has called attention to many of these same problems and has suggested, rather pessimistically, that efforts be instead concentrated on techniques designed to strengthen mechanisms of self-control: to develop procedures to persuade and so motivate the smoker that whenever and for whatever reason the impulse to smoke arises, he denies it motor expression. It is to be hoped that the impulses will become less intense, less painful to deny, and less frequent over the course of time.

I find his arguments compelling, but I would carry his pessimism one step further. In the present state of ignorance, I suspect that there are substantial numbers of heavy smokers whom techniques would be unable to motivate sufficiently even to try to quit smoking, or whose self-control mechanisms could not be strengthened sufficiently to allow them to give up smoking successfully for protracted periods of time. For such individuals there is, I believe, a less desirable but more realistically attainable goal: permitting the person to *smoke* to his heart's content, but developing techniques to help him switch to less noxious products, such as the new nontobacco cigarettes. For individuals whose smoking behavior is maintained by factors completely independent of the nicotine content of tobacco smoke, such as Tomkins' "habitual smokers," the substitution should, in principle, be relatively easy to effect. Conversely, to the extent that nicotine *is* involved, it would be more difficult for the individual to change to nontobacco products. However, it would seem to be more tolerable for such individuals to have to fight only one problem—nicotine deprivation— than a whole host of problems all at the same time.

In a subsequent paper Dr. Jarvik suggests that nontobacco cigarettes are smoked only by ex-smokers, and then for "not very long." This observation, as he points out, supports the position that psychological factors are not solely responsible for the maintenance of the cigarette habit. The observation certainly suggests that, for whatever reason, one cannot merely hand smokers nontobacco cigarettes and expect instant therapeutic success.

One factor responsible for the failure of cornsilk and lettuce cigarettes to attract loyal users may be that their taste is odious. After smoking one such product it occurred to me, in fact, that one might use them very effectively in an aversive-conditioning program. However, with repetition, many people come to tolerate quite quickly, if they do not actually come to enjoy, certain experiences that initially were literally distasteful. (Smoking "real" cigarettes is, after all, a pretty grim experience at first, and most drinkers will agree that they worked quite hard to acquire a taste for hard liquor.) This adaptation phenomenon suggests that, until the chemists help out by developing more palatable nontobacco products, there are techniques that behavioral scientists might develop to promote a tolerance of their taste.

A more critical factor in the lack of acceptance of nontobacco cigarettes by many smokers may be that as far as the nicotine component is concerned, switching to nicotine-free cigarettes is as abrupt a method of "kicking the habit" as stopping smoking altogether. "Cold turkey" techniques are not in general notably successful, and there is no reason to anticipate that an abrupt change from tobacco to nicotine-free cigarettes would be an exception.

Professor Logan proposes that a positive feedback loop is involved in responses to nicotine and nicotine deprivation. Steady smoking, he suggests, "produces a physiological need that gives rise to a psychological drive to smoke." Further, it "provides a kind of positive feedback situation in which the response produces events which, in turn, tend to lead to more of the same response." It should be possible, he argues, both quickly and painlessly to eliminate this intrinsic motivation to smoke by introducing procedures that gradually break the positive feedback loop. This type of shaping can be produced, he suggests, by gradually cutting down the number of cigarettes smoked or by reducing the number of puffs per cigarette. Interestingly enough, Logan is advancing the unusual argument that dependence on nicotine is relatively *easy* to eliminate and that it is the extrinsic factors contributing to the maintenance of smoking behavior that represent the therapeutic challenge.

One may disagree with the details of his analysis of the intrinsic factors involved in smoking and with his contention that the methods he suggests will wean the smoker from nicotine either quickly or painlessly. It does seem quite reasonable, nevertheless, to argue on a number of theoretical and empirical grounds that for many smokers a gradual reduction in nicotine consumption might have a greater probability of success in bringing about extended avoidance of nicotine than would abrupt cessation.

In principle it should be relatively easy to introduce gradual shaping procedures into the switch from tobacco to nontobacco cigarettes. One could simply make up a graded series of types of cigarettes in which the tobacco content is steadily decreased and, in compensatory fashion, the nontobacco content increased. (This procedure might also be helpful with bringing about tolerance of the taste of current tobacco substitutes.)

A number of practical decisions would have to be made if such a procedure were adopted. What would be the most advantageous number of steps to employ in the graded series, going from pure tobacco to completely tobacco-free cigarettes? How many days or hours—or how many cigarettes—should the smoker be asked to consume before changing to cigarettes in the next-lower step in the series? Should each individual be allowed to regulate his own rate of consumption—even though for some smokers this might result initially in an increase in rate in an attempt to keep nicotine intake at a relatively constant level? Or should steps be taken to prevent such an increase? These and other questions remain to be answered, but the broad rationale underlying the technique should be quite clear.

I strongly doubt that the method I have suggested would be a panacea, if only because not all individuals who declare their intentions to reform would be sufficiently motivated even to go through all the fuss and bother the regimen would entail. Further, many individuals could be expected to lack the willingness or ability to tolerate the repeated subjective discomfort that might be required to reduce their dependence on nicotine, even if done gradually.

But if Professor Logan's analysis of smoking behavior, as well as other similar types of psychological analyses, have any validity, this method should be at least as useful as many of our current techniques.

General Discussion

KORNETSKY opened the discussion by commenting on substitution mechanisms. Of all the people he has advised to switch from cigarettes to a pipe, only one successfully did so. Most of them bought a pipe or two; but despite the fact that they had real tobacco and were getting real nicotine, they eventually stopped smoking the pipe and went back to smoking cigarettes.

Smoking is a real challenge to the experimental psychologist; it moves him out of his rat laboratory and gives him a human problem to solve. Unfortunately it is a difficult one. He does not have much to say about how the habit was formed, but he is presented with an already established behavior whose acquisition he can only look at retrospectively. Now he is asked to extinguish the response, although he is ignorant of how it was acquired.

FERSTER commented on the tremendous influence of the animal learning laboratories both clinically and theoretically on the development of behavior therapy. He does not regard himself as a behavior therapist, although he often is taken for one.

The switch from the knowledge of the animal laboratory to its clinical application in therapy requires a philosophical and moral reorientation. This is the distinction between arbitrary and natural reinforcement. The therapist uses natural reinforcers. When it is said, "We can make a person stop smoking," the implication is that the motivation lies in the therapist rather than in the patient. If there is one rule in therapy, it is that the motives dealt with are in the patient and not in the therapist.

The skill of the therapist lies in observing and identifying the behavior of the patient carefully enough to be able to make use of motives already in his repertoire and to build on these. In discussing the alteration of smoking behavior, therefore, it is crucial to begin with the repertoire of the smoker and to avoid the notion of imposing something from the outside. There are some people who do not want to stop smoking and consequently will not.

GORDIS remarked that Spence had suggested the possibility of achieving abstinence by a gradual withdrawal through a decreasing dosage of nicotine provided in a series of substitute cigarettes. If the alkaloid involved in smoking bears any resemblance in its clinical manifestations to the opiates, he would be pessimistic about such an approach, since he doubted that there is any evidence indicating that making the withdrawal period from opiates more bearable by some device or another has any influence on the eventual relapse rate.

GORDIS, referring to the warning printed on the cigarette package, asked Logan whether punishment and the threat of punishment were synonymous. Thus a shock delivered to a subject is a punishment, but telling him he may get shocked is merely a threat. Do they have equal force in this situation? LOGAN replied that of course they do not have equal force, but that the threat of punishment is effective in suppressing behavior.

Concerning the reduction of dosage, GREEN volunteered the information that there is some data from ex-smokers indicating that before actually quitting there is a tendency to make changes in one's smoking behavior, such as changing from a nonfilter to a filter cigarette or reducing the number of cigarettes smoked. This action does not occur in all cases, but there is evidence in many cases of this decrease in ·dosage before quitting. The dosage change in shifting from nonfiltered to filtered cigarettes, however, may not result in changing the absolute number of cigarettes smoked. In general, most people stay within the same range of cigarettes smoked per day when changing from a higher dosage to a lower dosage cigarette. A few did increase, but approximately an equal number offset them by showing a decrease.

SCHUSTER offered some evidence from a few cases indicating that when subjects were shifted from cigarettes with a high nicotine and tar content to low ones, the frequency of cigarette smoking increased. He suggested that there are different types of smokers: some whose behavior is under the control of a variety of discriminative stimuli in the environment, and others whose behavior is controlled by the pharmacological effects of nicotine.

SMITH interjected that it might be possible to manipulate simultaneously the administration of nicotine both by cigarette and by a capsule. In this way a reduction in nicotine intake by changing the cigarette could be accomplished simultaneously with changes in the capsule. This method might result in a more sophisticated way of manipulating the pharmacological component of the process while trying to extinguish certain aspects of the psychological component. KORNETSKY pointed out, however, that the onset of effects with oral administration is much slower than with inhalation.

MENDELSON, after commenting on the unreliability of retrospective reports of consumption of alcohol, raised the question of the ultimate goal in the regulation of smoking behavior. Is the goal absolute abstinence, and is this reasonable? In the case of alcohol consumption, techniques for complete abstinence have been failures. Is there some way, based upon reasonable data, to set a socially acceptable norm of smoking? People might object that once you start smoking, you might keep on until you become addicted, but this does not happen with most social drinkers.

GREEN replied that there may be levels of alcohol consumption that are not dangerous to health, but that with cigarettes even ten per day shorten life expectancy; there is no safe dosage level with cigarettes. TOMKINS stated his recollection that under five per day there was no statistical evidence, and GREEN reiterated that at ten per day the evidence was clear.

GORDIS ended the discussion by reminding the conference that if there are to be firm data on the relationship between a person's alkaloid intake and his behavioral pattern in smoking, the amount of alkaloid in the person's body must be measured. All other intake measures are fallible. One might begin by measuring the amount of nicotine in the blood and urine. These may turn out not to be the relevant tissues, but something of this sort must be done to avoid constructing a whole edifice of invalid theory.

The Role of Nicotine in the Smoking Habit

MURRAY E. JARVIK

STATEMENT OF THE PROBLEM

ALTHOUGH a great deal of thought and effort has been devoted to the smoking habit, very little evidence exists concerning the relative role played by pharmacological and psychological factors. Since the smoking of hundreds of millions of people throughout the world now constitutes a recognized serious health problem, it is of some importance to elucidate the mechanisms underlying this habit. It might be well to define what is meant by smoking. Smoking is the inhalation into the mouth and respiratory system of the volatile products of combustion of burning tobacco.

Other plant products, such as opium and marijuana, have been smoked for a longer time than tobacco, but today tobacco smoking far exceeds all other kinds. Stimulation of the sense of smell by aromatic products of food, incense, and perfume may in some distant sense be related to smoking. The main problem this paper deals with, however, is why people will go out of their way to draw into their mouth and lungs smoke from a chopped-up burning plant. I think that the answer is psychopharmacological: that they have stumbled upon the most efficient way to bring high concentrations of the main alkaloid of tobacco—nicotine—to the brain. The evidence to support this hypothesis is only just beginning to accumulate. Totally nonpharmacological theories of smoking are still rather influential, and some of these will be described below.

Since such a vast proportion of mankind smokes today, it is not surprising to find great variations in smoking patterns. In all cases, however, there are at least three phases of the smoking habit: first an initiation phase, second a maintenance phase, and sometimes and increasingly so, a third discontinuation phase. These three phases may be repeated many times in a given individual. It is generally agreed that psychological factors are responsible for and precede the initiation of the habit and also must play a prominent role in the discontinuation of the habit. I want to examine the thesis, however, that pharmacological factors—and in particular, nicotine—play a very important role in the maintenance of the habit and in its resistance to discontinuation. Today opinions and speculations are far easier to find than facts, and I want to examine the evidence at hand and point the way to newer investigations of the role of nicotine.

Historical survey

It appears that tobacco smoking was introduced to Western civilization by Christopher Columbus (Lewin, 1931, 288), and it must rank in virtue somewhere between his discovery of America and the introduction (by his men) of syphilis into Europe. Columbus is said to have described the habit as follows: "I know of Spaniards who imitate this custom, and when I reprimanded the savage practice, they answered that it was not in their power to refrain from indulging in the habit. Although the Spaniards were extremely surprised by this peculiar custom on experimenting with it themselves they soon obtained such pleasure that they soon began to imitate the savage example." The habit, already widespread among the Indians of Central and North America, spread like wildfire throughout the countries of Europe. Up to this time the only kind of smoking that had occurred in Europe, Asia, and Africa had been opium and marijuana. During the sixteenth century tobacco was not only smoked but sniffed into the nose in the form of snuff; it was also chewed. For three centuries snuff was a very prevalent form of tobacco usage, and elaborate snuff boxes were used by monarchs during the eighteenth century. The popularity of these varying forms of tobacco usage point to some common factor responsible for these behaviors. Clearly respiratory stimulation, manipulation, orality, and spitting are not common factors.

Nicotine was first isolated from tobacco seeds by Posselt and Reiman in 1828. Although the first pharmacological studies were initiated by Orfila in 1843, the classical application of nicotine in pharmacology was made in 1889 by Langley and Dickinson who described the actions of the drug upon autonomic ganglia. Langley and Dickinson discovered that if an autonomic ganglion was painted with nicotine, responses to preganglionic stimulation but not to postganglionic nerve stimulation could be prevented. Certain nerves went through ganglia without synapsing and were unaffected by the nicotine block.

Nicotine is relatively unique among commonly used alkaloids in being derived from only one source, the leaves of the tobacco plant, *Nicotiana;* other alkaloids, such as caffeine, are found in a variety of plant sources. Interest in the physiological and psychological effects of tobacco has existed since the time of Columbus.

The tobacco habit was known to be strong from the beginning of its introduction to civilization, and it has been both reviled and praised for nearly five centuries. In the sixteenth century Pope Urban VIII excommunicated those who smoked or snuffed tobacco in the churches of Spain. In 1650 Pope Innocent X threatened with excommunication those who took snuff in St. Peter's in Rome. In Luneburg, Germany, in 1691 the death penalty was enforced against smoking. Throughout the centuries there has been much agitation about the use of tobacco, particularly by young people, yet despite such strong laws and heavy punishments the habit prospered.

In 1603 James I wrote in "Misocapnus" a strong condemnation of smoking. He imposed a high tax on tobacco and thereby improved his financial situation considerably. In 1652 tobacco cultivation in England was prohibited in order to aid the agriculture of the American colonies; the fruits of this decision influenced the economy of England and the United States to this very day.

In the seventeenth century in Turkey smoking was prohibited because it violated the laws of the Koran. The nose of a tobacco user was pierced, the stem of a pipe was passed through it, and he was ridden through the street on a donkey. Murad IV (1620) punished tobacco smoking with the death penalty, to be carried out in a form compatible with the Koran. In Persia and in Russia of that period smoking was punished by torture and death. Despite the severe punishment, smoking of tobacco continued at a great rate in Russia, and the death penalty was abolished by Peter the Great, who substituted a license to England to import tobacco into Russia.

On the other hand, tobacco had its champions. Molière said of tobacco that "it not only refreshes and cleanses the brain, but also leads the soul to virtue and teaches honesty." A Dutch physician, Bontekoe, at the same time said that "nothing is more necessary and beneficial to life and health than the smoke of tobacco. It gladdens the heart in solitude and relieves a sedentary life of all discomforts." For 500 years the battle has raged about whether the dangers of tobacco use exceed the pleasure and virtues of the habit. But evidence for danger to health has become increasingly clear during the last ten years, to the extent that the medical profession and the general public have begun to diminish their incidence of smoking.

Even though it has been known for more than 100 years that tobacco contains nicotine, a very potent alkaloid, the plant has never clearly been brought under the control of the Food and Drug Administration. This anomalous exception in the law stems from strong economic and political pressures. By contrast, the restrictions against the next-most common form of smoking in this country, marijuana, are extremely strong. But it is not easy to decide on a purely objective basis whether nicotine or tetrahydrocannabinol is a more toxic and dangerous drug.

The scientific study of smoking behavior has been largely neglected. During the latter part of the nineteenth century there were sporadic investigations of the effects of smoking and of nicotine on behavior, but these are not quite the same as the study of smoking. Rivers (1908) cites several experiments indicating that smoking has a deleterious effect upon human muscular activity. Palmen (1911) found that cigarette smoke first increased muscular work, but that fatigue set in more quickly. While psychomotor reactions have been reported to be improved (Hull, 1924, Johnson, 1918), steadiness is clearly impaired by smoking or nicotine (Fisher, 1927; Froeberg, 1920). The general impression is that the effects of smoking on motor efficiency is small and variable, but that it is almost always deleterious on activities involving fine movements. The effects of smoking or nicotine upon tests of mental efficiency were also small or equivocal, though they generally tended in the direction of impairment (Berry, 1917; Burnham, 1917; Bush, 1914; Carver, 1922; Hull, 1924). Larson, Haag, and Silvette (1961, 932) wrote: "Burnham's conclusion was that smoking decreases the ability to do mental work, but common experience seems to attest quite otherwise: men almost invariably light a cigarette *before* they commence mental work, and almost invariably *after* they finish physical work." The question of whether people smoke *because* of the influence smoking has upon their ability to work or on their reaction to work remains unexplored.

Nicotine is one of the few drugs in addition to alcohol and caffeine that shared the small stage of psychopharmacology before 1955. The few studies that were done, however, examined the effects of administered nicotine and did not seek to understand the possible rewarding properties of nicotine.

Types of smoking

A great number of epidemiological studies have been carried out to determine who smokes what and where (see Larson and Silvette, 1968; Royal College of Physicians,. 1962). Cigarette smoking still ranks far ahead of pipe smoking and cigar smoking although there has been a relative gain in the smoking of the latter two since the Surgeon General's Report gave them a better bill of health. As is shown in Table 7 in 1900 for each person in the United States over fifteen years of age only 49 cigarettes were consumed, as against 111 cigars. By 1962 the number of cigarettes per person had risen to 3,958, and cigars had

Table 7. Consumption of tobacco products per person aged 15 years and over in the United States for selected years, 1900–1962

Year	All tobacco, pounds	Cigarettes, number	Cigars, number	Pipe tobacco, pounds	Chewing tobacco, pounds	Snuff, pounds
1900	7.42	49	111	1.63	4.10	0.32
1910	8.50	138	113	2.58	3.99	.50
1920	8.66	611	117	1.96	3.06	.50
1930	8.88	1,365	72	1.87	1.90	.46
1940	8.91	1,828	56	2.05	1.00	.38
1950	11.59	3,322	50	.94	.78	.36
1960	10.97	3,888	57	.59	.51	.29
1961	11.15	3,986	56	.59	.51	.27
1962	10.85	3,958	55	.56	.50	.26

Source: Department of Agriculture, Economic Research Service. Reprinted from U. S. Public Health Service. 1964. *Smoking and health.* Report of the Advisory Committee to the Surgeon General of the Public Health Service. Washington, D.C.: U. S. Department of Health, Education, and Welfare. Public Health Service Publication 1103.

fallen to only 55. During the same period pipe-tobacco consumption fell from 1.63 to 0.56 pounds per capita, and chewing tobacco declined even more dramatically from 4.10 to 0.50 pounds. Snuff usage remained essentially the same (0.32 to 0.26). It is surprising to note that the number of snuff takers must be the same order of magnitude as pipe smokers today. During the last year (1968) the incidence of cigarette smoking or the number of cigarettes sold has fallen for the first time in history.

Smoking habits remain remarkably stable. K. P. Ball (1965) obtained epidemiologic data for more than 34,000 men and 6,000 women questioned in 1951, 1957, and 1960 and found that 75 per cent of these had not changed their method of smoking over nine years. Unfortunately, the same longitudinal data for the subsequent nine years is not available, and it might very well be different under the impact of antismoking publicity. Usually cigarette smoking is measured by the number of packs or number of cigarettes a smoker smokes each day. However, the rate and depth of puffing and the duration of smoking for each cigarette are also variables that must play an important role. For example, the average length of butts in American cities was 30.9 mm, compared to 18.7 mm for British discards. Cigarette-puff volume has generally averaged around 45 mm and puff duration approximately 2 sec. The number of puffs per cigarette ranges from 4 to 20.

Numerous attempts have been made to relate smoking patterns to personality or emotional factors. When this information is indisputably established, it will contribute something to the understanding of the role of nicotine. Matarazzo and Saslow (1960) summarized a large list of differentiating characteristics of smokers and nonsmokers (see Table 8). The 1962 Smoking and Health Report (U.S. Public Health Service, 1962) indicates that smokers are more restless, less dependable, and more neurotic than nonsmokers. Cigarette smokers are also more extroverted and pipe smokers more introverted than nonsmokers. The problem of cause and effect is a difficult one to solve, since it is conceivable that nicotine may influence the personality as it may influence the emotional state of an individual. Eysenck (1965) and collaborators indicated that extroverts indulge in smoking and overeating more than introverted individuals. Tomkins (1966) has indicated in his recent theoretical approach that smokers use tobacco to meet some deep need. He has classified them into four groups: habitual smokers; positive-affect smokers; negative-affect smokers; and addictive smokers. The habitual smokers presumably smoke just because the pattern has become established and is functionally autonomous (Allport, 1937). Positive-affect smokers require the stimulant action of smoking, whereas

Table 8. Means and ranges of smokers and nonsmokers

Variable	Psychiatric Patients (N = 40)		Student Nurses (N = 114) Females		University Undergraduates (N = 140) Females		Males	
	Non-smokers (N = 9)	Smokers (N = 31)	Non-smokers	Smokers	Non-smokers	Smokers	Non-smokers	Smokers
Socioeconomic Index:								
Mean	60.2	57.9	48.6	46.2	43.6	42.1	49.8	45.4
Range	44–73	14–77	11–73	11–77	11–71	11–73	11–77	11–73
IQ:								
Mean	93.6	98.8	117.6	118.4	110.9	109.2	107.9	109.2
Range	77–109	79–129	103–130	103–129	87–129	92–122	84–130	89–131
Anxiety level:								
Mean	28.9	25.9	12.3	14.8 °	12.0	15.3	11.0	14.7 °
Range	13–39	6–45	3–26	3–34	5–28	6–45	2–30	1–33
Psychosomatic Symptoms:								
Mean	12.1	13.9	6.3	8.2 °	3.7	6.1	3.3	3.9
Range	2–23	1–44	0–22	0–18	0–14	0–18	0–12	0–19
Cups of Coffee:								
Mean	2.8	4.2	0.9	2.6 †	1.5	2.7	1.0	3.5 †
Range	0–8	0–15	0–6	0–10	0–10	0–6	0–6	0–12
Liquor Score:								
Mean	1.22	2.06	1.0	1.2 °	1.3	1.5	1.5	2.2 †
Range	1–2	1–6	1–2	1–2	1–2	1–2	1–5	1–6

° Mean differences significant at the .05 level.
† Mean differences significant at the .001 level.

Reprinted with permission from Matarazzo, J. D., and G. Saslow. 1960. Psychological and related characteristics of smokers and nonsmokers. Psychological Bulletin, 57, 493–513.

negative-affect smokers require the sedative action. The apparent paradox is resolved by the supposition that these two groups of smokers simply react differently to nicotine or whatever it is in cigarettes that causes the effect they feel. The psychologically addicted person is a slave of his habit and is continually aware of not smoking. The existence and incidence of this behavior requires further investigation.

EVIDENCE FOR NICOTINE AS AN INCENTIVE

Indirect pharmacological actions of nicotine on peripheral structures

Most of the evidence for the role of nicotine in smoking is indirect and stems from various pharmacological literature spawned by this drug. Since Langley's day nicotine has been used as a tool in the study of the peripheral nervous system. It is now well known that acetylcholine has nicotinic actions that resemble those produced by nicotine (Goodman and Gilman, 1965). These are actions at the autonomic ganglia and the neuromuscular junction of striped voluntary muscle. Classically, nicotine first stimulates and then depresses. The peripheral actions of nicotine are now known to be rather complex in the intact organism because they are a product of the nicotinic cholinergic actions plus the powerful adrenergic effects produced by the release of catecholamines from their stores by nicotine.

In fact, the predominant effect of nicotine in the whole intact animal or human is sympathomimetic. It consists of an increase of pulse rate, blood pressure, and peripheral vasoconstriction; an increase in free fatty acids; a mobilization of blood sugar, and in short, the effects that might be expected from an increase in the level of catecholamines in the blood. There is also an impairment in reflexes (Domino and Baumgarten, 1968) and an arousing effect upon the electroencephalogram. Excitation of respiration occurs through stimulation of the chemoreceptors of the carotid body (Heymans, Bouckaert, and Dautrebande, 1931), but higher doses directly stimulate the medullary centers. High doses of nicotine—much higher than those encountered in smoking— result in convulsions. Nicotine produces nausea and vomiting, especially in novices. Increased motor activity of the intestines occurs that can be blocked by atropine.

The problem of whether nicotine produces its effect in a given case directly by stimulating receptors or indirectly by releasing other agents is a difficult one. The answer appears to be that there is always a complex interaction. The release of peripheral catecholamines, including epinephrine, from the adrenal medulla and norepinephrine from sympathetic nerve endings plays an important role in the peripheral cardiovascular, renal, and respiratory effects seen with this drug and also during smoking. Peripheral actions, for example, upon blood pressure may also be reflected in the activity of the brain. Conversely, actions upon the brain by which catecholamines and a variety of other substances are released may be reflected in the periphery. With this multiplicity of actions the paramount question arises of which actions contribute most to the incentive properties of nicotine. In other words, do people smoke cigarettes in order to get the nicotine into their respiratory systems, into their blood streams, or into their brains?

The mechanism whereby nicotine releases other substances remains a question of current interest. One method of determining whether the effect of nicotine on an organ or system is direct or indirect is to prerelease the substances that nicotine itself releases. Thus, if a rabbit is pretreated with reserpine, and norepinephrine is freed from its atria, then in the presence of atropine nicotine has no action on the rate or force of the heartbeat (Burn and Rand, 1958). The ability of nicotine to release substances was noted as early as 1912, when Dale and Laidlaw found that the pressor response of the cat for nicotine involved the release of epinephrine from the adrenal glands. It is possible that nicotine mimics acetylcholine in providing an initial link in the chain of events involved in stimulus-secretion coupling. As Douglas (1965) indicated, acetylcholine reacts with the plasma membrane of the secreting cell, producing an increased permeability to calcium ions, which arrive at some strategic site that initiates the process causing the release of transmitter substance. The ability of both acetylcholine and nicotine to release neurohumoral transmitters, particularly norepinephrine, may be prevented by ganglionic blocking agents, such as hexamethonium. It may be supposed that the action of nicotine is fairly specific and restricted to nicotinic cholinergic receptors like acetylcholine. At any rate, the releasing mechanism seems to be different from that seen with reserpine and tyramine, where a competition with the true transmitter (norepinephrine or 5-hydroxytryptamine) appears to be the basis of action (see Schievelbein and Werle, 1967).

Many of the well-known pharmacological effects of nicotine upon the organ systems of the body (the brain excluded) are the result of the release of catecholamines from peripheral stores. Indirect evidence for this mechanism has existed for some time. As Blackburn, Brozek, Taylor, and Keys (1962) indicated, smokers have a faster resting heart rate, a lower mean systolic and diastolic pressure, greater A-V oxygen difference, and a higher basal oxygen consumption, and they exhibit relatively less obesity than nonsmokers. Nicotine tends to produce a greater percentage increase in pulse rate than in blood pressure, but it does increase both variables (Herxheimer, Griffiths, Hamilton, and Wakefield, 1967; Roth, McDonald, and Sheard, 1945). According to Herxheimer et al. (1967), the effects of nicotine upon heart rate became apparent one to two minutes after inhalation.

Knapp et al. (1963) indicated that roughly twenty minutes after smoking, a gradual sympatheticlike constriction of the peripheral vasculature and acceleration of heart rate develops, then subsides. Lucchesi, Schuster, and Emley (1967) found that blood pressure, heart rate, and EKG showed changes following smoking and also following intravenous injection of nicotine. Skin temperature and finger volume measured by plethysmography both fall within five to ten minutes after cigarette smoking in normal individuals but not in heavy smokers with marked peripheral vascular disease.

Weatherby (1942) reported that smoking of a single cigarette by a habitual smoker results in an increase of 10 to 25 mm of mercury in the systolic and diastolic blood pressure. The pulse rate is increased 5 to 20 beats per minute, and the temperature of the skin of the finger drops 2 to 5 degrees (see Figure 2). Armitage (1965) has demonstrated

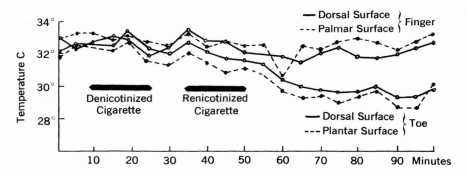

Figure 2. Temperature changes caused by smoking.

Reprinted with permission from Weatherby, J. H., 1942. Skin temperature changes caused by smoking and other sympathomimetic stimuli. *American Heart Journal, 24,* 17–30.

that the effects of both nicotine and tobacco smoke upon blood-pressure responses in cats are related to the release of catecholamines from the adrenal glands. Coffman (1967) has shown that the prior administration of reserpine or guanethedine to human subjects would antagonize the cutaneous vasoconstriction caused by tobacco smoking, presumably by preventing the usual actions of the catecholamines. Both Herxheimer et al. (1967) and Furey, Schaanning, and Spoont (1967) have shown that the effects on circulation produced by smoking tobacco are much greater than those brought about by smoking lettuce-leaf cigarettes.

A more direct approach to the problem has been taken by Kershbaum and Bellet and their collaborators (Kershbaum, Bellet, Jiminez, and Feinberg, 1966) who showed that urinary catecholamine excretion increased during smoking and increases even further with cigarettes than with cigars (Figure 3). There is a concomitant increase in free fatty acids as in mobilization. Kershbaum and Bellet (1964) showed that in dogs given nicotine daily for a six-week period there was a 50 per cent rise in the level of serum cholesterol. The implications for the etiology of atherosclerosis are evident. Kershbaum, Khorsandian, Caplan, Bellet, and Feinberg (1963) found that in patients who had undergone bilateral adrenolectomy the free fatty acid response to cigarette smoking was either minimal or absent. The effect of nicotine was also abolished when a ganglionic blocking agent, methaphan camphorsulfonate, was administered to the subjects.

Kershbaum, Pappajohn, and Bellet (1968) also found that tobacco smoking and nicotine administration to humans and animals caused an increase in the secretion of adrenocortical steroids. These authors raised the possibility that increased corticosteroids secretion might be due to enhanced corticotropin release resulting from nicotine-induced release of catecholamines. Another possibility is that nicotine may directly stimulate the hypothalamic pituitary pathways involved in the elaboration and secretion of adrenocorticotropic hormones.

The effects of nicotine upon diuresis may be either positive or negative, depending upon conditions. Nicotine may produce diuresis by inhibiting the secretion of antidiuretic hormones (DiPalma, 1965; Goodman and Gilman, 1965). On the other hand, in some patients the reverse effect occurs with antidiuresis following nicotine administration (Dalessio, 1969).

Effects of nicotine on the central nervous system

There are now a fair number of studies on the actions of nicotine upon the chemical, physiological, and electrical activity of the central nervous system (Murphree, 1967; Silvette, Hoff, Larson, and Haag, 1962). There is no question that the drug has powerful actions on the brain and spinal cord, but how these are connected with the smoking habit is

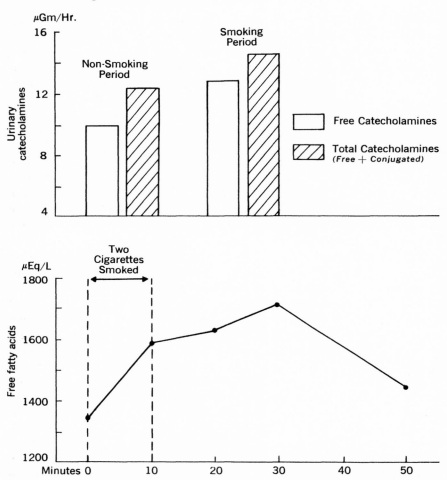

*Figure 3. Urinary catecholamine excretion and serum free fatty acid
levels after cigarette smoking in a normal man. FFA levels were
determined at the start of the 3-hour smoking period.*

Reprinted with permission from Kershbaum, A., S. Bellet, J. Jiminez, and
L. J. Feinberg, 1966. Differences in effects of cigar and cigarette smoking on
free fatty acid mobilization and catecholamine excretion. *Journal of the American
Medical Association, 195,* 1095–1098.

less clear. The rewarding effects of nicotine may be peripheral, central,
or a combination of the two. Nicotine regularly produces central stimulation, evidenced by activation of the electroencephalogram and by
convulsive seizures following high doses.

With carefully selected doses stimulant effects of nicotine may be

readily demonstrated in animals (Kuschinsky and Hotovy, 1943; Robustelli, 1963, 1966), and these effects resemble those of the amphetamines.

The same type of effect was observed when the drug was injected
into the ventricles (Armitage, Milton, and Morrison, 1966). In conscious
cats 2.5 to 10 micrograms of nicotine injected into the cerebral ventricles
through a Feldberg cannula produced blinking, vomiting, and twitching
of the ears, with facilitation of the pinna reflex. Following 30 to 100
micrograms, panting and salivation occurred, with meowing and urina-
tion and defecation. With 300 to 1,000 micrograms the result was
torticollis, ataxia, and blind charging, sometimes resulting in a clonic-
tonic convulson followed by recovery in about one-half hour. In anes-
thetized cats ear twitching, salivation, and labored respiration were
seen. There was usually a fall in arterial blood pressure within thirty
seconds after injection. It was necessary to wait thirty to forty-five
minutes to prevent cumulative effects.

Domino (1967) who has examined numerous effects of nicotine on
the central and peripheral nervous system concluded that "many of
the neuropharmacological and behavioral studies of nicotine, although
of academic interest, are clearly unrelated to tobacco smoking." Since
nicotine is one of the most venerable drugs studied in neuropharma-
cology, the literature describing its actions is very extensive (Silvette
et al., 1962). It is clear, however, as Domino points out, that although
the relationship of the well-known and lesser-known central effects
of small doses of nicotine upon the central nervous system to smoking
is still not clear, any theory of the causes of tobacco habituation must
take these actions into account.

The central stimulant actions of nicotine—including EEG activation,
tremor, and grand mal convulsions—can be antagonized by nicotinic
ganglionic blocking drugs, and particularly by mecamylamine (Stone,
Torchiana, Navarro, and Beyer, 1956). The activating effects of nicotine
have been noted in different ways by many investigators (Longo, Von
Berger, and Bovet, 1954). Support for the idea that there might be
nicotinic and muscarinic cholinergic receptors in the brain is afforded
by the work of Longo, Giuntina, and Scotti De Carolis (1967), who
showed that mecamylamine in doses of 0.5 to 1.0 mg/kg, which did
not affect the EEG of the rabbit, was nevertheless able to block convulsions produced by 1.5 mg/kg i.v. nicotine. Seizures may also be
induced by muscarinic drugs such as physostigmine and DFP, but these
are quite specifically antagonized by atropinelike drugs.

Domino (1967) found that in cats chronically implanted with brain
electrodes and intravenous catheters nicotine produced a relatively
unique effect. If the cats were sleeping naturally, it would produce a

behavioral and an EEG arousal, but this would be followed by a period involving an increase in incidence of activated sleep. It was possible to block these effects with 0.7 mg/kg of mecamylamine. Domino (1967) points out that the activating effects of nicotine are due in part to its ability to release vasopressin, angiotensin, epinephrine, and 5-hydroxytryptamine among other substances. However, the drug also produces a direct arousing effect upon the brain, which can be blocked by mecamylamine.

The review by Silvette et al. (1962) came to the same conclusions regarding the action of nicotine on the central nervous system as had been drawn years before by physiologists concerning its action on the peripheral nervous system. "Small doses of nicotine had a stimulating action on the central nervous system whereas large doses depressed." However, while small doses of nicotine cause arousal and stimulation characterized by desynchronization of the sleeping EEG, larger doses cause typical grand mal seizures. Tremor has been noted following nicotine administration to animals and man and has been ascribed to a direct action on the brain as well as the release of catecholamines. Furthermore, nicotine has a stimulating action at the neuromuscular junction. Other cholinergic drugs which produce tremor are arecoline (Holmstedt and Lundgren, 1967) and tremorine (Everett, Blockus, Shepperd, and Toman, 1956). Arecoline and tremorine produced tremor that can be antagonized by atropine demonstrating a muscarinic action. The nicotine tremor cannot be antagonized by atropine, but it presumably could be countered by nicotinic ganglionic blocking agents.

In low doses nicotine functions like its congener, lobeline. It causes reflex hyperpnea by stimulating the carotid and aortic bodies. Higher doses cause direct stimulation of the respiratory center, whereas still higher doses paralyze this center (Goodman and Gilman, 1965). Peripheral curarelike paralysis of the respiratory muscle also occur with high doses. The question still exists whether the tachycardia following nicotine is due to the action of catecholamines directly from the heart or rather to stimulation of the chemoreceptors in the aortic carotid bodies. A number of studies indicate that nicotine depresses the patellar reflex in both animals and man, while the flexor reflex is relatively unaffected (Domino and Baumgarten, 1968). It is known that the Renshaw cells are nicotinic cholinoceptive and might be responsible for these reflex effects of the drug.

All these peripheral physiological actions are at least involved if they are not causative of the smoking habit. Can it be that a rapidly beating heart or diminished reflexes feel so good that people go out of their way to elicit these responses? Or is the converse true—that the responses occur and may even be unpleasant, but that there are still some other actions of nicotine that make these bearable? Perhaps newer psychopharmacological studies could throw some light on this question.

Psychological actions of nicotine

If behavior involves an interaction with the environment, then the distinction between physiology and psychology can be said to occur at the skin surface. The study of sleep seems to straddle both physiology and psychology. As pointed out by Domino (1967), nicotine has a unique property of increasing REM sleep. Similar findings were reported by Jewett and Norton (1966). However, since even the heaviest smokers rarely smoke during sleeping periods, unless they suffer from insomnia, it is questionable whether these actions on REM sleep have any significance for the smoking habit. On the other hand, the stimulant properties of nicotine, the ability to produce arousal, may play a very real role in the incentive properties of the drug, as has been suggested by Tomkins (1966) and others.

The possibility that nicotine influences practically every sensory modality has been investigated, but no striking findings have emerged. Nicotine is surely not "hallucinogenic," like marijuana or lysergic acid diethylamide, and such sensory effects as are produced are weak or subtle.

Larson, Finnegan, and Haag (1950) found that cigarette smoking increased or facilitated flicker fusion frequency. On the other hand, Sheard (1946) found a decrease in light sensitivity of both rods and cones in a dark adaptation test, which persisted for 15 to 30 minutes after inhaling smoke from two standard cigarettes. No effects were observed following the smoking of nontobacco cigarettes. More recently CFF thresholds were found by Warwick and Eysenck (1963) to be raised, thus confirming the findings of Larson, Finnegan, and Haag (1950). However, Hirvonen et al. (1961, cited in Larson and Silvette, 1968) found a lowering of the fusion frequency of flicker following smoking.

Since cigarette smoke is taken into the mouth one might expect taste to be affected. Indeed Fischer, Griffin, and Kaplan (1963) found that smokers had a higher taste threshold for bitterness than nonsmokers. They felt that this factor led to smoking, but they might have equally as well concluded that smoking led to the increased threshold. Bronte-Stewart, Krut, and Perrin (1960) similarly found higher thresholds of bitter taste in smokers. Perhaps bitter nicotine masked other bitter tastes or maybe continual bitter stimulation resulted in habituation and desensitization. Sinnot and Rauth (1937) found that smokers have a higher threshold for sugar and salt than nonsmokers. However, Cooper, Bilash, and Zubek (1959) found that there was no significant difference in taste sensitivity between smokers and nonsmokers.

Wenusch and Schöller (1936) found that touch thresholds were higher in smokers than in nonsmokers, but that nonsmokers were more sensitive to the effects of cigarettes in raising the threshold. In any case, if changes in sensitivity to different types of stimuli are related to smoking, it is not known whether or how they influence smoking. If, indeed, impairment of perception is caused by smoking and if the causal relationship is perceived, one might expect this effect to act as a form of punishment that will diminish smoking. Clinical experience tells us that such punishment is ineffective. Furthermore, since even the punishment of intermittent claudication or of emphysema does not seem to discourage smokers, why should a slight dimming of vision or flattening of taste work? On the other hand, perhaps the improvement in flicker perception is sought by the smoker. Smoking in the blind has not been studied, although there is an allusion by Larson, Haag, and Silvette (1961, 534) that blind men might not enjoy smoking as much as the sighted. However, blindness presents a serious physical handicap to the smoker in manipulation, as well as being a fire hazard.

A number of authors have shown that nicotine causes stimulation and increased arousal in animals. It has a facilitative effect on conditioned avoidance behavior (Robustelli, 1963) and appetitive behavior (Morrison and Armitage, 1967). Bovet, Bovet-Nitti, and Oliverio (1966) found that nicotine produced a facilitating effect on avoidance conditioning in genetically pure strains of mice characterized by low nondrugged performance, whereas those that started with a high level of performance were impaired by nicotine.

The influence of nicotine upon animal behavior and learning has been reviewed extensively by McGaugh and Petrinovich (1965) and also by Larson, Haag, and Silvette (1961), Silvette et al. (1962) and Larson and Silvette (1968). Some investigators have found that nicotine injections or tobacco-smoke exposure reduce spontaneous activity in rodents, whereas others found that it stimulated activity. Species and dose effects were not usually well controlled. Other investigators found that nicotine injections or smoke inhalations impaired the ability of rats to run mazes. Simple illness can impair an animal's interest in food and its apparent learning ability. On the other hand, facilitation of learning is not so easily explained. Pechstein and Reynolds (1937) fumed rats with tobacco smoke and found that their learning capacity excelled those of control rats. Perhaps an amphetaminelike arousal may be produced by nicotine, and an animal that is more alert might be expected to learn more easily. An activating effect of nicotine might be as rewarding as an activating effect of caffeine or amphetamine.

One of the paradoxical effects of smoking is that individuals claim it relaxes them though nicotine has long yet been regarded as a stimulant drug. At the turn of the century a number of investigators (reported in Heimstra, Bancroft, and Dekock, 1967) found little effect of nicotine upon muscular fatigue. Finely coordinated movements are impaired by smoking presumably because of the tremor which is induced. Heimstra et al. (1967) discovered that cigarette smokers performed about as well as nonsmokers in a simulated driving task. However, performance was markedly impaired if cigarettes were taken away from them during the six-hour task. During this frustrating prolonged test, the most contented subjects were the smokers who were given cigarettes, and the most aggressive according to the Nowlis Mood Scale were the deprived smokers. In a somewhat different type of study Cooper et al. (1959) reported that chronic smokers performed less well in a test of endurance than did nonsmokers.

Tests of mental efficiency in humans have not given consistent results in deciding whether smoking has a deleterious effect or not (see Larson, Haag, and Silvette, 1961; Larson and Silvette, 1968). Hull (1924) found that pipe smoking caused nonsmokers to lose efficiency in speed of continuous mental arithmetic, while smokers showed a uniform gain. At any rate, the effects of smoking on mental efficiency appear to be very small, since there is great variability between different investigators. One of the problems is that smokers who are tested during a period of deprivation and nonsmokers who are given cigarettes or cigars to smoke are both in abnormal states. It is not surprising that each should do better when they are in their accustomed state of smoking or not smoking. However, the effects of smoking upon nonsmokers is much more comparable to the effects of other drugs on the abilities of naïve subjects.

There does seem to be some relationship between chronic smoking and scholarship and intelligence (cited in Larson and Silvette, 1968). Those with poorer grades or lower scores on intelligence tests tend to smoke more, but cause and effect relationships are not clear.

DIRECT EVIDENCE FOR NICOTINE AS AN INCENTIVE

The possibility that there is a rewarding substance in tobacco has been entertained since smoking was known. Since the discovery, more than a century ago, that the most powerful pharmacological component of tobacco is nicotine, the view has been often expressed that people who use tobacco are seeking the physiological effects of this alkaloid. Obvious as this thesis may seem, a number of alternative hypotheses have been suggested assuming that people smoke for reasons other than to obtain nicotine. These may be considered the sociological and psychological theories of smoking motivation, as contrasted with the pharmacological theory. Perhaps because it seems so obvious, very few studies have attempted to demonstrate that nicotine or something else in tobacco is a prime incentive. Three studies in man and two in animals with this psychopharmacological orientation will be examined in some detail.

The first published study in which the possible rewarding effects of nicotine were examined was by L. M. Johnston (1942). These were a series of rather nonsystematic observations of thirty-five volunteers, some of whom were smokers and others nonsmokers (numbers not given). Nicotine—1/50 of a grain (1.3 mg)—given hypodermically to nonsmokers was unpleasant and strange, light-headedness and "muzziness" appearing about five minutes after the injection and lasting about 15 minutes; "smokers almost invariably thought the sensation pleasant and, given an adequate dose, were disinclined to smoke for some time thereafter." As little as 1/40 of a grain (1.6 mg) is capable of producing toxic symptoms in nonsmokers, but 1/10 of a grain (6.5 mg) produced no untoward effects in heavy smokers. Toxic symptoms consisted of "swimminess," rapid and forcible cardiac action, nausea, vomiting, and syncope. The subjective sensation produced by one deep inhalation of cigarette smoke was said to resemble the intravenous injection of 1/500 to 1/750 of a grain (0.13 mg to 0.09 mg) of nicotine, and the latency of perception was about fifteen seconds, the duration only one or two minutes. Twelve strong puffs on a cigarette resembled the effect of 1/50 of a grain (1.3 mg) of nicotine injected hypodermically. Johnston found that the same effects could be mimicked by giving the drug orally, but in that case the latency of onset was prolonged. When 1/15 of a grain (4.3 mg) was dissolved in five ounces of water and swallowed, the characteristic sensation was noticed in about fifteen minutes. Some esophogeal irritation was noted with stronger solutions. One patient receiving this dose orally three times a day declared that it "steadied" her more than did phenobarbital. This observation is consonant with the usual reports of smokers that smoking relaxes them. Johnston (1942) found that three or four hypodermic injections of 1/50 of a grain (1.3 mg) of nicotine per day for about three weeks satisfied him more than smoking a cigarette, and he had feelings of deprivation when the injections were discontinued.

Finnegan et al. (1945) conducted a much better-designed study to examine the idea that nicotine may play a role in the cigarette habit. Twenty-four cigarette smokers were used, and a comparison was made of the rate at which they smoked their own cigarettes compared with low-nicotine cigarettes. Subjective reports were also taken. Further, the effects of a high-nicotine cigarette were studied.

Each subject smoked three kinds of cigarettes for a variable period of time. First they smoked their own cigarettes, and the number per day was counted. Next they smoked two cartons of cigarettes made from tobacco naturally low in nicotine but to which nicotine had been added, so that the nicotine content of the smoke per cigarette was 1.96 mg. This regimen was followed by at least four cartons of low-nicotine cigarettes that contained 0.34 mg of nicotine in the smoke of each cigarette. The length of time each cigarette was smoked is not clearly given. Although the results were not statistically analyzed, it appears that the people who did not miss the nicotine smoked more low-nicotine cigarettes. By contrast, those who complained smoked approximately the same number of low-nicotine cigarettes as their usual brands. The authors concluded, presumably from the fact that many subjects did not complain, that there are individuals in whom nicotine is not a factor in the cigarette habit (see Table 9).

It may be that the individuals who were able to endure the low-nicotine cigarettes without complaining nevertheless preferred the high-nicotine cigarettes; a comparative judgment was not requested. It may also be that the dose-response curve for the rewarding properties of nicotine is a logarithmic curve and that even though the nicotine content of the smoke was six times as large in the high-nicotine as in the low-nicotine cigarette, the subjective difference may not have been significant. Furthermore, the nicotine content of their own brands was presumably intermediate. No measures were taken of the subject's reactions to the high-nicotine cigarettes other than the number of cigarettes they smoked per day.

This experiment showed that subjects did not titrate the number of cigarettes smoked per day to keep the nicotine content constant. Of course there are other ways in which subjects might adjust the amount of nicotine they take in by varying the depth of inhalation and the length of the cigarette that they actually smoke (more nicotine is inhaled as the butt length gets shorter). As the authors themselves state, the number of subjects involved was too small to arrive at any definite conclusions concerning the reasons why some subjects seem to miss the nicotine whereas others do not.

Between 1945 and 1967 there are no published investigations dealing

Table 9. Role of nicotine in the smoking habits of 24 inveterate cigarette smokers

| Subject | Standard brands | Average daily consumption Experimental cigarettes | | | Degree to which nicotine was missed |
		Nicotine added (first period)	Low nicotine	Nicotine added (second period)	
L.H.	21.8	21.4	21.9	22.5	0
R.M.	20.7	24.2	31.5	20.3	0
S.N.	20.4	20.6	19.8	20.5	0
H.S.	ca. 60	ca. 60	ca. 75	ca. 60	0
J.B.	19.2	14.8	17.4	16.1	0
N.C.	19.4	18.9	20.1	21.3	0
(Means)	26.9	26.6	30.9	26.8 (Total)	6
A F.	24.0	23.8	22.3	18.9	°
S.H.	21.3	20.8	24.5	25.6	°
J.M.	19.3	19.1	36.2	23.9	°
G.O.	20.8	20.3	23.4	19.7	°
F.W	25.4	19.1	30.2	28.5	°
H.W.	23.4	28.9	22.7	26.6	°
(Means)	22.4	22.0	26.5	23.9 (Total)	6
J.F.	28.2	38.2	32.4	37.5	†
P.L.	24.5	27.2	28.5	23.1	†
F.P.	18.2	19.5	25.0	22.2	†
(Means)	23.6	28.3	28.6	27.6 (Total)	3
G.B.	25.5	17.0	27.7	20.7	‡
E.H.	22.1	25.5	28.5	30.3	‡
K.K.	25.1	27.3	26.4	27.4	‡
H.B.	25.3	28.4	25.8	24.2	‡
M.F.	21.4	25.8	24.8	28.6	‡
D.G.	34.4	27.6	27.0	26.7	‡
F.H.	28.8	24.4	26.7	25.4	‡
W.P.	21.0	21.6	16.1	19.3	‡
C.Z.	21.2	24.8	18.6	21.3	‡
(Means)	25.0	24.7	24.6	24.9 (Total)	9

0 Did not miss the nicotine.
° Mild initial dissatisfaction with low nicotine cigarettes.
† Definite temporary lack of satisfaction with low nicotine cigarettes.
‡ Definite and prolonged lack of satisfaction with low nicotine cigarettes.
Reprinted with permission from Finnegan, J. K., P. S. Larson, and H. B. Haag, 1945. The role of nicotine in the cigarette habit. *Science, 102,* 94–96.

with the influence of nicotine on smoking behavior. The paper by Lucchesi and collaborators is therefore both unique and of great importance (Lucchesi et al., 1967). When four volunteers—all smokers—received a blind intravenous infusion of nicotine amounting to 1 mg per hour for six hours, their smoking behavior was not altered significantly. When the rate of administration was increased to 2 to 4 mg/hr, a significant decrease in smoking frequency was obtained. Not only was the number of cigarettes decreased, but so was the average amount of each cigarette smoked. It would appear that different amounts of nicotine are needed to suppress smoking in different subjects.

Lucchesi et al. (1967) estimated that 4 mg/hr of nicotine is absorbed from smoking two standard cigarettes per hour. As can be seen from Table 10 the subjects did not completely compensate for the intravenous nicotine by cutting down the number of cigarettes smoked. Therefore, the total amount of nicotine under the combined conditions was greater than from cigarettes alone. One suggestion also made by Ejrup (1965) is that the local concentration of nicotine in the respiratory system is much higher than in the body and the smoker is seeking these local effects in part, if not entirely.

As is shown in Figure 4 the heart rate under the resting condition was low, representing either the depressant effect of eight hours of smoking deprivation or the lower heart rate that naturally occurs in the morning. Thereafter, when subjects were allowed to smoke freely, it can be seen that the heart rate increased. The superimposition of nicotine upon cigarette smoking resulted in an increase in heart rate,

Table 10. Comparison of average number of cigarettes consumed per six-hour session under saline control and drug conditions

	Saline control			Drug			
Subject	No. of sessions	Mean	± S.E.	No. of sessions	Mean	± S.E.	Level of significance
1	7	17.9	±0.72	7	14.4	±0.58	<0.005
2	4	7.0	±0	5	4.4	±0.24	<0.0005
3	6	7.3	±0.40	6	4.8	±0.48	<0.005
4	7	11.4	±0.52	5	8.2	±0.32	<0.005
5	5	6.7	±0.25	4	4.7	±0.25	<0.005

Reprinted with permission from Lucchesi, B. R., C. R. Schuster, and G. S. Emley, 1967. The role of nicotine as a determinant of cigarette smoking frequency in man with observations of certain cardiovascular effects associated with the tobacco alkaloid. *Clinical Pharmacology and Therapeutics, 8,* 789–796.

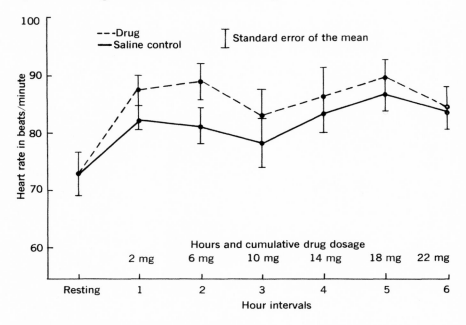

Figure 4. Mean heart rate per hour interval for 5 subjects under saline control and nicotine administration conditions.

Reprinted with permission from Lucchesi, B. R., C. R. Schuster, and G. S. Emley, 1967. The role of nicotine as a determinant of cigarette smoking frequency in man with observations of certain cardiovascular effects associated with the tobacco alkaloid. *Clinical Pharmacology and Therapeutics, 8,* 789–796.

with a remarkable parallelism between the two curves even with a dip at three hours. (Does this low represent lunch?) In Figure 5 it can be seen that while a diurnal increase in heart rate might account for some of the variations in smoking, nicotine must have accounted for part of the increase. When smoking was prohibited, the increase was significantly less than when it was permitted.

If the cardiovascular effects of smoking or nicotine are due to the release of catecholamines from stores, then a maximal or nearly maximal release obtained by the administration of additional nicotine would not be expected to have great effect. Presumably a smoker regulates his smoking behavior to elicit just the right response from the nicotine that is absorbed. Factors such as monetary cost and fatigue will limit the number of cigarettes smoked; but these are not likely to be important determinants of rate. On the other hand, the subjects used by Lucchesi et al. (1967) could have conceivably lowered

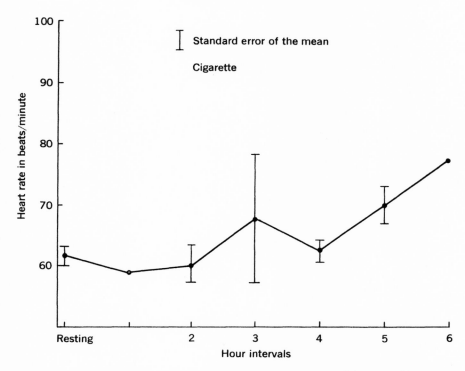

Figure 5. Mean heart rate per hour interval for one subject smoking one cigarette per hour for 3.5 hours. Each point represents 3 determinations.

Reprinted with permission from Lucchesi, B. R., C. R. Schuster, and G. S. Emley, 1967. The role of nicotine as a determinant of cigarette smoking frequency in man with observations of certain cardiovascular effects associated with the tobacco alkaloid. *Clinical Pharmacology and Therapeutics, 8,* 789–796.

the number of cigarettes they smoked to almost zero and still obtained the necessary amount of nicotine. If they did not do so, then clearly something other than nicotine kept them smoking. It was undoubtedly "habit" or secondary reinforcement, but the chances are they would have extinguished in time. But the fact that there *was* a decrease in smoking is at least compatible with the idea that nicotine functions as an incentive. It is also possible that the effect of the nicotine was nonspecifically depressing, and perhaps a barbiturate or chlorpromazine might have had the same effect. In any case, this experiment is good evidence that the nicotine feedback system is not very finely tuned.

A more direct test of the feedback incentive properties of nicotine was provided by Deneau and Inoki (1967). They implanted intravenous catheters in monkeys and allowed them to self-inject nicotine. At 10 micrograms/kg no monkey would self-administer nicotine, even though it was automatically injected with this dose once an hour. At 25 micrograms/kg all the monkeys self-administered nicotine. The average total dose ranged from 0.7 to 1.7 mg/kg and was very variable from day to day. At intervals of a month the doses were raised in an approximately logarithmic fashion to 50, 100, 200, 500, 1000, and finally 2000 micrograms/kg. Only one monkey continued to self-administer at the highest dose and received an average of 9.6 mg/kg and a maximum of 14.0 mg/kg nicotine.

The self-administration of a substance is necessary and sufficient to demonstrate that it has positive incentive value. Thus, food and water will be self-administered by subjects at certain times. Similarly certain drugs are rewarding in this same sense, and these include opiates, alcohol, barbiturates, amphetamines, and cocaine (but not phenothiazines, antihistamines, or many others). Humans will self-administer hallucinogenic agents—such as LSD, mescaline, psilocybin, and marijuana—but to my knowledge animals have not yet been trained to take these substances voluntarily.

Monkeys can, however, be trained to smoke cigarettes, and this behavior is the subject of study in a series of experiments in my laboratory (Jarvik, 1967). Perhaps half and maybe more of all monkeys can be trained to smoke. They are shaped by being taught to suck water out of a tube, whereupon a burning cigarette is substituted. Each monkey adopts a characteristic individualistic puffing pattern, and there is considerable day-to-day variation within as well as between monkeys. This situation is unlike that which prevails among humans, who have a characteristically stable daily smoking pattern. Thus far only a few monkeys have been used, and the initial shaping procedure has not been studied. It is my impression that acquisition is fairly rapid and levels off quickly.

Extinction has been studied, however, and it has been found that it is remarkably slow. This is true whether the animal is given hot air or just an empty tube. In Figure 6 can be seen some extinction curves; it demonstrates the persistence of the monkeys in puffing without the reinforcement of smoke. Poor extinction indicates that generalization will be great and discrimination poor in this situation. Hence performance with high- and low-nicotine cigarettes has not been compared. Even on the open market humans do not invariably pick the brand with the highest nicotine content, though the trend is in that direction. I think that a more promising approach will be to try to influence smoking

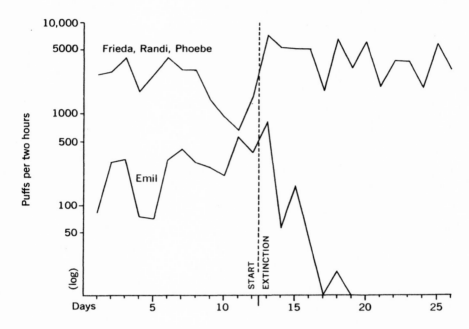

Figure 6. Extinction curves for puffing.

behavior with drugs, especially those known to influence nicotine or catecholamine action.

It is now known that animals will regulate their intake of drugs that are traditionally considered addicting, such as opiates, alcohol, cocaine, and amphetamine. Once a habit of taking these drugs is established, animals will attempt to keep the daily intake fairly constant (Pickens and Thompson, 1968; Thompson and Schuster, 1968; Weeks, 1962; Wikler and Pescor, 1967). The ability of an animal to keep the level constant indicates a good type of interoceptive discriminative control and also indicates that the factors underlying the need for the drug do not vary much. Deneau's experiment (Deneau and Inoki, 1967) and my own indicate that such a fine degree of control does not exist for nicotine.

NONNICOTINE FACTORS AS PRIMARY CAUSES FOR SMOKING

Arguments against the role of nicotine have rarely been based upon experiments. Bloedorn (1920) suggested that although oral administration of the active products of tobacco would be more efficient than smoking, smoking is the preferred route. The assumption is open to some question, since the blood levels of nicotine following inhalation are undoubtedly higher than following oral ingestion. Dixon (1921) argued that, though combustion destroyed most of the nicotine, it could not play a very important part in maintaining the habit; in fact, a very substantial amount of nicotine is inhaled with the smoke. During war time substitutes for tobacco have been smoked with apparent pleasure (Russ, 1955). Given free choice, however, tobacco is always preferred. Gies, Kahn, and Limerick (1921) pointed out that smokers do not tend to increase their dose—exactly the reverse of the situation that obtains among drug addicts. However, both assumptions may be wrong, since smokers do increase their dose up to an optimum, and drug addicts—for example, heroin addicts—do not invariably or indefinitely increase their dose.

Against the idea that nicotine plays an important role in smoking were the findings of Johnston (1942) that nonsmokers derived no pleasure from nicotine. Ejrup (1965) felt that people smoke to relieve the irritation of their respiratory tract; "the cigarette smoker scratches his itching bronchi with smoke." Von Ahn (1954, 112) found that an intravenous injection of nicotine was frequently unpleasant. Mulhall (1895) felt that smoking produced a pleasurable irritation of the respiratory tree. Larson, Haag, and Silvette (1961, 285) maintained that the cigarette break serves the purpose not only of getting nicotine, but also social aims. Bickford (1960) found that smoking a full cigarette produced as much activation on the electroencephalogram as smoking a regular cigarette. Hauser, Schwarz, Roth, and Bickford (1958) also obtained EEG effects from inhaling alone and concluded that nicotine was not necessary. Rosenberg (1959) felt that the movements involved in smoking were the real incentives, rather than nicotine. J. A. C. Brown (1963) concluded that not nicotine but taste was the goal of smoking.

The Surgeon General's Report (U.S. Public Health Service, 1964, 34 and 354) considered the habitual use of tobacco as based primarily on psychological and social causes. These authors state: "undoubtedly, the smoking habit becomes compulsive in some heavy smokers, but the drive to compulsion appears to be solely psychogenic since physical dependence does not develop to nicotine or to other constituents of tobacco."

A survey of purely psychological explanations of smoking has been given by Larson, Haag, and Silvette (1961) and Larson and Silvette (1968). Most of these views are purely speculative. The oral component has been stressed by psychoanalysts, and Freud in 1905 compared smoking to thumbsucking and considered it an oral autoerotic manifestation of deprivation of sucking at the breast. Jacobs, Knapp, et al. (1965) and Jacobs, Anderson, et al. (1966) and also Schubert (1965) used interviews and questionnaires to assess personality factors; all came to the conclusion that smokers did have personality characteristics different from those of nonsmokers. In particular they were characterized by arousal-seeking, a state compatible with the known effects of nicotine. Jacobs, Knapp, et al. (1966) felt that smokers were seeking specific stimulation of the oral and respiratory zones and that they exhibited "oral attitudes, particularly an underlying feeling of deficit, along with the fanstasy of having been frustrated by nurturant figures in childhood" and thus developed an "oral preoccupation with putting things in the mouth, such as by excessive drinking, chewing, biting or sucking." Furthermore, smokers looked for the sympathomimetic effects of cigarettes to keep them in a state of excitement or activation. This circumstance explains why heavy smokers are more rebellious, impulsive, and danger-seeking.

It should be pointed out that personality theories are not incompatible with pharmacological theories. Psychological determinants have also been postulated for other drug habits, including heroin and alcohol. I am arguing that nicotine is necessary through not perhaps sufficient for the maintenance of the smoking habit. A nicotine-free cigarette should satisfy oral needs, and studies with such a cigarette should clarify the problem.

IS SMOKING AN ADDICTION TO NICOTINE?

The question of whether smoking represents an addiction to nicotine is both terminological and comparative. The idea of "addiction" is generally not favored by those who work with "illegal" drugs, such as opiates and barbiturates. Avoiding the controversy at this point, the question is simply whether smoking is or can be as strong a habit as heroin-taking or alcoholism. It is not easy, particularly in human beings, to measure the strength of an incentive. If one asks how much money a person is willing to pay for a cigarette as compared to a "fix" of heroin, one is immediately aware of the difficulty in comparison: one purchase is legal and the other is not.

A traditional method of testing an incentive is to determine how much unpleasantness an animal will endure in order to obtain his goal. A commonly used technique was the obstruction box (Warden,

1931), which measured the amount of electric shock an animal would tolerate to get food, water, a sexual partner, or its child. Another method is to study how hard an animal will work for a given reward. Since cigarettes are relatively cheap, it is not necessary to work terribly hard to obtain them. It is conceivable that a very heavy smoker would "walk a mile for a Camel." During World War II in Europe people would go to incredible lengths to obtain cigarettes, collecting butts from the gutters, resorting to prostitution, and bartering their meager food supplies for cigarettes (Brecher, 1969).

At any rate, cigarette smoking shares with heroin taking the elaboration of goal-directed behavior, a strong habit, a strong instrumental or operant conditioned response. The stimulus in each instance is highly reinforcing. In the heroin habit, however, the reinforcing agent has been precisely identified, and the user knows what it is as well as anyone. The cigarette smoker, on the other hand, is not at all sure what, if any, substance he is working for, though it is hard for me to doubt that the essential reinforcer is nicotine.

It used to be thought that tolerance and physical dependence were essential ingredients of addiction. It is now known that a substance can be highly reinforcing when little or no tolerance or physical dependence has developed. Nicotine surely has less of either of these characteristics than any of the opiates.

An extremely influential and authoritative definition of addiction is that adopted by the Committee on Drug Addiction of the National Research Council (1960) and subsequently by the World Health Organization (1964), which stated that "addiction is a state of periodic or chronic intoxication, detrimental to the individual and society produced by the repeated administration of a drug; its characteristics are a compulsion to take the drug and to increase the dose, with the development of psychic and sometimes physical dependence on the effects of the drug, so that the development of compulsion to continue the administration of the drug becomes an important motive in the addict's existence" (Goodman and Gilman, 1965, 134). Subsequent difficulties with this definition caused the World Health Organization to recommend that the term "addiction" be dropped. It is unlikely that this recommendation will be followed, even though attempts are being made here and there. Jaffe (1965, 258) suggests that drug addiction be defined as "a behavioral pattern of compulsive drug users, characterized by overwhelming involvement with the use of the drug, the securing of its supply, and a high tendency to relapse after withdrawal." The trouble with this definition is that it is difficult to quantify the terms "compulsive" or "overwhelming." I would modify and simplify this definition to: "Drug addiction is a behavioral pattern characterized by a tendency to obtain and introduce into the body quantities of a drug to achieve pleasurable effects." It is apparent that the last phrase makes this statement more of a theory than a definition. Like Jaffe, I do not feel that drug addiction requires either physical dependence or tolerance, though in some cases these may occur.

The term "addiction" has come to have some derogatory connotations, but the air of moral condemnation surrounding it is not nearly as bad as that which surrounds the newer term, "drug abuse." The latter is a moralistic term describing drug usage that "deviates from the approved medical or social patterns within a given culture" (Jaffe, 1965). If abuse depends on social approval, it would be necessary to ask whether approval is indicated by the statistical average of the ratings of the number of the community or by laws passed by their representatives and implemented by various agencies. The use of contraceptive pills may well be considered drug abuse by some.

The Surgeon General's report on Smoking and Health (U.S. Public Health Service, 1962) made a strong distinction between drug addiction, such as heroin taking, and drug habituation, such as tobacco smoking. Since that time the World Health Organization has dropped the use of the term "addiction," and the distinction has become less clear. Most recently smoking has been called a "psychic dependence," but this term does not offer any advantage over the older term "addiction," and in fact, the spiritualistic connotations of the term "psychic" offer a distinct disadvantage.

It is clear, however, that some degree of tolerance and physical dependence to nicotine develop in heavy smokers. Although longitudinal studies of the development of tolerance are lacking, it is clear that nausea and malaise experienced by novice smokers soon pass away. It is known that cigarette smokers have more efficient enzymes for destroying coal-tar derivatives than do nonsmokers. It would not be surprising to find that the rate of metabolism of nicotine was enhanced in smokers as well.

Physical dependence is measured by a withdrawal or abstinence syndrome. Is there a *withdrawal syndrome* that accompanies the cessation of smoking? Obviously if there is, one would expect it to be greater in heavy smokers than in light smokers. Goodman and Gilman (1965) note that cigarette withdrawal is associated mainly with craving and restlessness, since smoking dependence is primarily psychic and does not have the constitutional basis of narcotic addiction. In fact, a variety of withdrawal or abstinence signs and symptoms have been reported (Larson, Haag, and Silvette, 1961). The signs have been mainly cardiovascular and gastrointestinal. A fall in pulse rate has often been noted. It has also been noted that following surgery heavy smokers have a higher incidence of intestinal ileus, and that this can be cured by forcing them to smoke. Head (1939) reported that upon rising in the morning, after eight hours of deprivation, his pulse and respiration were slow, blood pressure and basal metabolism were low, and salivary secretion was markedly increased. After smoking one cigarette, all these functions returned to normal. In any case, the withdrawal symptom that persists the longest, even for years, is the craving for a smoke.

A number of studies have indicated that there is substance to the popular idea that weight gain occurs on stopping smoking. Overeating might be considered a withdrawal effect. For example, 246 out of 333 ex-smokers reported that they gained weight when they stopped smoking (Hammond and Percy, 1958).

To be sure, many smokers stop without any complaints except craving, and there seems to be considerable individual variability in this respect. It is clear that the "cold turkey" type of collapse following opiate withdrawal does not occur with nicotine withdrawal. Notwithstanding this fact, the smoking habit may be just as difficult to break as the opiate habit.

IS THERE A CONSTITUTIONAL PREDISPOSITION TO SMOKE?

It has frequently been asked whether alcoholics or heroin addicts have something peculiar about their body chemistry that makes them susceptible to the habit. The tobacco companies have been interested in demonstrating that there is a genetic tendency to smoke that might be related to a tendency to develop cancer. The first point appears to have been demonstrated, because there is a higher concordance for smoking between identical twins than for fraternal twins or sibs (Fisher, R. A., 1959; Shields, 1962). The relationship of smoking to body types is still controversial (Livson and Stewart, 1965; Seltzer, 1965).

SECONDARY REINFORCEMENT AND SMOKING

Glucose is undoubtedly a reinforcing stimulus, but it is not perceived as such by an organism even as sophisticated as man. Instead, one perceives a potato or a piece of bread or a grape, and these visual stimuli are reinforcing. But the starch or sucrose is digested, and the glucose reaches the glucostatic mechanism, where it sets in motion the chain of events that facilitates behavior associated with the procurement of glucose-yielding food. But dietetic artificially sweetened non-nutritive foods and beverages are popular because the stimuli associated with real sugar have themselves acquired reinforcing value—they are secondary or higher-order reinforcers (Kimble, 1961; Reynolds, 1968). The same situation undoubtedly holds for cigarettes. Nicotine is undoubtedly the primary reinforcing agent in tobacco. But it is not easily perceived, while everything else about cigarettes is.

During the initiation of the smoking habit in a teenager, the role of nicotine must be crucial. At this stage the nicotine is strongly reinforcing, and the pleasurable novelty keeps the smoker going. The maintenance of the habit is quite different than the initiation. A heavy smoker has achieved a certain momentum and will go out of his way to obtain his cigarettes. It is my opinion that although smoking may be initiated by nonpharmacological factors, they come into play immediately. The same is true of heroin addiction, glue sniffing, barbiturate addiction, and alcoholism, among other drug habits. The reinforcing effects of nicotine must be substantial, but all the behavior that goes along with getting the nicotine into the system is repeated over and over again and soon becomes secondarily reinforcing. Since a smoker of a pack a day takes about 60,000 puffs a year, all of them accompanied by the same kind of movement and stimuli, it is not surprising that secondary reinforcement becomes very strong. Kimble (1961) has pointed out that the strength of the secondary reinforcement is proportional to the number of times the secondary reinforcing stimulus is primarily reinforced. Extinction to the secondary reinforcement takes longer and longer following more frequent association.

It is quite evident that secondary reinforcement plays an important role in other drug habits, such as opiate addiction. Spragg (1940) noted that a chimpanzee exhibiting withdrawal signs while being deprived of morphine showed temporary relief when he was injected with saline in the same way that he had previously received morphine. Conversely, Jaffe (1965) reports that "narcotics addicts often report that they feel sensations very similar to withdrawal symptoms (including an intense craving for drugs) when they return to situations where drugs are available."

Nevertheless psychological factors alone cannot be responsible for the maintenance of the smoking habit. If they were, then nicotine-free tobacco or nontobacco cigarettes would have a greater success; yet it is known that Cubebs, cornsilk, and lettuce cigarettes are smoked only by ex-smokers, and then not for very long. Opinions are nevertheless divided, and there are those who feel that smoking is a purely psychological habit, similar to playing a musical instrument or painting.

Cigarette filters present a serious problem to the nicotine theory because they lower the amount of nicotine that penetrates to the smoker. Yet the percentage of filtertip cigarettes used has increased from 0.6 in 1950 to 54.6 in 1962. Why do smokers use them? First of all, not all smokers adopt them. Secondly, the use of filters is a response to antismoking publicity as well as to cigarette advertising. Third, the smoker compensates for the filter by applying more negative air pressure to the cigarette. Furthermore, the filters do remove tars, phenols, and other irritating substances that are presumably not reinforcing. Nonetheless, the use of filters is a paradox, since they represent an obstruction between the smoker and his goal.

CONFLICT AND SMOKING

Patterns of behavior are maintained by a balance between reward and punishment. Animals will subject themselves to fatigue and danger to obtain food or sex, and so will man. For the vast majority of mankind, earning one's daily bread means enduring unpleasant labor. Some incentives, such as oxygen or water, are easy to obtain, but others, such as honey or pearls, require some risk, and sometimes the price is just too high. Smoking presents a picture of conflict between the pleasure of nicotine reinforcement and the punishment of disease, crime, and moral condemnation.

It is quite clear that smoking itself produces pain as well as pleasure; but the pain is long delayed, so much so that it is difficult even for scientists to make the association (Cohen and Heimann, 1962). Today it is clear that cigarette smoking causes cancer of the lung, mouth, tongue, larynx, and pharynx; that it plays a role in atheroscleratic disasters, including myocardial infarction and cerebrovascular accidents; its role as a causative factor in peripheral vascular disease has long been known; respiratory troubles, such as bronchitis and emphysema, are caused by smoking; peptic ulcer and cancer of the stomach seem to be causally related as is cancer of the bladder; smoking seems to play a role in tobacco amblyopia. It is surprising that the fear of these diseases is not enough to deter and stop people from smoking, but even after they have the diseases and are dying from them, they frequently cannot stop. Some people claim that they can stop and start anytime they want with the greatest of ease, whereas others experience excessive difficulty. It must be that the strength of the habit is vastly different among individuals.

It is clear that fear can be a powerful deterrent to drug usage. The fact that heroin is illegal or the fiction that LSD causes selected chromosomal damage or the association between butter and atherosclerosis keeps people from using these substances. Health propaganda is beginning to make people stop smoking, just as the fear of pregnancy and syphilis has a deterrent effect upon sexual activity.

The cure of smoking depends primarily on fear today. Moral condemnation has never played a great role except in conversion to certain religious groups, such as the Seventh Day Adventists or Mormons. People stop smoking today because they are afraid of growing ill or dying. Only when the fear is strong enough to counteract the pleasure of smoking will they stop. It appears that the most successful cures result from a combination of social pressure and willpower—the same factors involved in curbing obesity.

If nicotine is the primary reinforcer, then some form of drug treatment should be effective in curbing smoking. Substitution therapy with lobeline has been tried (Edwards, 1964a; Merry and Preston, 1963), but with a notable lack of success. However, administration of nicotine ought to work. This method has been tried only by Johnston (1942). M. M. Miller (1941) has reported that amphetamine is useful in curbing smoking. One might expect chlorpromazine to be equally useful. But nerve-shattering life-threatening fear is probably the best counter-incentive to nicotine.

SPECULATIONS ON MECHANISM OF NICOTINE
ACTION IN SMOKING

In 1960, at a conference on cadiovascular effects of nicotine and smoking, Dr. J. H. Burn said: "It seems to me extremely likely that the pleasure of smoking is derived in part from the release of norepinephrine from its store in the brain by nicotine, the release giving an increased feeling of cheerfulness and a sense of relief from fatigue." Nicotine is known to release catecholamines from their stores in the periphery, and it is reasonable to assume the same action would occur in the brain. On the other hand, Westfall, Fleming, Fudger, and Clark (1967) could observe no changes in brain epinephrine following injections 0.5 and 1.0 mg/kg i. p. nicotine. Changes were observed, however, in whole mouse brain and rat diencephalon. The authors emphasized, however, that measurement of amines in a whole brain area could very easily mask a response taking place in a small restricted area.

The catecholamine-releasing property of nicotine must be considered in conjunction with the catecholamine theory of emotion (Schildkraut and Kety, 1967). This theory assumes that catecholamine activity in the brain, particularly norepinephrine but possibly also dopamine and epinephrine, might be responsible for sustaining feelings of well-being. Antidepressant drugs are known to elevate levels of catecholamines, although they influence other chemicals in the brain as well (Jarvik, 1965). Amphetamine is capable of improving the mood under certain circumstances.

The demonstration by Olds and Milner (1954) that certain areas in the brain can function as centers for the reinforcement or reward if they are electrically stimulated has led to a great deal of work on central mechanisms of reinforcement. Stein and Seifter (1962) have demonstrated that drugs can influence self-stimulation in animals and that the most intensely rewarding points in the brain are distributed along the medial forebrain bundle (see Figure 7), which is the principal diencephalic pathway of ascending noradrenergic fibers. Some drugs facilitate self-stimulation—for example, monamine oxidase inhibitors and amphetamine—and are known to either release catecholamines or to facilitate their release. On the other hand, drugs that inhibit self-stimulation deplete the brain of catecholamines (reserpine, alpha-methyl paratyrosine) or block adrenergic transmission (chlorpromazine) (Wise and Stein, 1969). Stein and Wise (1967) have demonstrated that rewarding electrical stimulation of the medial forebrain bundle releases norepinephrine and its metabolites into solution perfused through the hypothalamus and amygdala.

More recently these same investigators have demonstrated that suppression of self-stimulation occurs in rats who have had electrodes implanted in the medial forebrain bundle if norepinephrine synthesis is inhibited (Wise and Stein, 1969). The enzyme dopamine-beta-hydroxylase is inhibited by systemic administration of disulfiram or intraventricular administration of diethyl dithiocarbamate. The suppressed behavior could be reinstated by intraventricular injections of l-norepinephrine but not d-norepinephrine. Intraventricular administration of dopamine and serotonin were ineffective. The implication is that norepinephrine acts by disinhibiting efferent fibers in the amygdala and that thus norepinephrine is inhibitory itself, but the net result is facilitation of behavior. Nicotine may operate like amphetamine to release norepinephrine from its stores in the brain and thereby produce an improvement in mood and reinforcement of behavior associated with its administration.

The results of releasing brain norepinephrine depends upon the interaction between positive and negative feedback mechanisms. The interaction between such mechanisms would mean that an inverted U-shaped curve with an optimum level of stimulation ought to exist. If

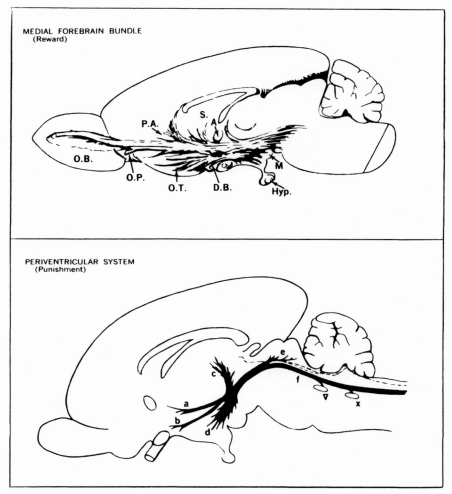

Figure 7. Upper. Diagram representing medical forebrain bundle (the presumed substrate of reward mechanism) in a generalized and primitive mammalian brain. Some abbreviations are: A., Anterior commissure; D.B., Nucleus of the diagonal band; M., Mammillary body; S., Septum. Lower. Similar diagram representing the periventricular system of fibers (presumed substrate of punishment mechanism). Some abbreviations are: b., Anterior hypothalamus; c., Thalamus; d., Posterior hypothalamus; e., Tectum.

Reprinted with permission from Le Gros Clark, W. E., J. Beatte, G. Riddoch, and N. M. Dott, 1938: *The Hypothalamus*. Edinburgh: Oliver and Boyd.

the peak is very high, then potentiation of smoking ought to occur with treatments that facilitate the release of norepinephrine. Thus, amphetamine and nicotine ought to synergize with one another. Treatments that impair the release of norepinephrine should result in a decreased effectiveness of nicotine to produce a reward. The effects of learning complicate the picture because, if an animal performs a response that ordinarily produces a given level of reward, his memory of this fact may cause him to work harder, not less hard, when the same actions produce less reward. This disappointment effect may be related to what has sometimes been called cognitive dissonance. In other words, the ability of an animal to titrate its reward to a certain level and then stop depends upon the interaction of negative and positive feedback systems. On the one hand, one might predict that amphetamine would substitute for stimuli produced by food or nicotine, and it seems to work that way for food. The evidence on smoking is less clear. M. M. Miller (1941) felt that amphetamine was effective in curing smoking, and in any case it removed the pleasure from the habit.

In summary then, the evidence from millions of people proves that smoking can become a very strong habit, difficult to break. The evidence to date is compatible with the idea that nicotine is the essential ingredient in tobacco responsible for developing and maintaining the habit. It is proposed that nicotine produces reinforcing effects by stimulating reward mechanisms in the brain, very likely by causing or facilitating the release of norepinephrine at these centers.

Comments on Paper by Jarvik
CHARLES R. SCHUSTER

As Dr. Jarvik has aptly stated, we are here today to discuss why people go out of their way to draw smoke from a chopped-up burning plant into their mouths and lungs. I believe he has presented a very convincing argument that the ultimate answer to this question is that the inhalation of tobacco smoke is the most efficient means of bringing high concentrations of the alkaloid nicotine to the brain. Phrased in behavioral terms, it could be said that smoking behavior is reinforced by the pharmacological effects of nicotine. Given the assumption that nicotine can act as a positive reinforcer, stimuli associated with the act of smoking can acquire conditioned reinforcing properties that help to maintain the behavior in strength. This conclusion receives support from previous research, in which we have been able to demonstrate that stimuli associated with the administration of morphine acquire very strong conditioned reinforcing properties (Schuster and Woods, 1968). A further and perhaps more insidious source of reinforcement for smoking is derived from the fact that this behavior can become linked as a member of a chain of responses that is ultimately reinforced by events totally independent of the act of smoking. Since the receipt of the reinforcer is not contingent upon the act of smoking, we can refer to this act as a form of "superstitious" behavior. For example, as I sat here writing this discussion, I was smoking. Although the completion of this manuscript was not dependent upon the act of smoking, it is such a strongly linked member of the chain of my writing behavior that I find myself unable to write unless I am free to smoke. It can be said, therefore, that my writing behavior is dependent upon smoking. To the extent that smoking has become a member of a large number of chains in my behavioral repertoire, I am psychologically dependent upon smoking. Any attempts to aid people in breaking their smoking habit, I believe, must take these sources of nonpharmacological reinforcement into account.

For the past three years Dr. Benedict Lucchesi and I have been investigating the effects of various drugs on cigarette-smoking behavior. Dr. Jarvik has very adequately reviewed our work showing that the intravenous infusion of nicotine diminishes the frequency and amount of cigarettes consumed (Lucchesi, et al., 1967). It is important to note that the subjects of this experiment were unaware that we were studying cigarette-smoking behavior and did not know of the drug being administered. Further, they did not express any motivation to stop smoking at the time of the experiment. Subsequent to our work with nicotine, we investigated several other drugs that have been suggested as aids in helping people break their smoking habit. I would briefly like to report on the results of these investigations. The drugs we tested were lobeline, d-amphetamine, and meprobamate. All three of these drugs had been used previously in smoking clinics. The assumption that nicotine is the reinforcer for smoking behavior has led to the suggestion that lobeline, an alkaloid with similar pharmacological activity and showing cross-tolerance to nicotine, might be effective in helping people to stop smoking. At the present time there are several preparations containing lobeline that have been marketed as aids for people who want to stop or limit their smoking. As Dr. Jarvik has stated, however, the literature is contradictory as to the effectiveness of lobeline in this regard. Reports range from lobeline's being highly effective (Dorsey, 1936; Rapp, et al., 1959; Rapp and Olen, 1955) to its being no more effective than a placebo (Research Committee of the British Tuberculosis Association, 1963; Scott et al., 1962). In our study we administered buffered lobeline in dosages of 2 and 4 mg three times daily for seven consecutive days. This dosage regimen is recommended by the manufacturer of commercially available lobeline tablets. In comparison to a seven-day control period, in which the subjects received placebo medication, lobeline produced no changes in the frequency or amount of cigarettes consumed in each daily test session. Meprobamate, a mild tranquilizer, has been used to diminish anxiety in people who are attempting to stop smoking. The underlying assumption is that smokers tend to smoke when they become anxious. We have tested dosages of 400 and 800 mg of meprobamate and found that it produced no change in cigarette-smoking behavior. At the higher dosage subjects did complain of drowsiness and lethargy. The anorexic agent, d-amphetamine, has been prescribed to smokers who are afraid of gaining weight when they stop smoking. When given dosages of 5 and 10 mg of d-amphetamine, the subjects in our experiment increased their cigarette-smoking frequency by about 25 per cent. This increased smoking, however, was probably a result of a nonspecific stimulant effect of the drug, since the subjects were observed to be more loquacious and active.

The results with d-amphetamine are of particular importance in relationship to Dr. Jarvik's hypotheses that nicotine's reinforcing efficacy is based upon its ability to release central stores of norepinephrine. As Dr. Jarvik has stated, amphetamine's behavioral effects are as well based upon its ability to release norepinephrine. It is therefore difficult for me to understand why cigarette smoking should be increased by the administration of amphetamine. One might assume that there should be at least some "satiation" of the central reinforcing mechanisms by amphetamine, leading to a diminished need for nicotine intake. Obviously more direct measures of these brain biochemical events are needed to resolve the questions.

The failure of our research to find a drug that suppresses cigarette smoking behavior, other than nicotine, is depressing. However, it should not lead to a curtailment of such research. Other drugs that affect the ability of nicotine to release central stores of norepinephrine remain to be investigated. If drugs can be found that are safe, are easily administered, and block the reinforcing effects of nicotine, they may prove to be a valuable adjunct to behavioral modification techniques in aiding the smoker to break this habit.

General Discussion

PREMACK opened the discussion by questioning Jarvik's suggestion that nicotine in the blood gets to the amygdala (a positive reinforcing center) and releases norepinephrine that produces the reward or reinforcement; his objection was on the grounds that this facilitating effect, originally found by Stein, depended upon the previous injection of a norepinephrine suppressant. He refused to accept Jarvik's explanation that this result was due to the fact that the optimal amount was already present.

MENDELSON brought up some findings from Lexington to indicate that in addictions with an acute, severe abstinence syndrome there is growing evidence for some prolonged alteration in such matters as cardiac function. Abstinence may have an acute facet with the added presence of physiological changes, which may last a long time, a sort of "memory" of the addiction process that "locks in" the addiction.

KNAPP reported an early study of his in which the abrupt termination of smoking produced a drop in pulse rate and blood pressure. The subjective findings were more variable but suggested a mild physical dependency, qualitatively different from that produced by other drugs, something like the withdrawal symptoms from amphetamine; but these are minor, with lethargy and some sleepiness. The effect is not catastrophic.

He then pointed out the possible analogy with depression; in that case evidence seems to be emerging of some disruption of central catecholamines particularly affecting the store of norepinephrine. This finding adds plausibility to Jarvik's norepinephrine theory. Nicotine might periodically increase the store of norepinephrine in the brain. The acute withdrawal phase in smoking, then, might be expected to resemble a depression. This hypothesis prompted HUNT to call for a more specific definition of depression, since the acute nicotine-withdrawal reaction he once experienced had none of the usual experiential aspects of depression such as sorrow, but was more of a washed-out, flat, "bushed" feeling that he had often experienced after an experimental injection of adrenalin or following prolonged and heavy physical exertion. KNAPP agreed that any signs of sadness or any urge to cry were not present in many withdrawal reactions and that the subjective impressions often did include an uncomfortable feeling of being slowed down.

BALTER proposed that nicotine, like cocaine, might have a fast metabolism and that when taken directly into the lungs it might produce very rapid action with rapid reinforcement and possibly rapid withdrawal effects. But SCHUSTER objected, noting that as far as rapid withdrawal effects were concerned, the peripheral measures he used (heart beat, blood pressure, and respiration) did not show any cyclical variation. Once the individual had the first cigarette of the day, the levels increased and were then maintained at the new level.

BALTER then suggested that in looking for drug substitutes, researchers ought to cease looking for a perfect match and be guided instead by the concept of goodness of fit. He pointed out that even methadone, which currently serves as a satisfactory replacement for heroin, does not duplicate the total pattern of heroin. Some patients are reported to supplement it with the amphetamines, perhaps for the rush and excitement involved.

GORDIS interjected that, while it would not be proper to equate nicotine with heroin, there was much that could be learned from the methadone story. The situation with opiate addiction, before the advent of the methadone treatment, had many of the same features here discussed in connection with smoking, particularly as far as the reinforcing conditions were concerned.

Opiates were taken in a certain social milieu with some ritualization. There was missionary activity in the peer group. The psychoanalysts became involved in the psychodynamics of addiction, and the sociologists discussed it in terms of an antidote to the horrors of slum life or as a buffer against the pain of being black or Puerto Rican. All sorts of external reinforcers were present, like those described in the case of tobacco smoking. Just as in the case of tobacco, the various behavior therapies have been a failure. No amount of psychoanalysis and no amount of conditioning has made any serious dent in the use of opiates. Nor did the various psychopharmacological treatments prove effective.

What is common to both opiate and tobacco addiction? There is a common element of compulsive drug-seeking behavior. In opiate addiction, and perhaps in tobacco smoking, there is a compulsive and repetitive seeking to introduce some foreign substance into the body.

Another aspect must be remembered: the person who has abstained from opiates, even for a long time, is not the same as a person who has never had them at all. The abstainer from narcotics is not the same as a narcotic virgin, and this fact has actual physical and pharmacological consequences. He is a different organism, and there is evidence that the changes continue over long periods of time.

Fortunate circumstances led to Dr. V. P. Dole's discovery of the usefulness of methadone as a substitute drug for heroin. It was already in use as a drug for the short-term transition between drug use and detoxification. Gradually it became clear that the pharmacology of methadone in a prior heroin user differed from its pharmacology in a novice patient. It suppressed the craving for heroin and blocked its euphoric effect without having any detrimental action on physiological or psychological functions. Moreover, under methadone treatment the patients were able to live normal, productive, and socially acceptable lives.

It is not unusual for some of the patients, after the methadone treatment has been instituted, to go out into the streets, back to their original social setting—perhaps back to Harlem—and try heroin again. The experience is invariably disappointing because the pleasure previously found in heroin is no longer found. Subsequent visits to old neighborhoods result in the patient's watching others using heroin but not using it himself—a behavior his friends in the same social milieu find very surprising. They cannot understand how the patient can refuse heroin.

GORDIS pointed out a lesson here: that all of the alleged reasons for drug addiction—such as its shielding the individual against a hostile and discriminatory environment and its providing him with a ritualized social experience—suddenly lose importance once the narcotic craving had been attacked with a drug that seems to be specific.

The analogy with tobacco is still dubious, and some differences must be noted. The narcotic agent in smoking is not known. It may be nicotine, or it may be some other chemical constituent of the tobacco. The disruption of a smoker's life is minimal compared to the social catastrophe of opiate addiction. The dangers of smoking are not necessarily due to the addicting properties of the cigarette. The substance causing lung cancer or chronic bronchitis may not be the same one responsible for the compulsive drug seeking. Nevertheless, many of the lessons from the methadone program are worth keeping in mind.

KORNETSKY reaffirmed his belief that nicotine is the primary agent in smoking and that in some fashion it furnishes reinforcement for the behavior. He then mentioned the fact that the papers had exemplified two different approaches, Jarvik talking about the primary reinforcement effect of nicotine and Logan talking about drive reduction. SCHUSTER replied that he saw no incompatibility in the two viewpoints. In his opinion the most conceivable solution is that there is intermittent reinforcement by nicotine, with the bulk of the maintenance of the behavior attributable to conditioned reinforcers—the whole chain of behavior in lighting up a cigarette and the attendant stimuli associated with these.

There seemed to be no serious disagreement, and the discussion moved to MENDELSON's concluding remarks. He suggested that the commonality in all drug usage is its production of some rather sudden changes in the state of the organism. The nature of the reinforcement could be a change in state reflected through a change in cardiac rate, a change in the mobilization of peripheral resistance, and the like. These may be produced by the release of catecholamines and an enhancement of catecholamine metabolites. With the cessation of substance use, there might be a fall below base line, the drive for the drug constituting an attempt on the part of the organism to reestablish a base line or an above-base line state. This hypothesis suggests that the search concentrate on some agent producing a peripheral adrenergic response.

Part Three
An Overview

A Sociologist's Point of View

EDGAR F. BORGATTA

I AM going to begin with some comments on our own research. We are in part replicating with a national sample the study that was carried out in a specific West Coast area. We did borrow a few questions from the West Coast study, as I think they did from us, and some overlapping data will therefore result. But the data will have to do not merely with the use of the psychotropic drugs, but with smoking and some other aspects of behavior as well.

The problem remains that we did not use our own survey organization, and it has resulted in such difficulties as the fact that possibly 45 per cent of the population (males) turns out to be 30 per cent according to the sample collected, and that the method of data collection and a few other minor questions of this sort will have to be dealt with, but we will overcome—because, as everybody knows, research professors can always find a way out of data inadequacies. But the fact is that we will have some replicating data that are not tied to a particular city which has some very unique characteristics in terms of being involved with drugs, and possibly we will have data on such things as smoking behavior.

The comments that I have to make are a little scattered, but let me assert that examining the habit mechanisms in smoking behavior is an important topic. The habit mechanisms are important in the development of a theory that allows us to understand individual behavior; I doubt that any of us will quarrel with this. But we do have to recognize that there are different ways of approaching these aspects of knowledge in developing a "predictive science." If I recall correctly, this is one of the definitions of psychology.

What models are to be used depends upon what predictions are to be made. The learning models that have been presented and discussed are very interesting, but they are provocative at various points because they are designed ordinarily to be tested in a laboratory. They are not necessarily well tested in the laboratory, because of the very severe limitation that the parameters tying the various propositions together are not specified. The result is that most of the experimentation is really designed to establish whether a certain input has a consequence, not what the magnitude of the consequence is for a certain input, nor the nature of the parameters, nor the interactions within parameters—at least for a moderately large set of propositions. The models tend, therefore, to be very simplified (or possibly oversimplified), even when designed to correspond to a laboratory-oriented science, and when one starts to take the analogy from these theories into the field, there are all kinds of problems.

As I said, the problems are not necessarily bad. They may be provocative in a sense that is useful. I spoke with Dr. Logan about the proposition that arose from his reference to the cigarette package, which can be summarized as follows: if the person starts to smoke in the presence of the negative message, he will be more committed to smoking; and I suggested that if that were correct, then the alternative would be correct—that if the person had not smoked in the presence of the positive message, he would be more committed not to smoke. I maintain that this is provocative because it should raise questions about the operation of advertising and other media in the concerns with the manipulation of smoking behavior in the whole population.

Concerning whether I agree with both of those statements, I am not sure. No message reaches the population singularly; there is also a milieu besides the single message, and the experiences of an individual have some sort of cumulative content, which is not necessarily identifiable into separate units in the sense that would be the case in a theory of learning that has been tested in the laboratory.

It is also very difficult for me to handle some of these concepts because, for example, notions are reverted to in some anecdotal descriptions of critical incidence and threshold. And since I am a little concerned with historical analysis, I know how history is described, and I find it very difficult to believe that history is really *causal* in its handling of the variables. Therefore I find it very difficult to believe that the anecdotes are really providing the causal sequences inferred in them.

Then, if the progress is from some of the more formal theories of learning to the softer theories—which I would identify with a tradition coming through James Mark Baldwin, Charles Horton Cooley, George Herbert Mead, and others—concepts of socialization arise. It is very difficult to call someone like George Herbert Mead anything but a behaviorist, but the fact of the matter is that the model is a generalized one that essentially describes by analogies what is involved rather than by specification. And so, for example, the difference between George Herbert Mead and Baldwin and Cooley is really that Mead had access to the conditioning analog, which became available, I believe, in 1902, after Baldwin's and Cooley's major works. The description is quite seductive, but if that model is formulated into a set of propositions to be tested and examined in the laboratory, there is more than a little difficulty. If there is no difficulty, it is hard to explain why in some forty years there have not been many laboratory tests of Mead's work, and indeed very little field examination of the propositions.

What I am indicating here is that there are some types of models that tend to be nonempirical in nature—that is, very difficult to validate and very difficult to examine through scientific paraphernalia. There certainly are some other excellent examples, where it is even easier to see what difficulties arise. For example, in sociology there is an orientation or a group of people concerned with what is called functional analysis. In functional analysis certain things are specified as "functional"; then some analysts go on to specify even what is "dysfunctional," but what they start with is functional. *This means that they have to set up a system.* Within the system they then go on to describe what is a functional prerequisite, and this definition constitutes the theory. The problem is that there are no relationships specified between the so-called functional prerequisites; there is no variable specification; and there are all the difficulties of having an excellent set of words that are "meaningful" to some but really do not convey knowledge in the usual scientific sense.

Examining the model of habit requires—from my point of view, at least—more concern possibly with the specification of whether one is dealing with the acquisition of the habit or the maintenance of the habit, if not for theoretical reasons, then at least for practical reasons. For example, mention is made of the place of substitution in the learning model dealing with the problem of habit. If the same model is then applied to the acquisition of the habit, someone should raise the question: "What is smoking the substitution for?" This was really not raised except by inference to some of the concomitants of the acquisition of smoking behavior. If there is a learning model that states that in the process of learning three elements are necessary, one of which is the situation, the other the incentive, and the third the drive, then if one alters the patterns in some way, one is left with the drive. The drive must be taken into account. This fact also has to be taken into account in the original acquisition. The point is that in many of these models the acquisition of the behavior may not be the same problem as the maintenance of the behavior, and the reason I emphasize this point is that it does raise the question of what variables are involved in the acquisition of the behavior and also in the maintenance of the behavior. It may not be one single thing which is being substituted for another, but it may be one thing in a complex of many that is being altered, or some other changes may be occurring, so that another condition is arrived at.

And this point is anticipating one of my other comments. I did want to also raise this question of the study of the mechanisms in terms of where the change is applied. Is it to be applied in the sense of an individual prediction—that is, the model of the individual and how he changes; or is this to be applied in the sense of a type of regression of what is the set of regularities that one would anticipate to occur in a population? In the former case one has to deal with the problem of specification of all conditions of the individual. In the latter case, one has to deal essentially with the specification of the conditions in the population. This does not imply at all that these things are incompatible; but they are different problems from the point of view of the handling of the data, and they possibly also raise a problem of manipulation.

This conference made the transition very easily from dealing with the problem of how a person acquires the smoking habit, without stating whether he wants to or not, to dealing with the problem of how he gets rid of the habit when he wants to, or at least when he says he wants to. All kinds of interesting questions can be explored about what is meant when a man says he wants to get rid of the habit. In terms of individual prediction, is one concerned with whether or not people get rid of the habit independently or whether they want to get rid of the habit? Certainly in a statistical sense, if one is dealing with the manipulation of the entire system and dealing with individuals as units within that system—rather than dealing with the individual as a system—the concern must be with the problem of definition at that level.

I think that the emphasis on extrinsic and intrinsic factors is again an important matter for concern, and attention must be given them. But there are many possible stratifications of the variables. I think that the question of whether or not variables can be classified as manipulable rather than not manipulable is of interest, and among the manipulable variables those that are viable as manipulable in the society are also of concern, because the concern is with a restricted system. Many things that can be manipulated abstractly are not open to such action for reasons of civil liberties, civil rights, or legal and other circumstances. There is an old saying among sociologists that one of the reasons that sociology is not a predictive science is that it is not possible to set up the kinds of experiments that would allow researchers to check the hypotheses they would like. And if they could, the society would probably be one no one would like. There are, therefore, some dilemmas in terms of how the science is advanced.

I am going to refer just a little bit to the research that we have in process rather than give results. I do want to note that our social-psychological science has a very poor record for involvement in what is called social experimentation—that is, large-scale manipulation—and with the input and circumstances that can be described as "noise in the system." I have been involved in a few of these, and they are usually identified as evaluative research. Most such "experiments" tend to be relatively unproductive of what is known as positive findings. This lack of results is embarrassing to several therapeutic and "helping" professions. The rationalizations often advanced for negative findings are more plausible sometimes than at other times.

We did one experiment that is reported in the book I recently edited with Robert R. Evans (Borgatta and Evans, 1968). In that volume we reported that a follow-up after four or five months found that a very focused and, I think, relatively ingenious educational and informative propaganda campaign had virtually no effects in the dissuasion of smoking on the campus. We were extremely nervous about this finding because it did not really gibe with the kinds of events we wanted. But we did propose that it might be too early at that time to examine the findings; we went back after roughly sixteen months following the educational campaign and did a follow-up again, and we found that by this time there was a significant effect, though not a large one.

This led us to speculate: *Why?* The speculation leads to the notion that arrival at college is a critical period in people's lives, they are subject to many stimuli, they receive many "messages." There are many ways in which they sort them, and in these circumstances possibly the messages cannot take an immediate effect; they have to take effect as they are sorted out. *This reasoning is not explanation;* it is post-hoc speculation. The fact of the matter is that we do have an example of an effect that did show up somewhat later, and our post-hoc "throng" is vague and general. I think that this form of research may have to be resorted to more often, and it is not independent from the questions of what mechanisms are involved. There is some opportunity for controlling who the individuals are in the experiments and a certain knowledge of the circumstances from which they proceed. And indeed, there are some interesting aspects of this particular study because a number of effects converged to produce the so-called significant findings.

People who had hesitated to smoke hesitated to smoke differentially if they had received the message. People who were beginning smokers stopped smoking differentially if they received the message; further, the persons who were supposedly heavy smokers also received the message and differentially stopped smoking. The effect was therefore not a unique one associated with particular groups; this fact leads to more questions than answers. It does happen that these data are from large samples, with rich data from fairly good instruments. It is to be hoped, therefore, that some information on manipulation will emerge. But in the complexity of the situation, I hope that it is appreciated that this is almost trivial information by comparison with descriptive longitudinal information dealing with the relationship among the variables in the population.

An alternate set of analyses is possible for so-called natural data or data in a regression sense that falls in the economics or econometrics literature, in the sociological literature, and in a few other areas, into a category now called path analysis and causal inference. These analyses may serve a little bit better in regression analysis and the problems of inference. The hope may provide just a little bit more purchase on ordering models and in causal inference and dealing with some of the problems of analysis. And I would maintain that if we are really interested in the mechanisms that operate in smoking behavior, which now divorces this as a separate topic for analysis rather than the more abstract one of habit mechanisms, we may need to have more of this descriptive kind of information.

The Effects of Prolonged Alcohol Ingestion on the Eating, Drinking, and Smoking Patterns of Chronic Alcoholics

NANCY K. MELLO AND
JACK H. MENDELSON

EIGHT subjects were observed during periods of experimentally induced intoxication of one to three months. Subjects controlled the amount and frequency of their alcohol consumption and cigarette smoking by working at a simple operant task: 1,000 responses on a portable button box earned a single poker chip, which could be spent to obtain a single cigarette or a single ounce of bourbon. Each operant box contained a separate counter for alcohol and for cigarettes, and the subject could work for only one at a time. Points earned were exchanged for poker chips once each day, at 8:00 A.M. The major behavioral findings were as follows:

1. Subjects tended to work for one or two days until they earned enough chips to drink for two or three days. Subjects rarely worked while they were drinking, and they maintained a pattern of discrete working and drinking intervals over three months. During the twenty-four to thirty-six hour abstinent intervals subjects showed partial-withdrawal signs of mild to moderate tremor of the extremities. Partial-withdrawal signs were frequently observed during the falling phase of

the blood-alcohol curve. The encapsulated spree-work pattern may most closely resemble episodic drinking in real life.

When the same subjects were given unrestricted access to alcohol, they drank more consistently than during the period when the amount available was determined by their work output. Although cyclical fluctuations in overall intake occurred; subjects drank at least twenty ounces of bourbon each day and did not intersperse drinking with periods of abstinence. The average blood-alcohol level maintained was higher in two subjects and lower in a third subject. In each instance, however, blood-alcohol levels were relatively more stable throughout the drinking period.

2. The combined daily caloric intake from food (2,000 calories) and alcohol averaged between 4,000 and 5,000 calories over a three-month period. However, no subject showed an increase in weight, and one subject lost weight during the study. These data challenged the notion that calories in alcohol are equivalent to and substituted for calories in food. The interaction of alcohol and diet will be examined in future studies.

3. There was an approximate correlation between the drinking-working cycles and the smoking-working cycles. However, subjects worked less consistently for cigarettes than for alcohol. Three of the four subjects smoked appreciably less during the drinking period than during the before- and after-alcohol periods. However, smoking cycles usually corresponded to drinking cycles.

During the period of unlimited access to alcohol all subjects stopped working for cigarettes after the first one or two days of drinking, and they did not resume working once their accumulated cigarette supply was exhausted.

These data indicate that during inebriation alcoholics decline to work at a simple task, even to obtain such a desirable commodity as cigarettes. These data probably illustrate relative aversiveness of the task rather than the relative potency of alcohol and cigarettes as reinforcers.

General Discussion

As THE final discussion opened some of the members of the conference asked whether or not the remaining hour should be devoted to drawing up a plan of behavior modification that the American Cancer Society could use to guide its efforts in controlling smoking. Unfortunately some strong disagreement arose as to the type of model to be used. MATARAZZO interceded to remind the group that the purpose of the conference was not to draft a course of action, but to provide for an interchange of ideas among people of varied interests and backgrounds. The aim was the increase of individual understanding through the exchange of individual knowledge. Increased understanding and intellectual involvement were at issue, rather than guide lines for immediate action. HUNT drew an analogy with Eric Bentley's comments at Columbia on student activism. Bentley defined the "unliberated university" as a place for deliberation and learning, a place where students can make themselves ready for action, with action and reform to come later, outside the university. Despite these comments the participants devoted some time to the problem of social control of smoking behavior.

LOVEJOY felt that the antismoking campaign to date has been a step-by-step procedure that encourages habituation to the threat of punishment. There were increasingly more confident charges: smoking is carcinogenic. These were followed by rebuttals: it is not. As the information about the dangers of smoking increased, the pressure against smoking was maintained, but people became used to the bombardment in repeated doses of threats of increasingly severe punishment. Habituation tends to set in, and the threat loses its impact. It might be wise to stop for a few months all the continuing spot announcements on radio and television and the other publicity and then suddenly to reenter with an intensified, massive campaign using every possible medium and instrument. The people who have relaxed and become comfortable in their smoking habits would then be faced with a sudden and massive threat.

TOMKINS pointed out that with the first big push against smoking cigarettes, sales dropped dramatically but then rose again. GREEN noted, however, that in the past year actual manufacturing had decreased, despite the fact that the population had risen and despite the fact that the age-mix changes in the population would favor an increase in smoking, since the people who were dying included many, like older women, who had never smoked. The increase in twenty-one-year-olds, a group that is more likely to smoke, would suggest that the consumption of cigarettes should be going up, while instead it is leveling off. Blitz effects do occur—sharp drops in smoking when the pressure against it gets strong—but there also is a steadier, long-term, very gradual decrease.

BALTER remarked that in one sense the generation of people smoking now is damned. The pressure is merely kept on in hope. There is real hope with the children, however. Here Balter felt that a neutral approach would work best, rather than reliance on authority and punishment.

He felt that material could be introduced into the school curriculum under the general rubric of all kinds of drugs and their effects (not necessarily their abuse) on the body; and that the topic of smoking could be included in this neutral framework. The child would not be in the situation of being told what to do or what not to; there would be no chance for rebellion. He would be exposed to information that will have an impact. The time might come when children will be putting down their elders for smoking.

KORNETSKY entered in to make several points. There are peer groups now in some high schools who condemn smoking. He then stressed that the marijuana smoker usually begins as a cigarette smoker. Finally, he mentioned socioeconomic status as a factor, and GREEN stated that the greatest percentage of smokers comes from the group earning $5,000 to

$6,000 annual income. Education is also a factor; after grammar school, the more education, the less smoking; with the rate of quitting also much higher at higher educational levels.

BORGATTA, as a sociologist, commented that as the culture is changed its values tend to change, and by paying attention to those aspects that influence the general values of the society one might be able to alter behavior patterns over time. He jokingly remarked that if he told Frank Logan that Ph.Ds are less likely to smoke, the statement would have less impact than the information that people who are educated are less likely to smoke: the latter makes it a matter of values.

MENDELSON, continuing on the theme of shaping public attitudes, commented on influencing drinking practices, an area where his policy has been to provide the most rational information to the public, allowing them to make their own decisions about their behavior. Material is being supplied to secondary schools around the country, aimed at the bright adolescent who can look at drinking behavior and know what the consequences of a drinking problem can be, but there is no attempt to push him toward a position.

MENDELSON then returned to the problem of drive reduction and the nature of reinforcers, noting that the drive-reduction model did not seem to fit many alcohol patterns. He felt the alcoholic consuming large quantities was not effecting anxiety reduction, was not alleviating depression, but actually was moving into a dysphoric state. The simple paradigm that one does something because it makes him feel good does not apply here. He next suggested that social facilitation through alcohol may not be concordant with tension reduction. It is actually easier to find a reduction of tension associated with cessation of drinking; when something bad happens, the alcoholic turns off rather than turning on. MATARAZZO interrupted to ask if Mendelson thought that an arousal model might be better than a reinforcement or drive-reduction model and received a positive answer. BALTER stated his belief that Mendelson was not saying that drinking was not instrumental, but rather that it was not understood what instrumental function it serves.

People search out, they try a variety of things, but what they fix on is a choice behavior. To understand choice behavior some factor involving selective preference is needed to explain why some people prefer some drugs to others.

LOVEJOY added that more should be known about the successful quitters. Did they terminate abruptly or did they taper off?

TOMKINS came in here to discuss his affect types. The positive-affect smoker, who smokes relatively little anyway, can give it up easily if he believes that smoking is bad for him. Characteristically he is a person who is well-controlled and who maximizes positive affect in general and knows how to coax it out of the world.

The negative-affect smoker is primarily controlled by his negative-affect state, which is unpredictable. When he feels good, he may say, paradoxically and without insight, "You know, I don't really feel the urge to smoke." But when it is suggested that he give the habit up, he anticipates much misery and thinks, "I can give it up, but how can I keep from backsliding?" After a withdrawal program he tends later to return to smoking. So he goes, off again and on again.

Smoking addicts are quite different. They go through hell in quitting, but once they are successful, they usually remain abstainers. The relationship between cessation and maintenance of cessation is extremely complex.

TOMKINS went on to say that not all behavior is instrumental. Some may be simply a concomitant of a highly activated state. There are nonlearning aspects of behavior; it is not an all-or-none choice. One does not have to reject learning models in order to extend the range of phenomena examined in smoking and drinking behavior.

At this point the conference closed. To add a touch of summary and integration, the editor wishes to quote from a letter he received from FRANK LOGAN some time after the meeting:

> As I came away from the conference, I felt we could summarize the results as indicating the sources of conflict surrounding smoking. There are at least three identified sources of avoidance tendencies: it is expensive and inconvenient, it indicates some personal lack of control, and it is potentially hazardous to health. At the same time there are also at least three identified sources of approach tendencies: smoking becomes intrinsically addicting, it may serve secondary needs of the individual such as rebellion, and it may be primarily rewarding through biochemical action of nicotine. As you well know, dealing with conflict is not easy, and I would hope the results of the conference would be the stimulation of research, particularly aimed at preventive therapy. There are ideas and principles in the basic psychology of learning that could help direct such research.

References

ALLPORT, G. W. 1937. *Personality*. New York: Holt.
———— 1961. *Pattern and growth in personality*. New York: Holt.
———— 1968. Six decades of social psychology. In S. Lunstedt (ed)., *Higher education in social psychology*. Cleveland, Ohio: The Press of Case Western Reserve University.
AMERICAN CANCER SOCIETY. 1963. *Cigarette smoking and lung cancer*. New York: American Cancer Society.
———— 1964. *Can we help them stop?* Chicago: American Cancer Society, Illinois Division.
ANGUS, MONICA. 1963. Stop. *Canadian Nurse*, 59, 653–655.
ARMITAGE, A. K. 1965. Effects of nicotine and tobacco smoke on blood pressure and release of catecholamines from the adrenal glands. *British Journal of Pharmacology and Chemotherapy*, 25, 515–526.
ARMITAGE, A. K., A. S. MILTON and C. F. MORRISON. 1966. Effects of nicotine and some nicotine-like compounds injected into the cerebral ventricles of the cat. *British Journal of Pharmacology and Chemotherapy*, 27, 33–45.
BACHMAN, D. S. 1964. Group smoking deterrent therapy. *General Practice*, 30, 86–89.

——— 1966. Personal communication.

BAER, D. J. 1966. Scholastic aptitude and smoking attitude and behavior of college males. *The Journal of Psychology, 64,* 63–68.

BALL, K. P. 1965. First year's experience in anti-smoking clinic. *British Medical Journal, 5451,* 1651–1653.

BALTIMORE CITY HEALTH DEPARTMENT. 1963. Smoking and lung cancer: A new approach. *Baltimore Health News, 40,* 145–150.

——— 1964. Report on anti-smoking project. *Baltimore Health News, 41,* 45–47.

BARTLETT, W. A., and R. W. WHITEHEAD. 1957. The effectiveness of meprobamate and lobeline as smoking deterrents. *Journal of Laboratory and Clinical Medicine, 50,* 278.

BECK, I. FLORA. 1953. The use and abuse of tobacco. *Lancet, 265,* 392–397.

——— 1955. "Minor" addictions, *Lancet, 268,* 1266.

BELL, R. G. 1961. Tobacco withdrawal symptoms. *Applied Therapeutics, 4,* 1028.

BERELSON, B., and G. A. STEINER. 1964. *Human behavior: An inventory of scientific findings.* New York: Harcourt, Brace.

BERGLER, E. 1946. Psychopathology of compulsive smoking. *Psychiatric Quarterly, 20,* 297–321.

BERKSON, J. 1958. Smoking and lung cancer: Some observations on two recent reports. *Journal of the American Statistical Association, 53,* 28–38.

BERNE, E. 1964. *Games people play.* New York: Grove.

BERNSTEIN, D. A. 1968. The modification of smoking behavior. Evanston, Illinois: Northwestern University, unpublished doctoral dissertation.

——— 1969. The modification of smoking behavior: A review. *Psychological Bulletin, 71,* 418–440.

BERRY, C. S. 1917. Effects of smoking on adding. *Psychological Bulletin, 14,* 25–28.

BICKFORD, R. G. 1960. Physiology and drug action: An electroencephalographic analysis. *Federation Proceedings, 19,* 619–625.

BLACKBURN, H. W., J. BROZEK, H. L. TAYLOR, and A. KEYS. 1962. Cardiovascular and related characteristics in habitual smokers and nonsmokers. In G. James and T. Rosenthal (eds.), *Tobacco and health.* Springfield, Illinois: C. C. Thomas.

BLOEDORN, W. A. 1920. The barbarous custom of smoking. *Medical Record and Annals, 97,* 185–188.

BORGATTA, E. F., and R. R. EVANS. 1968. *Smoking, health, and behavior.* Chicago: Aldine Publishing Company.

BOVET, D., F. BOVET-NITTI, and A. OLIVERIO. 1966. Effects of nicotine on avoidance conditioning of inbred strains of mice. *Psychopharmacologia, 10,* 1–5.

BRECHER, E. 1969. Personal communication.

BRECHER, RUTH, and E. BRECHER. 1964. *Smoking—the great dilemma.* Washington, D.C.: Public Affairs Pamphlet No. 361, The Public Affairs Committee.

BRONTE-STEWART, B., L. H. KRUT, and M. J. PERRIN. 1960. The relationship of smoking to ischaemic heart disease. *South African Medical Journal, 34,* 511–512.

BROWN, C. T. 1964. Tobacco addiction: A further inquiry. *Military Medicine, 129,* 637–640.

BROWN, J. A. C. 1963. The nature and treatment of smoking. *Medical World, 98,* 187–192.

BROZEK, J., and O. KEYS. 1957. Change of body weight in normal men who stop smoking cigarettes. *Science, 125,* 1203.

BURN, J. H. 1960. Cardiovascular effects of nicotine and smoking. Part II. Pharmacological actions of nicotine and tobacco smoke. The action of nicotine on the heart. *Annals of the New York Academy of Sciences, 90,* 70–73.

BURN, J. H., and J. RAND. 1958. The action of nicotine on the heart. *British Medical Journal, 1,* 137–139.

BURNHAM, W. H. 1917. The effect of tobacco on mental efficiency. *Pedagogical Seminary, 24,* 297–317.

BUSH, A. D. 1914. Tobacco smoking and mental efficiency. *New York Medical Journal, 99,* 519–527.

CAIN, A. H. 1964. *The cigarette habit: An easy cure.* Garden City, New York: Doubleday.

CAMPBELL, D. T., and J. C. STANLEY. 1966. *Experimental and quasi-experimental designs for research.* Chicago: Rand McNally.

CAMPBELL, K. A. 1965. A smoker's clinic. *Medical Officer, 114,* 116–117.

CANNELL, C. F., and J. MacDONALD. 1956. The impact of health news on attitudes and behavior. *Journalism Quarterly, 33,* 315–323.

CARLIN, A. S., and H. E. ARMSTRONG, JR. 1968. Aversive conditioning: Learning or dissonance reduction? *Journal of Consulting and Clinical Psychology, 32,* 674–678.

CARNEY, R. E. 1967. Sex chromatin, body masculinity, achievement motivation and smoking behavior. *Psychological Reports, 20,* 859–866.

CARTWRIGHT, ANN, F. M. MARTIN, and J. G. THOMSON. 1960. Efficacy of an anti-smoking campaign. *Lancet, 1,* 327–329.

CARVER, D. J. 1922. The immediate psychological effects of tobacco smoking. *Journal of Comparative Psychology, 2,* 279–302.

CATTELL, R. B., and S. KRUG. 1967. The personality factor profile peculiar to the student smoker. *Journal of Counseling Psychology, 14,* 116–121.

CHRISTIANO, C. J., R. D. JONES, and S. V. ZAGONA. Psycho-social correlates of smoking behavior and attitudes for a sample of Anglo-American, Mexican-American, and Indian-American high school students. Prepublication received from the National Clearinghouse for Smoking and Health.

CLAWSON, T. A. 1964. Hypnosis in medical practice. *American Journal of Clinical Hypnosis, 6,* 232–236.

COAN, R. W. 1967. Research strategy in the investigation of personality correlates. In S. V. Zagona (ed.), *Studies and issues in smoking behavior.* Tuscon: The University of Arizona Press.

216   References

COFFMAN, J. D. 1967. The attenuation by reserpine on guanethidine of the cutaneous vasoconstriction caused by tobacco smoking. *American Heart Journal, 74,* 229–234.

COHEN, J., and R. K. HEIMANN. 1962. Heavy smokers with low mortality. *Industrial Medicine and Surgery, 31,* 115–120.

COLBY, K. M. 1964. Psychotherapeutic process. *Annual Review of Psychology, 15,* 347–370.

COMMITTEE ON DRUG ADDICTION AND NARCOTICS, National Academy of Sciences. 1960. Minutes of 21st Meeting, January.

COOPER, R. M., I. BILASH, and J. P. ZUBEK. 1959. The effect of age on taste sensitivity. *Journal of Gerontology, 14,* 56–58.

CRUICKSHANK, A. 1963a. The anti-smoking clinic. *Lancet, 2,* 353–354.

————— 1963b. Smokers advisory clinic: Ministry of health final report on the initial clinic. *Monthly Bulletin of the Ministry of Health, 22,* 193–194.

DALE, C. L. 1964. A report on the 5-day plan to help adult smokers stop smoking. In *Can we help them stop?* Chicago: American Cancer Society, Illinois Division.

DALE, H. H., and P. B. LAIDLAW. 1912. The significance of the suprarenal capsule in the action of certain alkaloids. *Journal of Physiology, 45,* 1–26.

DALESSIO, D. J. 1969. Nicotine and the antidiuretic hormone. *Journal of the American Medical Association, 207,* 954.

DALZELL-WARD, A. J. 1964. The development of anti-smoking clinics in the United States. In *Can we help them stop?* Chicago: American Cancer Society, Illinois Division.

DAVIS, F. 1956. Extracts from a report on "Cigarette smoking motivation study." London Research Services Ltd., Tobacco Research Council, Glen House, Stag Place.

DAY, C. W. 1959. Fear-reduction and cigarette marketing. *Studies in Public Communication* (Committee on Communication, University of Chicago), 2, 48–54.

DENEAU, G. A., and R. INOKI. 1967. Nicotine self-administration in monkeys. *Annals of the New York Academy of Sciences, 142,* 277–279.

DENSEN, P. M., B. DAVIDOW, H. E. BASS, and ELLEN W. JONES. 1967. A chemical test for smoking exposure. *Archives of Environmental Health, 14,* 865–874.

DiPALMA, J. R. 1965. Introduction; Brief history in Part I, Modern approaches to pharmacology. In J. R. DiPalma (ed.), *Drill's pharmacology in medicine.* New York: McGraw-Hill.

DIXON, W. E. 1921. The tobacco habit. *Lancet, 2,* 1071.

DOLLARD, J., and N. E. MILLER. 1950. *Personality and psychotherapy: An analysis in terms of learning, thinking, and culture.* New York: McGraw-Hill.

DOMINO, E. F. 1967. Electroencephalographic and behavioral arousal effects of small doses of nicotine: A neuropsychopharmacological study. *Annals of the New York Academy of Sciences, 142,* 216–244.

DOMINO, E. F., and A. M. BAUMGARTEN. 1968. Effects of smoking cigarettes of differing nicotine content on the human patella. *Federation Proceedings,* 27, 219.

DORSEY, J. L. 1936. Control of the tobacco habit. *Annals of Internal Medicine,* 10, 628–631.

DOUGLAS, W. W. 1965. 5-Hydroxytryptamine and antagonists; polypeptides-angiotensin and kinins. In L. S. Goodman and A. Gilman (eds.), *The pharmacological basis of therapeutics.* New York: Macmillan.

DUBITZKY, M., and J. SCHWARTZ. 1968. Ego-resiliency, ego-control, and smoking cessation. *Journal of Psychology,* 70, 27–33.

DULANEY, D. E., JR. 1962. The place of hypotheses and intentions: An analysis of verbal control in verbal conditioning. In C. W. Eriksen (ed.), *Behavior and awareness.* Durham, North Carolina: Duke University Press.

EDWARDS, G. 1964a. Double-blind trial of lobeline in an anti-smoking clinic. *Medical Officer, 111,* 158–160.

———— 1964b. Hypnosis and lobeline in an anti-smoking clinic. *Medical Officer, 111,* 239–243.

EJRUP, B. 1964. Treatment of tobacco addiction: Experiences in tobacco withdrawal clinics. In *Can we help them stop?* Chicago: American Cancer Society, Illinois Division.

———— 1965. The role of nicotine in smoking pleasure, nicotinism, treatment. In U. S. Von Euler, *Tobacco alkaloids and related compounds.* New York: Pergamon Press.

ERIKSEN, C. W. (ed.). 1962a. *Behavior and awareness.* Durham, North Carolina: Duke University Press.

———— 1962b. Figments, fantasies, and follies: A search for the subconscious mind. In C. W. Eriksen (ed.), *Behavior and awareness.* Durham, North Carolina: Duke University Press.

ESTES, W. K. 1967. Reinforcement in human learning. *Technical Report* No. 125, December 20. Institute for Mathematical Studies in the Social Sciences, Stanford University.

ESTRIN, ELIZABETH, and DOROTHY QUERRY. 1965. A no-smoking project for ninth and tenth grades. *Journal of School Health,* 35, 381–382.

EVANS, R. R. 1967. Smoking behavior among University of Wisconsin freshmen. *Report to Laymen.* Madison: American Cancer Society, Wisconsin Division.

EVANS, R. R., E. F. BORGATTA, and G. W. BOHRNSTEDT. 1967. Smoking and MMPI scores among entering Freshmen. *Journal of Social Psychology,* 73, 137–140.

EVERETT, G. M., E. E. BLOCKUS, I. M. SHEPPERD, and J. P. TOMAN. 1956. The production of tremor and a Parkinson-like syndrome by 1-4 dipyrrolidine-2-butyne, "Tremorine." *Federation Proceedings,* 15, 420.

EYSENCK, H. J. 1963. Smoking, personality and psychosomatic disorders. *Journal of Psychosomatic Research,* 7, 107–130.

———— 1965. *Smoking, health, and personality.* London: Weidenfeld and Nicolson.

EYSENCK, H. J., M. TARRANT, M. WOOLF, and L. ENGLAND. 1960. Smoking and personality. *British Medical Journal, 1,* 1456–1460.

FEATHER, N. T. 1962. Cigarette smoking and lung cancer: A study of cognitive dissonance. *Australian Journal of Psychology, 14,* 55–64.

———— 1963. Cognitive dissonance, sensitivity, and evaluation. *Journal of Abnormal and Social Psychology, 66,* 157–163.

FERSTER, C. B., J. I. NURNBERGER, and E. B. LEVITT. 1962. The control of eating. *Journal of Mathetics, 1,* 87–109.

FINNEGAN, J. K., P. S. LARSON, and H. B. HAAG. 1945. The role of nicotine in the cigarette habit. *Science, 102,* 94–96.

FISCHER, R., F. GRIFFIN, and A. R. KAPLAN. 1963. Taste thresholds, cigarette smoking, and food dislikes. *Medicina Experimentalis, 9,* 151–167.

FISHER, R. A. 1959. *Smoking—the cancer controversy.* Edinburgh: Oliver and Boyd.

FISHER, V. E. 1927. An experimental study of the effects of tobacco smoking on certain psychophysical functions. *Comparative Psychology Monographs, 4,* No. 19.

FORD, S., and F. EDERER, 1965. Breaking the cigarette habit. *Journal of the American Medical Association, 194,* 139–142.

FRANKS, C. M., R. FRIED, and BEATRICE ASHEM. 1966. An improved apparatus for the aversive conditioning of cigarette smokers. *Behavior Research and Therapy, 4,* 301–308.

FRIEDMAN, M., and R. H. ROSENMAN. 1959. Association of specific overt behavior pattern with blood and cardiovascular findings. *Journal of the American Medical Association, 169,* 96–106.

FROEBERG, S. 1920. Effects of smoking on mental and motor efficiency. *Journal of Experimental Psychology, 3,* 334-346.

FUREY, S. A., J. SCHAANNING, and S. SPOONT. 1967. The comparative effects of circulation of smoking tobacco and lettuce leaf cigarettes. *Angiology, 18,* 218–223.

FURNAS, J. C. 1938. *So you're going to stop smoking.* New York: Simon and Schuster.

GADOUREK, I. 1965–1966. Drinking and smoking habits and the feeling of well-being. *Sociologia Neerlandica, 3* (Winter), 28–43.

GIES, W. J., M. KAHN, and O. V. LIMERICK. 1921. The effect of tobacco on man. *New York Medical Journal, 113,* 809–811.

GLASER, R. 1969. Preprint to appear in *The encyclopedia of educational research* (4th ed.). New York: Macmillan.

GOODMAN, L. S., and A. GILMAN. 1965. *The pharmacological basis of therapeutics.* New York: Macmillan.

GOULD, W. L. 1953. Use of a lozenge to curb smoking appeal. *General Practice, 7,* 53–54.

GRAFF, H., V. B. O. HAMMETT, and N. BASH. 1966. Results of four anti-smoking therapy methods. *Pennsylvania Medical Journal, 69,* 39–43.

GREENE, R. J. 1964. Modification of smoking behavior by free operant conditioning methods. *Psychological Record, 14,* 171–178.

GREENO, J. G. 1968. *Elementary theoretical psychology.* Reading, Massachusetts: Addison-Wesley.

GUILFORD, JOAN. 1966. *Factors related to successful abstinence from smoking: Final report.* Los Angeles: American Institutes for Research.

HAENSZEL, W., M. B. SHIMKIN, and H. P. MILLER. 1956. *Tobacco smoking patterns in the United States.* Public Health Monograph No. 45. Washington, D.C.: U.S. Public Health Service.

HAMMOND, E. C. 1962. The effects of smoking. *Scientific American, 207,* 3–15.

HAMMOND, E. C., and CONSTANCE PERCY. 1958. Ex-smokers. *New York State Journal of Medicine, 58,* 2956–2959.

HAUSER, H., B. E. SCHWARZ, G. ROTH, and R. G. BICKFORD. 1958. Electroencephalographic changes related to smoking. *Electroencephalography and Clinical Neurophysiology, 10,* 576.

HEAD, J. R. 1939. The effects of smoking. *Illinois Medical Journal, 76,* 283–287.

HEATH, C. W. 1958. Differences between smokers and nonsmokers. *American Medical Association Archives of Internal Medicine, 101,* 377–388.

HEIMSTRA, N. W., N. R. BANCROFT, and A. R. DEKOCK. 1967. Effects of smoking upon sustained performance in a simulated driving task. *Annals of the New York Academy of Sciences, 142,* 295–307.

HEISE, J. G. 1962. *The painless way to stop smoking.* Manhasset, New York: Channel Press.

HERXHEIMER, A., R. L. GRIFFITHS, B. HAMILTON, and M. WAKEFIELD. 1967. Circulatory effects of nicotine aerosol inhalation and cigarette smoking in man. *Lancet, 2,* 754–755.

HESS, CATHERINE. 1964. New York City's stop smoking program. In *Can we help them stop?* Chicago: American Cancer Society, Illinois Division.

HEYMANS, C., J. J. BOUCKAERT, and L. DAUTREBANDE. 1931. Sinus carodidien et reflexes respiratoires. III. Sensibilité des sinus carotidiens aux substances chimiques. Action stimulante respiratoire reflexe du sulfure de sodium, du cyanure de potassium, de la nicotine et de la lobeline. *Archives Internationales de Pharmacodynamie et de Therapie, 40,* 54–91.

HOCHBAUM, G. M. 1964. A critique of psychological research on smoking. Symposium, American Psychological Association Convention: September.

HOFFSTAEDT, E. G. W. 1964a. Anti-smoking campaign. *Medical Officer, 111,* 59–60.

———— 1964b. The use of lobeline in the treatment of smokers. *Medical Journal of Australia, 1,* 288.

HOINVILLE, G. W., and H. W. BIGGS. 1966. Establishing smoking habits in retrospect. *The Statistician, 16,* 23–43.

HOLMSTEDT, B., and G. LUNDGREN. 1967. Arecoline, nicotine and related compounds. Tremorgenic activity and the effect upon brain acetylcholine. *Annals of the New York Academy of Sciences, 142*, 126–142.

HOMME, L. E. 1965. Control of coverants, the operants of the mind. *The Psychological Record, 15*, 501–511.

HORN, D. 1964. Brief description of the experimental course for the control of cigarette smoking. In *Can we help them stop?* Chicago: American Cancer Society, Illinois Division.

———— 1969. Smokers self-testing kit, Part II. Washington, D.C.: National Clearinghouse for Smoking and Health, U.S. Department of Health, Education, and Welfare.

HORNE, T. 1963. Smoking and health. *Journal of School Health, 33*, 451–456.

HULL, C. L. 1924. The influence of tobacco smoking on mental and motor efficiency. *Psychological Monographs, 33*, No. 150.

HUNT, W. A., and JANE FLANNERY. 1938. Variability in the affective judgment. *American Journal of Psychology, 51*, 507–513.

JACOBS, M. A., L. S. ANDERSON, E. CHAMPAGNE, N. KARUSH, S. J. RICHMAN, and P. H. KNAPP. 1966. Orality, impulsivity and cigarette smoking in men: Further findings in support of a theory. *Journal of Nervous and Mental Diseases, 143*, 207–219.

JACOBS, M. A., P. H. KNAPP, L. S. ANDERSON, N. KARUSH, R. MEISSNER, and S. J. RICHMAN. 1965. Relationships of oral frustration factors with heavy cigarette smoking in males. *Journal of Nervous and Mental Diseases, 141*, 161–171.

JAFFE, J. H. 1965. Drug addiction and drug abuse. In L. S. Goodman and A. Gilman (eds.), *The pharmacological basis of therapeutics.* New York: Macmillan.

JAMES, W. H., A. B. WOODRUFF, and W. WERNER. 1965. Effect of internal and external control upon changes in smoking behavior. *Journal of Consulting Psychology, 29*, 184–186.

JANIS, I. L., and L. MANN. 1965. Effectiveness of emotional role-playing in modifying smoking habits and attitudes. *Journal of Experimental Research in Personality, 1*, 84–90.

JANIS, I. L., and J. C. MILLER. 1968. Factors influencing tolerance for deprivation. In National Clearinghouse for Smoking and Health, *Directory of on-going research in smoking and health.* Arlington, Virginia: U.S. Public Health Service.

JANIS, I. L., and R. F. TERWILLIGER. 1962. An experimental study of psychological resistance to fear arousing communication. *Journal of Abnormal and Social Psychology, 65*, 403–410.

JARVIK, M. E. 1965. Drugs used in the treatment of psychiatric disorders. In L. S. Goodman and A. Gilman, (eds.), *The pharmacological basis of therapeutics.* New York: Macmillan.

———— 1967. Tobacco smoking in monkeys. *Annals of the New York Academy of Sciences, 142*, 280–294.

JEFFREYS, MARGOT, M. NORMAN-TAYLOR, and GWEN GRIFFITHS. 1967. Longer-term results of an anti-smoking educational campaign. *Medical Officer*, *117*, 93–95.

JEWETT, R. E., and S. N. NORTON. 1966. Effects of some stimulant and depressant drugs on sleep cycles of cats. *Experimental Neurology*, *55*, 463–474.

JOHNSON, O. J. 1918. Effects of smoking on mental and motor efficiency. *Psychological Clinic*, *12*, 132–140, 230–235.

JOHNSTON, L. M. 1942. Tobacco smoking and nicotine. *Lancet*, 2, 742.

———— 1952. Cure of tobacco smoking. *Lancet*, *263*, 480–482.

KAUFMAN, W. 1954. Correspondence: How to help patients stop smoking. *Journal of the American Medical Association*, *155*, 338.

KERSHBAUM, A., and S. BELLET. 1964. Cigarette smoking and blood lipids. *Journal of the American Medical Association*, *187*, 32–36.

KERSHBAUM, A., S. BELLET, J. JIMINEZ, and L. J. FEINBERG. 1966. Differences in effects of cigar and cigarette smoking on free fatty acid mobilization and catecholamine excretion. *Journal of the American Medical Association*, *195*, 1095–1098.

KERSHBAUM, A., R. KHORSANDIAN, R. F. CAPLAN, S. BELLET, and L. J. FEINBERG. 1963. The role of catecholamines in the free fatty acid response to cigarette smoking. *Circulation*, *28*, 52–57.

KERSHBAUM, A., D. J. PAPPAJOHN, and S. BELLET. 1968. Effect of smoking and nicotine on adrenocortical secretion. *Journal of the American Medical Association*, *203*, 275–278.

KEUTZER, CAROLIN S. 1967. Behavior modification of smoking: A review, analysis, and experimental application with focus on subject variables as predictors of treatment outcome. Eugene: University of Oregon, unpublished Doctoral Dissertation.

KEUTZER, CAROLIN S., E. LICHTENSTEIN, and H. L. MEES. 1968. Modification of smoking behavior: A review. *Psychological Bulletin*, *70*, 520–533.

KIMBLE, G. A. 1961. *Hilgard and Marquis' conditioning and learning*. New York: Appleton-Century-Crofts.

KIMELDORF, C., and P. J. GEIWITZ. 1966. Smoking and the Blacky orality factors. *Journal of Projective Techniques and Personality Assessment*, *30*, 167–168.

KNAPP, P. 1962. American psychiatric association conference report on studies of cigarette smoking. *The New York Times*, May 11, *18*, 3.

KNAPP, P., C. M. BLISS, and H. WELLS. 1963. Addictive aspects in heavy cigarette smoking. *American Journal of Psychiatry*, *119*, 966–972.

KOENIG, K. P., and J. MASTERS. 1965. Experimental treatment of habitual smoking. *Behavior Research and Therapy*, *3*, 235–243.

KOPONEN, A. 1960. Personality characteristics of purchasers. *Journal of Advertising Research*, *1*, 6–12.

KRAMER, J. C., R. A. BASS, and J. E. BERECOCHEA. 1968. Civil commitment for addicts: The California program. *American Journal of Psychiatry, 125,* 816–824.

Kuschinsky, G., and R. Hotovy. 1943. Über die zentral erregende Wirkung des Nicotins. *Klinische Wochenschrift, 22,* 649–650.

Lader, M., and N. Sartorius. 1968. Anxiety in patients with hysterical conversion symptoms. *Journal of Neurology, Neurosurgery and Psychiatry, 31,* 490–495.

Lane, J. P. 1961. Smokers' reactions to a television program about lung cancer: A study of dissonance. *Dissertation Abstracts, 21,* 2812–2813.

Lane, N. E., A. Oberman, R. E. Mitchell, and A. Graybiel. 1966. The thousand aviator study: Smoking history correlates of selected physiological, biochemical, and anthropometric measures. Washington: Bureau of Medicine and Surgey, MF022.03.02-5007.11, NASA Order R-136, April 27.

Langley, J. N., and W. L. Dickinson. 1889. On the local paralysis of peripheral ganglia, and on the connexion of different classes of nerve fibers with them. *Proceedings of the Royal Society, 46,* 423–431.

Larson, P. S., J. K. Finnegan, and H. B. Haag. 1950. Observations on the effect of cigarette smoking on the fusion frequency of flicker. *Journal of Clinical Investigation, 29,* 483–485.

Larson, P. S., H. B. Haag, and H. Silvette. 1961. *Tobacco: Experimental and clinical studies.* Baltimore: Williams and Wilkins.

Larson, P. S., and H. Silvette. 1968. *Tobacco: Experimental and clinical studies. Supplement 1.* Baltimore: Williams and Wilkins.

Lawton, M. P. 1962. A group therapy approach to giving up smoking. *Applied Therapeutics, 4,* 1025–1028.

————— 1967. Group methods in smoking withdrawal. *Archives of Environmental Health, 14,* 258–265.

Lawton, M. P., and R. W. Phillips. 1956. The relationship between excessive cigarette smoking and psychological tension. *American Journal of Medical Science, 232,* 397–402.

Le Gros Clark, W. E., J. Beatte, G. Riddoch, and N. M. Dott. 1938. *The Hypothalamus.* Edinburgh: Oliver and Boyd.

Leone, L. A., H. Musiker, M. Albala, and W. McGurk. 1967. A study of the effectiveness of the smoking deterrence clinic. Providence: Rhode Island Hospital (mimeographed).

Leventhal, H., and Patricia Niles. 1964. A field experiment on fear arousal with data on the validity of questionnaire measures. *Journal of Personality, 32,* 459–479.

Levin, M. 1959. Perceived risk in smoking: An exploratory investigation. *Studies in Public Communication, 2,* 54–60 (Committee on Communication, University of Chicago).

Lewin, L. 1931. *Phantastica: Narcotic and stimulating drugs: Their use and abuse.* (Translated from the 2nd German edition by P. H. A. Wirth.) New York: E. P. Dutton and Co.

Lichtenstein, E., and Carolin S. Keutzer. 1969. Experimental investigation of diverse techniques to modify smoking: A follow-up report. *Behavior Research and Therapy, 7,* 139–140.

LICHTENSTEIN, E., CAROLIN S. KEUTZER, and K. H. HIMES. 1969. Emotional role-playing and changes in smoking attitudes and behavior. Submitted for publication.

LICHTENSTEIN, E., A. F. POUSSAINT, S. H. BERGMAN, T. JURNEY, and R. SHAPIRO. 1967. A further report on the effects of the physician's treatment of smoking by means of a placebo. *Diseases of the Nervous System, 28,* 754–755.

LILIENFELD, A. M. 1959. Emotional and other selected characteristics of cigarette smokers and nonsmokers as related to epidemiological studies of lung cancer and other diseases. *Journal of the National Cancer Institute, 22,* 259–282.

LINDSLEY, O. R. 1959. Reduction in rate of vocal psychotic symptoms by differential positive reinforcement. *Journal of the Experimental Analysis of Behavior, 2,* 269.

———— 1963. Direct measurement and functional definition of vocal hallucinatory symptoms. *Journal of Nervous and Mental Diseases, 136,* 293–297.

LIVSON, N., and L. H. STEWART. 1965. Morphological constitution and smoking. A further evaluation. *Journal of the American Medical Association, 192,* 806–808.

LONDON, S. J. 1963. Clinical evaluation of a new lobeline smoking deterrent. *Current Therapeutic Research, 5,* 167–175.

LONGO, V. G., F. GIUNTINA, and J. SCOTTI DE CAROLIS. 1967. Effects of nicotine on the electroencephalogram of the rabbit. *Annals of the New York Academy of Sciences, 142,* 159–169.

LONGO, V. G., G. P. VON BERGER, and D. BOVET. 1954. Action of nicotine and of the "ganglioplegiques centraux" on the electrical activity of the brain. *Journal of Pharmacology and Experimental Therapeutics, 111,* 349–359.

LUBLIN, I. 1968. Some problems in the aversive conditioning of cigarette addicts. San Diego, California. Paper read at the meeting of the Western Psychological Association.

LUCCHESI, B. R., C. R. SCHUSTER, and G. S. EMLEY. 1967. The role of nicotine as a determinant of cigarette smoking frequency in man with observations of certain cardiovascular effects associated with the tobacco alkaloid. *Clinical Pharmacology and Therapeutics, 8,* 789–796.

MANDLER, G. 1967. Verbal learning. In *New directions in psychology, III.* New York: Holt.

MANN, L. 1966. The effects of emotional role playing on smoking attitudes and habits. *Dissertation Abstracts, 26,* 4104–4105.

MARSTON, A. R., and R. McFALL. 1968. Behavioral modification of smoking. In National Clearinghouse for Smoking and Health, *Directory of on-going research in smoking and health.* Arlington, Virginia: U.S. Public Health Service. 1960.

MATARAZZO, J. D., and G. SASLOW. 1960. Psychological and related characteristics of smokers and nonsmokers. *Psychological Bulletin, 57,* 493–513.

MATARAZZO, J. D., G. SASLOW, and E. N. PAREIS. 1960. Verbal conditioning of two response classes; some methodological considerations. *Journal of Abnormal and Social Psychology, 61,* 190–206.

MAUSNER, B. 1966. Report on a smoking clinic. *American Psychologist, 21,* 251–255.

MAUSNER, B., and E. PLATT. 1968. The natural history of cigarette smoking. Privately circulated draft. Glenside, Pennsylvania: Beaver College.

MCARTHUR, C., E. WALDRON and J. DICKINSON. 1958. The psychology of smoking. *Journal of Abnormal and Social Psychology, 56,* 267–275.

MCDONALD, R. L., 1965. Personality characteristics, cigarette smoking, and obstetric complications. *Journal of Psychology, 60,* 129–134.

MCFALL, R. M. 1969. The effects of having subjects monitor their smoking behavior. Chicago: Paper given at the Midwestern Psychological Association meeting, May 8.

MCFARLAND, J. W. 1965. Physical measures used in breaking the smoking habit. *Archives of Physical Medicine and Rehabilitation, 64,* 323–327.

MCFARLAND, J. W., H. W. GIMBEL, W. A. J. DONALD, and E. J. FOLKENBERG. 1964. The 5-day program to help individuals stop smoking. *Connecticut Medicine, 28,* 885–890.

MCGAUGH, J. L., and L. PETRINOVITCH. 1965. Effects of drugs on learning and memory. *International Review of Neurobiology, 8,* 139–196.

MCGRADY, P. 1960. *Cigarettes and health.* Public Affairs Pamphlet 220A. The Public Affairs Committee.

MCNAMEE, H. B., NANCY K. MELLO, and J. H. MENDELSON. 1968. Experimental analysis of drinking patterns of alcoholics; concurrent psychiatric observations. *American Journal of Psychiatry, 124,* 81–87.

MEES, H. L. 1966. Placebo effects in aversive control; a preliminary report. Paper read at joint Washington State-Oregon Psychological Association meeting.

MERRY, J., and G. PRESTON. 1963. The effect of buffered lobeline sulphate on cigarette smoking. *Practitioner, 190,* 629–631.

MILEY, R. A., and W. G. WHITE. 1958. Giving up smoking. *British Medical Journal, 1,* 101.

MILLER, M. M. 1941. Benzedrine sulphate in the treatment of nicotinism. *Medical Record, 153,* 137–138.

MILLER, N. E. 1969. Learning of visceral and glandular responses. *Science, 163,* 434–445.

MONK, MARY, M. TAYBACK, and J. GORDON. 1965. Evaluation of an anti-smoking program among high school students. *American Journal of Public Health, 55,* 994–1004.

MOODIE, W. 1957. Smoking, drinking, and nervousness. *Lancet, 2,* 188–189.

MORRISON, C. F., and A. K. ARMITAGE. 1967. Effects of nicotine upon the free operant behavior of rats and spontaneous motor activity of mice. *Annals of the New York Academy of Sciences, 142,* 268–276.

MOSES, F. M. 1964. Treating smoking habit by discussion and hypnosis. *Diseases of the Nervous System, 25,* 184–188.

MULHALL, J. C. 1895. The cigarette habit. *Transactions of the American Laryngological Association, 17,* 192–200. Reprinted in *Annals of Ontology, Rhinology, and Laryngology,* 1943, 52, 714–721; and in *New York Medical Journal,* 1895, 62, 686–688.

MURPHREE, H. B. (ed.) 1967. The effects of nicotine and smoking on the central nervous system. *Annals of the New York Academy of Sciences, 142,* 1–333.

National Clearinghouse for Smoking and Health. 1967a. *Bibliograhy on smoking and health.* Arlington, Virginia: United States Public Health Service.

——— 1967b. *Directory of on-going research in smoking and health.* Arlington, Virginia: United States Public Health Service.

——— 1968. *Directory of on-going research in smoking and health.* Arlington, Virginia: United States Public Health Service.

NICHOLS, J. R., and S. HSIAO. 1967. Addiction liability of albino rats: Breeding for quantitative differences in morphine drinking. *Science, 157,* 561–563.

NOLAN, J. D. 1968. Self-control procedures in the modification of smoking behavior. *Journal of Consulting and Clinical Psychology, 32,* 92–93.

OBER, D. C. 1966. The modification of smoking behavior. Urbana: University of Illinois, Unpublished doctoral dissertation.

OCHSNER, A. 1964. Aids in the discontinuance of smoking. In *Can we help them stop?* Chicago: American Cancer Society, Illinois Division.

OLDS, J., and P. MILNER. 1954. Positive reinforcement produced by electrical stimulation of septal area and other regions of rat brain. *Journal of Comparative and Physiological Psychology, 47,* 419–427.

ORFILA. 1851. Memoire sur la nicotine et sur la conicine. *Annales d'Hygiène Publique, Industrielle, et Sociale, 45,* 147–230.

ORNE, M. 1962. On the social psychology of the psychological experiment: With particular reference to demand characteristics and their implications. *American Psychologist, 17,* 776–783.

PALMEN, E. 1911. Über die Einwirkung des Tabakrauchens auf die körperliche Leistungsfähigkeit. *Skandinavisches Archiv für Physiologie, 24,* 187–196.

PAUL, G. L. 1966. *Insight vs. desensitization in psychotherapy.* Stanford, California: Stanford University Press.

——— 1968. A two year follow-up of systematic desensitization in therapy groups. *Journal of Abnormal Psychology, 73,* 119–130.

——— In press. Behavior modification research: Design and tactics. In C. M. Franks (ed.), *Assessment and status of the behavior therapies and associated developments.* New York: McGraw-Hill.

PECHSTEIN, L. A., and W. R. REYNOLDS. 1937. The effect of tobacco smoke on the growth and learning behavior of the albino rat and its progeny. *Journal of Comparative Psychology, 24,* 459–469.

PICKENS, R., and T. THOMPSON. 1968. Self-administration of amphetamine and cocaine by rats. Reports from Research Labs, Department of Psychiatry, University of Minnesota, No. PR–66–4, 1966. Reported in T. Thompson, and C. R. Schuster, *Behavioral pharmacology.* Englewood Cliffs, New Jersey: Prentice-Hall.

PLAKUN, ARLENE L., J. AMBRUS, I. BROSS, S. GRAHAM, M. L. LEVIN, and C. A. ROSS. 1966. Clinical factors in smoking withdrawal: Preliminary report. *American Journal of Public Health, 56,* 434–441.

PLAUT, T. F. A. 1967. *Alcohol problems: A report to the nation.* New York: Oxford University Press.

POUSSAINT, A. F., S. H. BERGMAN, and E. LICHTENSTEIN. 1966. The effects of physician's smoking on the treatment of smokers. *Diseases of the Nervous System, 27,* 539–543.

POVORINSKII, V. A. 1962. Psychotherapy in smoking. In R. B. Winn (ed.), *Psychotherapy in the Soviet Union.* New York: Grove Press.

POWELL, J., and N. AZRIN. 1968. The effects of shock as a punisher for cigarette smoking. *Journal of Applied Behavior Analysis, 1,* 63–71.

PREMACK, D. 1963. Rate differential reinforcement in monkey manipulation. *Journal of Experimental Analysis of Behavior, 6,* 81–89.

———— 1965. Reinforcement theory. In D. Levine (ed.), *Nebraska symposium on motivation.* Lincoln: University of Nebraska Press.

PYKE, SANDRA, N. McK. AGNEW, and JEAN KOPPERUD. 1966. Modification of an over-learned maladaptive response through a relearning program: A pilot study on smoking. *Behavior Research and Therapy, 4,* 197–203.

QUINN, R. P. 1961. Cranberries, cigarettes, cancer, and cognitive dissonance. *American Psychologist, 16,* 409.

RAAB, W., and H. KRZYWANEK. 1965. Cardiovascular sympathetic tone and stress response related to personality patterns and exercise habits: A potential cardiac risk and screening test. *American Journal of Cardiology, 16,* 42–53.

RAPP, G. W., B. T. DUSZA, and L. BLANCHET. 1959. Absorption and utility of lobeline as a smoking deterrent. *American Journal of the Medical Sciences, 237,* 287–292.

RAPP, G. W., and A. A. OLEN. 1955. Critical evaluation of lobeline based smoking deterrent. *American Journal of the Medical Sciences, 230,* 9–14.

RAYMOND, M. J. 1964. The treatment of addiction by aversive conditioning with apomorphine. *Behavior Research and Therapy, 1,* 287–291.

Research Committee of the British Tuberculosis Association. 1963. Smoking deterrent study. *British Medical Journal, 2,* 486–487.

RESNICK, J. H. 1968a. Effects of stimulus satiation on the over-learned maladaptive response of cigarette smoking. *Journal of Consulting and Clinical Psychology, 32,* 501–505.

———— 1968b. The control of smoking behavior by stimulus satiation. *Behavior Research and Therapy, 6,* 113–114.

REYNOLDS, G. S. 1968. *A primer of operant conditioning.* Glenview, Illinois: Scott, Foresman, and Company.

RIVERS, W. H. R. 1908. *The influence of alcohol and other drugs on fatigue.* London: Edward Arnold.

ROBUSTELLI, F. 1963. Azione della nicotina sull'apprendimento del ratto nel labirinto. *Lincei, Rendiconti, Clase di Scienze Fisiche, Matematiche e Naturali, 34,* 703–709.

———— 1966. Azione della nicotina sul condizionamento di salvaguardia di ratti di un mese. *Lincei, Rendiconti, Classe di Scienze Fisiche, Matematiche e Naturali, 40,* 490–497.

ROSENBERG, A. 1954. Tobak—et socialt problem. *Ugeskrift for Laeger, 116,* 858–860.

ROSENHEIM, M. 1962. Can drugs stop smoking? *Prescriber's Journal, 2,* 79–80.

ROSS, C. A. 1964. Report on smoking withdrawal. In *Can we help them stop?* Chicago: American Cancer Society, Illinois Division.

ROTH, GRACE M., J. B. McDONALD, and C. SHEARD. 1945. The effect of smoking cigarettes and the intravenous administration of nicotine on the heart and peripheral blood vessels. *Medical Clinics of North America, 29,* 949–957.

The Royal College of Physicians of London. 1962. *Smoking and health.* New York: Pitman Publishing Company.

RUSS, S. 1955. *Smoking and its effects.* London: Hutchinson's Scientific and Technical Publications.

RUTNER, I. T. 1967. The modification of smoking behavior through techniques of self-control. Wichita, Kansas: Wichita State University, unpublished master's thesis.

RYLE, A. 1962. Smoking and neurosis. *British Medical Journal, 1,* 1344.

SALBER, E. J., and J. ROCHMAN. 1964. Personality differences between smokers and nonsmokers. *Archives of Environmental Health, 8,* 459–465.

SANFORD, N., H. WEBSTER, and M. FREEDMAN. 1957. Impulse expression as a variable of personality. *Psychological Monographs, 71,* No. 440.

SCHACTER, S. 1968. Obesity and eating. *Science, 161,* 751–756.

SCHIEVELBEIN, H., and E. WERLE. 1967. Mechanism of the release of amines by nicotine. *Annals of the New York Academy of Sciences, 142,* 72–82.

SCHILDKRAUT, J. J., and S.S. KETY. 1967. Biogenic amines and emotion. *Science, 156,* 21–30.

SCHUBERT, D. S. P. 1959. Personality implications of cigarette smoking among college students. *Journal of Consulting Psychology, 23,* 376.

———— 1965. Arousal seeking as a central factor in tobacco smoking among college students. *International Journal of Social Psychiatry, 11,* 221–225.

SCHUSTER, C. R., and J. H. WOODS. 1968. The conditioned reinforcing effects of stimuli associated with morphine reinforcement. *International Journal of the Addictions, 3,* 223–230.

SCOTT, G. W., A. G. C. COX, K. S. MACLEAN, T. M. L. PRICE, and N. SOUTH-WELL. 1962. Buffered lobeline as a smoking deterent. *Lancet, 1*, 54–55.

SELTZER, C. C. 1965. Morphological constitution and smoking. *Journal of the American Medical Association, 194*, 98.

SHEARD, C. 1946. The effects of smoking on the dark adaptation of rods and cones. *Federation Proceedings, 5*, 94.

SHIELDS, J. 1962. *Monozygotic twins brought up apart and brought up together.* London: Oxford University Press.

SHRYOCK, H. 1965. *Mind if I smoke?* Mountain View, California: Pacific Press Publishing Association.

SIBLEY, R. F. 1966. A method for studying the effect of induced attitude inconsistency on behavior change. Buffalo State University of New York at Buffalo, unpublished Doctoral Dissertation.

SILVETTE, H., E. C. HOFF, P. S. LARSON, and H. G. HAAG. 1962. The actions of nicotine on central nervous functions. *Pharmacological Reviews, 14*, 137–173.

SINNOT, J. J., and J. E. RAUTH. 1937. Effect of smoking on taste thresholds. *Journal of General Psychology, 17*, 151–153.

SKINNER, B. F. 1948. "Superstition" in the pigeon. *Journal of Experimental Psychology, 38*, 168–172.

———— 1953. *Science and human behavior.* New York: Macmillan.

SMITH, G. M. 1967. Personality correlates of cigarette smoking in students of college age. *Annals of the New York Academy of Sciences, 142*, 308–321.

———— 1969a. between personality and smoking behavior in preadult subjects. *Journal of Consulting and Clinical Psychology,* in press.

———— 1969b. Personality correlates of in Puerto Rican high school students. Unpublished; available from author on request.

Smoking Deterrent Study. 1963. *British Medical Journal, 2*, 486–487.

SOLOMON, R. L., and L. C. WYNNE. 1954. Traumatic avoidance learning: The principles of anxiety conservation and partial irreversibility. *Psychological Review, 61*, 353–385.

SPRAGG, S. D. S. 1940. Morphine addiction in chimpanzees. *Comparative Psychology Monographs, 15*, No. 132.

STEIN, L., and J. STEIFTER. 1962. Muscarinic synapses in the hypothalamus. *American Journal of Physiology, 202*, 751–756.

STEIN, L., and C. D. WISE. 1967. Release of hypothalamic norepinephrine by rewarding electrical stimulation or amphetamine in the unanesthetized rat. *Federation Proceedings, 26*, 651.

STEWART, L., and N. LIVSON. 1966. Smoking and rebelliousness: A longitudinal study from childhood to maturity. *Journal of Consulting Psychology, 30*, 225–229.

STONE, C. A., M. L. TORCHIANA, A. NAVARRO, and K. H. BEYER. 1956. Ganglionic blocking properties of 3-methyl-amino-isocamphane hydrochloride (mecamylamine): A secondary amine. *Journal of Pharmacology and Experimental Therapeutics, 117*, 169–183.

STRAITS, B. C. 1965. Sociological and psychological correlates of adoption and discontinuation of cigarette smoking. University of Chicago (mimeographed).

———— 1966. The discontinuation of cigarette smoking: A multiple discriminant analysis. Paper presented at the annual meeting of the American Sociological Association.

———— 1967. The discontinuation of cigarette smoking: A multiple discriminant analysis. In S. V. Zagona (ed.), *Studies and issues in smoking behavior*. Tuscon: The University of Arizona Press.

STRAITS, B. C., and L. SECHREST. 1963. Further support of some findings about the characteristics of smokers and nonsmokers. *Journal of Consulting Psychology*, 27, 282.

SWARTZ, H., and A. COHEN. 1964. Clinical evaluation of smokurb as a smoking deterrent. *Current Therapeutic Research*, 6, 290–296.

SWINEHART, J. W., and J. C. KIRSCHT. 1966. Smoking: A panel study of beliefs and behavior following the PHS report. *Psychological Reports*, 18, 519–528.

THOMAS, C. B. 1960. Characteristics of smokers compared with nonsmokers in a population of healthy young adults, including observations on family history, blood pressure, heart rate, body weight, cholesterol and certain psychologic traits. *Annals of Internal Medicine*, 53, 697–718.

THOMPSON, D. S., and T. R. WILSON. 1966. Discontinuance of cigarette smoking: "Natural" and with "therapy." *Journal of the American Medical Association, 196*, 1048–1052.

THOMPSON, T., and C. R. SCHUSTER. 1968. *Behavioral pharmacology*. Englewood Cliffs, New Jersey: Prentice-Hall.

TIGHE, T. J., and R. ELLIOTT. 1967. Breaking the cigarette habit: Effects of a technique involving threatened loss of money. Washington, D.C.: Paper read at American Psychological Association Meeting.

TOCH, H., T. ALLEN, and W. LAZER. 1961. Effects of cancer scares: The residue of the news impact. *Journalism Quarterly*, 38, 25–34.

TODD, G. F., and J. T. LAWS. 1959. The reliability of statements about smoking habits. In *Tobacco Manufacturers Standing Committee Research Paper* (2nd edition), Great Britain: Tobacco Manufacturers Standing Committee.

TOMKINS, S. S. 1966. Psychological model for smoking behavior. *American Journal of Public Health*, 56, 17–20.

TOOLEY, J. T. 1968. Behavioral strategies for the control of smoking. In National Clearinghouse for Smoking and Health, *Directory of on-going research in smoking and health*. Arlington, Virginia: U.S. Public Health Service.

TURLE, G. C. 1958. An investigation into the therapeutic action of hydrooxyzine (atarax) in the treatment of nervous disorders and the control of the smoking habit. *Journal of Mental Science, 104*, 826–833.

UNDERWOOD, B. J. 1957. *Psychological research.* New York: Appleton-Century-Crofts.

U.S. *News and World Report.* 1965. Smoking scare? What's happened to it. January 11, 38–41.

U.S. Public Health Service. 1962. *Smoking and health.* Report of the Advisory Committee to the Surgeon General of the Public Health Service. Washington, D.C.: U.S. Department of Health, Education, and Welfare.

———— 1964. *Smoking and health.* Report of the Advisory Committee to the Surgeon General of the Public Health Service. Washington, D.C.: U.S. Department of Health, Education, and Welfare. Public Health Service Publication 1103.

VALLANCE, T. R. 1940. Suggestibility of smokers and nonsmokers. *Psychological Record, 4,* 138–144.

VAN PROOSDIJ, C. 1960. *Smoking.* London: Elsevier.

VELDMAN, D. J., and O. H. BROWN. 1969. Personality and performance characteristics associated with cigarette smoking among college freshmen. *Journal of Consulting and Clinical Psychology, 33,* 109–119.

VERPLANCK, W. S. 1962. Unaware of where's awareness: Some verbal operants—notates, monents, and notants. In C. W. Eriksen (ed.), *Behavior and awareness.* Durham, North Carolina: Duke University Press.

VON AHN, B. 1954. *The acute effect of tobacco-smoking and nicotine on the electrocardiogram—especially during induced hypoxia. A clinical and experimental investigation.* Uppsala: Appelbergs Boktryckeri AB.

VON DEDENROTH, T. E. A. 1964a. The use of hypnosis with "tobaccomaniacs." *The American Journal of Clinical Hypnosis, 6,* 326–331.

———— 1964b. Further help for the "tobaccomaniac." *The American Journal of Clinical Hypnosis, 6,* 332–336.

WARDEN, C. J. 1931. *Animal motivation: Experimental studies on the albino rat.* New York: Columbia University Press.

WARWICK, K. M., and H. J. EYSENCK. 1963. The effects of smoking on the CFF threshold. *Life Sciences, 4,* 219–225.

WATNE, A. L., R. L. MONTGOMERY, and WANDA W. PETTIT. 1964. A cigarette information program. *Journal of the American Medical Association, 188,* 872–874.

WEATHERBY, J. H. 1942. Skin temperature changes caused by smoking and other sympathomimetic stimuli. *American Heart Journal, 24,* 17–30.

WEATHERLEY, D. 1965. Some personality correlates of the ability to stop smoking cigarettes. *Journal of Consulting Psychology, 29,* 483–485.

WEEKS, J. R. 1962. Experimental morphine addiction: Method for automatic intravenous injections in unrestrained rats. *Science, 138,* 143–144.

WENUSCH, A., and R. SCHÖLLER. 1936. Über den Einfluss des Rauchens auf die Reizschwelle des Drucksinnes. *Medizinische Klinik, 32,* 356–358.

WESTFALL, T. C., R. M. FLEMING, MARY F. FUDGER, and W. G. CLARK. 1967. Effect of nicotine and related substances upon amine levels in the brain. *Annals of the New York Academy of Sciences, 142,* 83–100.

Subject Index

INTANGIBLE HERITAGE AND
THE MUSEUM

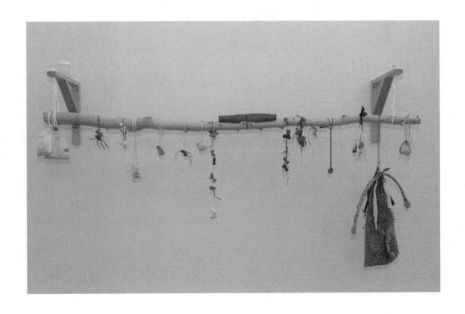

Critical Cultural Heritage Series
Series Editor: Beverley Butler
Part of the University College London Institute of Archaeology Publications Series,
published for the Institute by Left Coast Press, Inc.
General Series Editor: Ruth Whitehouse
Founding Series Editor: Peter Ucko

The aim of this Critical Cultural Heritage series is to define a new area of research
and to produce a set of volumes that make a radical break with the existing canon
of cultural heritage texts. In a fundamental shift of perspective, Jacques Derrida's
rallying call to "restore heritage to dignity" inspires both a re-examination of the
core question of what constitutes cultural heritage and an engagement with the
ethical issues that shape the possible futures of this research area.

The series is intended to be of transformative value in creating new agendas within cultural heritage discourse, using individual texts as building blocks.
Central to the project is a re-alignment of cultural heritage studies through a
wider scholarship committed to disrupting the Eurocentrism which underpins
current theory and practice and through a contemporary "politics of recognition"
that is concerned with articulating new, alternative or parallel characterisations of
heritage value. The aim is to centre cultural heritage studies within a wider concern for the preservation of human dignity and justice and to use these alternative
discourses as a resource for future action, thereby creating a proactive, responsive
and just future for both cultural heritage studies and heritage practice.

Volume 9: Shaila Bhatti, *Translating Museums: A Counterhistory of South Asian
Museology*
Volume 8: Marilena Alivizatou, *Intangible Heritage and the Museum: New
Perspectives on Cultural Preservation*
Volume 7: Charlotte L. Joy, *The Politics of Heritage Management in Mali: From
UNESCO to Djenné*
Volume 6: Layla Renshaw, *Exhuming Loss: Memory, Materiality, and Mass
Graves of the Spanish Civil War*
Volume 5: Katharina Schramm, *African Homecoming: Pan-African Ideology
and Contested Heritage*
Volume 4: Mingming Wang, *Empire and Local Worlds: A Chinese Model of
Long-Term Historical Anthropology*
Volume 3: Dean Sully, Ed., *Decolonizing Conservation: Caring for Maori
Meeting Houses outside New Zealand*
Volume 2: Ferdinand de Jong and Michael Rowlands, Eds., *Reclaiming Heritage:
Alternative Imaginaries of Memory in West Africa*
Volume 1: Beverley Butler, *Return to Alexandria: An Ethnography of Cultural
Heritage Revivalism and Museum Memory*

Information on these titles and other volumes in the UCL Institute of Archaeology
Series can be obtained from the Left Coast Press, Inc. (www.LCoastPress.com).

INTANGIBLE HERITAGE AND THE MUSEUM

New Perspectives on Cultural Preservation

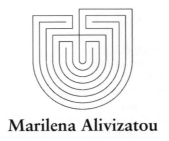

Marilena Alivizatou

Walnut Creek, California

LEFT COAST PRESS, INC.
1630 North Main Street, #400
Walnut Creek, CA 94596
http://www.LCoastPress.com

ISBN 978-1-61132-150-0 hardcover
ISBN 978-1-61132-151-7 paperback
eISBN 978-1-61132-152-4 institutional eBook
eISBN 978-1-61132-533-1 consumer eBook

Library of Congress Cataloging-in-Publication Data:

Alivizatou, Marilena.
Intangible heritage and the museum : new perspectives on cultural preservation / Marilena Alivizatou.
   p. cm. — (Critical cultural heritage series. University College London institute of archaeology publications series ; v.8)
 Includes bibliographical references.
  ISBN 978-1-61132-150-0 (hardback : alk. paper) — ISBN 978-1-61132-151-7 (pbk. : alk. paper) — ISBN 978-1-61132-152-4 (institutional eBook) — ISBN 978-1-61132-533-1 (consumer eBook)
 1. Ethnological museums and collections. 2. Cultural property—Protection.
 3. Cultural property—Government policy. 4. Museums—Management.
 5. Museums—Administration. 6. World Heritage areas. I. Title.
   GN35.A48 2012
   305.80074—dc23
                        2011052999

Printed in the United States of America

♾™ The paper used in this publication meets the minimum requirements of American National Standard for Information Sciences—Permanence of Paper for Printed Library Materials, ANSI/NISO Z39.48–1992.

Cover image: Ceremonial Room Offerings (detail). National Museum of the American Indian, Smithsonian Institution (Image no. 20120411). Photo by R. A. Whiteside.

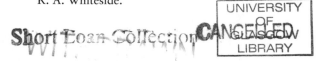

For my parents

Contents

Illustrations

Acknowledgments

This book is the outcome of a research on intangible heritage that began in 2003. My initial interest in this topic grew out of earlier studies of folk culture in Greece, my country of origin, and the role of museums in its preservation. Conducting an internship at UNESCO in 2004 highlighted the truly global dimensions of intangible heritage. Raised in a country where the idea of heritage is usually associated with remains of the classical past, I was very interested in examining the processes through which peoples' ways of life, beliefs, and traditions were recognised as heritage, and what this meant in terms of cultural identity and preservation. The museum, as a cultural archive but also a social space experiencing important transformations over the last decades, emerged as the ideal site to explore these questions. My research journey that started in 2003 took me from Greece, France, and the UK to New Zealand, Vanuatu, the United States, and more recently Qatar and Thailand. The chapters that follow narrate this journey and present the findings of my research with the hope of contributing to the growing academic dialogue on intangible heritage, but also to the work of students and professionals in the fields of heritage and museums.

Many people and institutions have contributed to my research over the last years. I would like to thank the State Scholarships Foundation of Greece, the University of London Central Research Fund, the UCL Graduate School, and the UCL Institute of Archaeology for financing my research. My sincere thanks go to Dr. Beverley Butler for her guidance, endless support, and critical feedback over the last eight years, and Dr. Graeme Were for his thoughtful recommendations and encouragement. At the Institute I am thankful to Prof. Stephen Shennan and Judy Medrington for their continued support and to the Institute's Publications Committee, in particular to Marion Cutting. For feedback, advice, and discussions that were central to the development of many ideas expressed in the next pages I wish to thank Prof. Michael Rowlands, Prof. Nick Stanley, Kathy Tubb, Prof. Patrick Boylan, Prof. Maurice Godelier, Dr. Daphne Voudouri, Dr. Alexander Bauer, Dr. Paul Basu, Dr. Alexandra Denes, Dr. Paritta Chalermpow Koanantakool, Prof. Peter Davis, Dr. Christina Kreps, Dr. Kate Hennessy, and Dr. Michelle Stefano. I would also like to thank Mitch Allen, Stefania Van Dyke, and Stefania De Petris at Left Coast Press.

Special thanks also go to those who enabled and facilitated my research in New Zealand, Vanuatu, UK, France, and the United States. In New Zealand, I am grateful to the late Seddon Bennington, Aaron Brown, Stephanie Gibson, Arapata Hakiwai, Erana Hemmingsen, Karl Johnstone, Kolokesa Mahina-Tuai, Sean Mallon, Eric Ngan, Rhonda Paku, Roma Potiki, Turei Reedy, Lucy Arthur, Maruhaeremuri Sterling, Awhina Tamarapa, and Megan Tamati-Quennell. In Vanuatu, my thanks go to Ralph Regenvanu, Marcelin Abong, Jean Tarisesei, Martha Kaltal, Jacob Kapere, Jimmy Takaronga Kuautonga, Eddie Hinge Virare, and Lissant Bolton. In Washington, Richard W. West, José Barreiro, Howard Bass, Karen Fort, Ann McMullen, Jim Pepper Henry, John Beaver, Terry Snowball, and Gaby Tayac received me warmly at the National Museum of the American Indian. Special thanks to Patricia Nietfeld at the Cultural Resources Center in Suitland and Johanna Gorelick at the George Gustav Heye Center in New York. My thanks also go to Richard Kurin, James Early, Atesh Sonneborn, Olivia Cadavel, and Diane N'Diaye at the Smithsonian Center for Folklife and Cultural Heritage in Washington. At the Horniman, I would like to thank Janet Vitmayer, Margaret Birley, Louise Bacon, Andrew Willshire, and Victoria Brightman. Special thanks to Hassan Arero. In Paris, my thanks go to Stéphane Martin, Philippe Peltier, Christine Hemmet, Anne-Christine Taylor, Hélène Joubert, Madeleine Leclair, Sophie Mercier, and Emmanuel Désveaux for sharing their opinions about their work at the musée du quai Branly. At UNESCO, I would like to thank Katerina Stenou, Rieks Smeets, Cesar Moreno, David Stehl, Isabel Vinson, Tim Curtis, and Mania Yiannarakis.

I would also like to thank the postgraduate cultural heritage and museum studies students and undergraduate anthropology students for the stimulating discussions we have had in the last years.

Finally, this book would have not been written without the unfailing support and love of my family, friends, and above all my husband, Michael.

Chapter 1

Intangible Heritage and the Museum

Preserving material objects is not the only way to conserve a heritage.

—David Lowenthal (1985:384)

In October 2003, after almost three decades of international negotiations on how best to protect folk cultures and traditions (see Seitel 2001; Aikawa 2004, 2009), the General Conference of UNESCO adopted the Convention for the Safeguarding of Intangible Cultural Heritage. Largely drawing on Japanese and Korean post-Second World War laws as well as the structure and terminology of the 1972 Convention Concerning the Protection of World Cultural and Natural Heritage, the 2003 Convention brought intangible heritage into the international scene. In so doing it shifted interest from historical monuments, archaeological sites, and natural parks to living traditions, embodied skills, and oral expressions. Informed by an anthropological understanding of culture, this new concept of intangible heritage has come to encompass all those practices—including rituals, tales, performing arts, crafts, and ceremonies—that are transmitted orally from the past and act as symbols of identity in the present.

Thinking institutionally about cultural heritage in terms not only of a sensu stricto materiality but also of human knowledge, belief, and practice has been widely heralded as a more inclusive and people-oriented approach (see Matsuura 2004; Smith and Akagawa 2009). This has been further expressed in the widespread use of the term on an international level, but also in the active endorsement of the 2003 Convention and relevant programmes by states that had not been well represented in the World Heritage Convention of 1972—an instrument that has often been criticised as Eurocentric (Munjeri 2004, 2009). But the emergence of intangible heritage in the global scene has raised complex questions: Is the institutionalisation of culture as intangible heritage a hegemonic and universalising project? Does intangible heritage mask the bureaucratisation

Intangible Heritage and the Museum: New Perspectives on Cultural Preservation by Marilena Alivizatou, 15–26. ©2012 Left Coast Press, Inc. All rights reserved.

or "thingification" (Byrne 2009:229) of peoples' lifeways? How is the dichotomy between the tangible and the intangible to be approached?

The aim of this book is to provide a critical examination of intangible heritage on both conceptual and practical levels. To this end, my work explores intangible heritage not only in the international sphere of cultural diplomacy, but also, via a more grounded approach, in the complexities of twenty-first-century heritage and museum practice. This is pursued through multi-sited fieldwork research (Marcus 1995) in order to investigate local negotiations of intangible heritage in specific museums and heritage institutions across the North and South. These are the National Museum of New Zealand Te Papa Tongarewa in Wellington, the Vanuatu Cultural Centre in Port Vila, the National Museum of the American Indian in Washington and New York, the Horniman Museum in London and the musée du quai Branly in Paris. Discussed widely as contemporary spaces of cultural representation and museological innovation (see Simpson 1996; Bolton 2003; Kreps 2003; Shelton 2003; Message 2006; Clifford 2007; de l'Etoile 2007a, 2007b; Phillips 2007; Price 2007, 2010), these five "zones of contact and conflict" (see Clifford 1997) provide unique insights to the above questions.

At the centre of this book is an examination of cultural preservation: the effort to protect, conserve, or safeguard the traces of past for the future, which constitutes a key narrative of modernity (Lowenthal 1985, 1998; Nora 1989; Smith 2006). Inherent in this is an underlying notion of authenticity, which implies that cultural heritage, either in the form of buildings, objects, or oral expressions, is an original manifestation of the past in the present and therefore needs to be preserved intact for future generations. This is particularly problematic for the area of oral culture, as it hints at processes of cultural stagnation and ossification. One of the objectives of my research then is to critically examine the idea of cultural preservation and explore new approaches to heritage authenticity and cultural transmission. By examining modern preservationism in the context of erasure and transformation, I argue for a more fluid and flexible understanding of culture, heritage, and traditions. The idea is to think beyond concepts of decay, salvage, and loss and engage with cultural change as a new heritage value. To this end, chapter 2 brings under scrutiny recent debates in heritage studies, public archaeology, and anthropology to problematise further the idea of a heritage of destruction and change.

A parallel aim is to question the idea of the museum as a repository of material culture, a space dedicated to the preservation and display of artefacts and specimens. Engaging with intangible heritage calls for a people-centred museology and provides a conceptual framework for rethinking contemporary museum work and the relation between the tangible and the intangible (see Kurin 2004a, 2004b; Svensson 2008; Kreps 2009). Whilst historically museums have been seen as temples of knowledge primarily concerned with collections of objects (Bennett 1995; Duncan 1995), a more recent critique has argued for a museological humanisation and civic reorientation (Kreps 2003, 2009; Ames 2006; Butler 2006; Smith 2006). In this context, intangible heritage emerges as a parallel framework for reimagining the museum, its collections and role as a public institution. This raises the issue of community or participatory museology (Karp et al. 1992; Peers and Brown 2003; Watson 2007), and brings up ideas of cultural inclusion and dialogue that are further problematised in the context of the five museums.

In the last decades, a period defined by Ruth Phillips as "the second museum age" (2005), museums have emerged as public and dialogic spaces, where practices of representation and interpretation are carefully planned and often shared. The participation of community groups in museum work has meant that oral histories and traditional knowledge and beliefs are gradually incorporated in official museum narratives, until recently the exclusive product of scientific explanations by museum professionals (see Cruickshank 1992; Whiteley 2002). As a consequence, the didactic voice of the modernist museum is replaced by notions of multivocality and dialogue that challenge ideas of linearity and objectivity (see Hooper-Greenhill 2000:151–153). Yet this hints at a new exclusivity inherent in the power of self-representation, as groups that had historically been marginalised are now actively involved in museum work (see Zimmerman 2010). Chapter 3, for example, explores issues of community empowerment in Te Papa Tongarewa's Maori and community galleries. Similarly, chapter 5 investigates the narrative of the inaugural exhibitions produced by twenty-four Native American tribes at the National Museum of the American Indian. The celebratory tone of many of these exhibitions, combining local lore, oral history, and traditional belief, is increasingly criticised as unscientific and even propagandistic, hinting that grassroots voices of intangible heritage are often entangled in political narratives. This then invites a more critical examination of the relationship between museums and their communities (see Ames 1999; Boast 2011).

Since the adoption of the 2003 Convention, intangible heritage has been the subject of a significant academic dialogue (see Ruggles and Silverman 2009; Smith and Akagawa 2009; Lira and Amoeda 2010). Under scrutiny has come not only its emergence in the context of UNESCO (Nas 2002; Hafstein 2004, 2009; Alivizatou 2007, 2008a), but also its broader impact on actual cultural practices and practitioners (de Jong 2007; Hafstein and Bendix 2009). Valdimar Hafstein, for example, has examined its intellectual origins in folklore studies, anthropology research, and intellectual property debates, but also in the cultural preservation framework of Japan and Korea (2004). One of Hafstein's main arguments is that selection and exclusion are key characteristics of intangible heritage. In resonance with Barbara Kirshenblatt-Gimblett (2004), he underlines the role of modern capitalism and cultural economies of tourism in the construction of a global context for intangible heritage (Hafstein 2009). Michael Brown has further problematised the 2003 Convention in relation to the broader debate on the ownership of cultural property (2005). Underlining the paradoxical situation of protecting local cultural expressions through international safeguarding measures, he raises the question of whether intangible heritage is a "resource of all of humanity" or belongs to its community of origins (2005:49), an idea that has also been discussed by Ferdinand de Jong in his examination of the heritagisation of the Kankurang masquerade in Senegal and Gambia (2007). Critical of UNESCO's proclamation of the masquerade in 2005 as a Masterpiece of the Oral and Intangible Heritage of Humanity, de Jong explores how this new regime of visibility impacts on the actual performance by local communities. His critique forms part of a broader literature that problematises the impact of global heritage processes and is further explored in chapter 2 (see also Byrne 1995; Kreps 2003; Smith 2006; Butler 2007; de Jong and Rowlands 2007; Labadi and Long 2010; Joy 2011).

Building on this relatively recent academic dialogue, my research examines intangible heritage in the context of contemporary museology. As museums are moving towards a more dynamic engagement with communities and extend their activities beyond the preservation and display of collections, intangible heritage is gradually adopted as a new field of action. This creates space to examine how different museums engage with the intangible in their practice and how they perceive their preservation role with regards to living and not only material culture.

A MUSEOLOGY OF INTANGIBLE HERITAGE

Although intangible heritage is a relatively recent concept, museums and cultural bodies have long been concerned with the preservation of oral traditions and folk cultures. "The break marked by the disappearance of peasant culture" (Nora 1989:7) that followed the Industrial Revolution in nineteenth-century Western Europe meant that ways of life embedded in tradition and old custom were gradually abandoned. It is this break between past and present, the separation between the old and the new, that led to the foundation of modern sites of memory, spaces, events, and objects acting as mechanisms that perpetuate and preserve the memory of the past (Nora 1989). These sites of memory or *lieux de mémoire*—museums, archives, parades, registers, and commemorative ceremonies—marked the rise of modern historical consciousness, a collective awareness that the past is a separate entity and that certain aspects of it ought to be preserved for the future. New institutions were thus gradually founded to keep the memory of the past alive. The birth of the public museum in nineteenth-century Europe and North America is part of this project (Hooper-Greenhill 1992; Bennett 1995).

However, the museology of the past did not include only objects and specimens, but also broader lifeways and traditions. Skansen, in Sweden, is widely regarded as one of the first in a series of open-air museums built before the First World War to present, on the one hand, vernacular buildings and farmsteads and, on the other, rural and traditional ways of life, cultural practices, festivities, music, and crafts (Oliver 2001). Artur Hazelius (1833–1901), the founder of Skansen, lived at a time when large parts of the rural population of Sweden were moving to industrial zones and urban areas, and it was felt that Swedish peasant and folk culture (tangible and intangible) was disappearing. Skansen—with its rebuilt cottages and houses; the associated objects, furniture, and tools; but also the folk celebrations, festivities, and demonstrations—expressed a romanticised version of the past that was a marker of national identity and could provide future generations with a sense of roots and continuity. In this sense, it was the forerunner of open-air museums, institutions not only concerned with the preservation of artefacts and treasures, but also with the broader cultural and social environment in which they exist, including a sense of place and locality.

The idea that the past is embedded in space and cultural practice took further shape in the mid-twentieth century with the development of "ecomuseums." Based on similar ideas of identity as being rooted in place and tradition, the rise of ecomuseums in France saw the transformation of old buildings and sites and deserted industrial facilities into cultural spaces concerned with preserving the memory of local communities. Conceptualised by Georges Henri Rivière, the propagator of the French *nouvelle muséologie* (1989), and museologist Hugues de Varine, ecomuseums shifted interest from museums for objects to museums for communities by emphasising the institution's social responsibility and connection with local groups (Davis 1999). In 1971 the first ecomuseum was founded in Creusot-Montceau, in the French department of Bourgogne (see http://www.ecomusee-creusot-montceau.com). A central aim of the project was to connect different areas of the same territory and celebrate its nineteenth-century industrial past (Gob and Drouguet 2003:39). Of value were not so much the relics of the disused industrial sites as the spirit of the place, the habits, customs, and traditions of the community; in other words, expressions that bridge the tangible-intangible dichotomy (Boylan 2006). A fundamental prerequisite for the success of an ecomuseum in France was, thus, the participation of the local community that would sustain and inform its practice (Gob and Drouguet 2003:40). The development of ecomuseums in France and gradually around the world can be seen as a response to a museum practice inherited from the nineteenth century and primarily concerned with the display of collections for urban or elite audiences (see Bourdieu and Darbel 1989). In this context, several local museums and cultural centres representing Indigenous, ethnic, or minority groups were founded in the latter part of the twentieth century to represent communities that had been excluded from larger and more prominent cultural establishments (see Karp et al. 1992; James 2005).

The focus on community engagement and participation has been further reflected in the work museums undertook to connect with a wider and previously marginalised public. Shifting interest from objects to audiences was one of the key themes of the "new museology" movement in the 1990s (Vergo 1989; MacDonald 2006) and a central topic of the agenda on social inclusion (Sandell 2002). Museum and community partnerships vary enormously and may include consultation with local communities, local schools, and religious or ethnic groups as part of wider outreach, education, or exhibition projects (see Karp et al. 1992; Sandel 2002; Watson 2007). A significant part of the literature, however, is particularly concerned with partnerships between museums and what is widely referred to as "source communities" (see Clifford 1997; Peers and Brown 2003), the first owners and makers of museum pieces from outside Europe and for the last century the subject of many museums and exhibits (Ames 1992; Nederveen Pieterse 1997). James Clifford's discussion of the museum as a "contact zone" has been a central theme in negotiating the relationship between museums and Indigenous groups (1997). Talking mostly about encounters between museums and American Indian groups, Clifford notes how museums are being transformed through partnerships with communities and further describes the museum as a site of conflict and negotiation. Similarly, Ruth Phillips, speaking from a Canadian perspective, explains how ideas of negotiation and dialogue are central features of this "second museum age" (2005).

The transformation of late nineteenth- and early twentieth-century museums from authoritative institutions to "contact zones" (Clifford 1997) or "interactive theatres" (Phillips 2005) largely took place within the social and political mobilisations that marked the end of the twentieth century, like the civil rights and the Indigenous peoples movements (Niezen 2003). In the field of heritage and museums, this led for example to the adoption of the Native American Grave Protection and Repatriation Act (NAGPRA) by the U.S. Senate in 1990, or the establishment in 1992 of the Canadian Task Force on museums, which underlined the need to respect and take into consideration the beliefs, opinions, and claims of Native groups, but also led to different controversies surrounding claims for repatriation (Simpson 1996; Hubert and Fforde

2005; Nash and Colwell-Chanthaphonh 2010). The 1992 Draft Declaration on the Rights of Indigenous People by the United Nations, which formed the basis for the development of the 2007 Declaration, further intensified claims of Native groups and communities over land and self-determination, leading several critics to challenge the foundations of Native cultural property arguments (see Kuper 2003).

The above developments had important ramifications in museum work. The participation of Native groups in the international human rights scene brought Indigenous preoccupations and concerns to the fore and led to the establishment of museum-like cultural centres run and funded by Indigenous communities around the world (Mead 1983; Clifford 1988; Stanley 1998, 2007; Hendry 2005; Coody Cooper and Sandoval 2006; Kasarherou 2007). As several critics have argued, most museums established in Africa, Asia, and the Pacific as part of colonial processes had little to do with the preoccupations and interests of local people (see Appadurai and Breckenridge 1992 and Bharucha 2000 for South Asia; Konare 1995 for West Africa; Bolton 2003 for Vanuatu; Kreps 2003 for Indonesia; McCarthy 2007 for New Zealand). With decolonisation, the museum as a colonial construct is gradually reinvented to serve local audiences, often inviting new ways for defining the institution, its functions, and its responsibilities (see Kreps 2011).

Against this backdrop, intangible heritage emerges as a postcolonial narrative of community development. Christina Kreps, for example, has related intangible heritage to the empowerment of Indigenous knowledge and the humanisation of museums (Kreps 2003, 2007, 2009), whereby voices and practices that had been historically overlooked now become central to the development of new museological paradigms of valuing and caring for the past. "Indigenous curation," the preservation and interpretation of Indigenous collections by Indigenous peoples, emerges therefore as an expression of intangible heritage, which ultimately liberates culture from the oppressive, exclusive, and authoritarian articulations of Western museology (see Stanley 1998; Kreps 2003, 2009).

MULTI-SITED RESEARCH: MUSEUM ETHNOGRAPHY

Intangible heritage has thus been related to a postcolonial reinvention of museum practice centred on providing a space for cross-cultural communication. This creates a new context for a museology that is not only about the preservation of collections, but rather more ambitiously is also about the safeguarding of traditional knowledge and the expression of local identity. The question that is raised, then, is how this broad institutional narrative that emerged primarily within the context of global heritage politics is actually translated in contemporary museum practice. In pursuing this global and local investigation, a more grounded ethnographic approach reveals further negotiations. The relatively recent trend of museum and heritage ethnographies (see Price 1989, 2007; Handler and Gable 1997; MacDonald 2002; Kreps 2003; Basu 2007; Butler 2007; Joy 2011; Bhatti 2012) has provided new approaches to the investigation of museum and heritage cultures. Researchers increasingly employ ethnographic methods, such as interviews and participant observation, to investigate closely the operations of heritage institutions and peoples. Often their aim is to analyse the concerns and values of different constituencies and propose a critical reading of more dominant narratives.

Drawing on different sources, including museum policies, curatorial work, exhibitions, collections, activities, and public events, this study investigates the multiple translations of intangible heritage in contemporary museum practice as recorded during my research, from 2006 to 2008. This required a complete immersion in the museum environment, public indoor and outdoor spaces, exhibitions, museum theatres, shops and cafeterias, collection stores, conservation labs, staff offices, and meeting rooms. Overall data consist of transcribed interviews conducted between 2006 and 2008 or notes from unrecorded discussions (in cases where informants opposed the use of voice recorder), photographs of displays, panels, labels, video clips of events and performances, field notes with recollections of specific stories, as well as a variety of museum ephemera such as brochures, maps, leaflets, and publications of limited circulation.

Conducting fieldwork research in different museum localities and against UNESCO's global heritage framework has been an exercise in multi-sited ethnographic research, a methodology that is increasingly used in the social sciences (Marcus 1995; Hannerz 1998, 2003). For Marcus, this is a "mobile ethnography" that is "designed around chains, paths, threads, conjunctions, or juxtapositions of locations," and "in which the ethnographer establishes some form of literal, physical presence, with an explicit, posited logic of association or connection among sites" (1995:105). As such, it is "an exercise in mapping terrain" rather than a "holistic representation" that does not work in "the dualistic 'them–us' frame of conventional ethnography, but requires considerable more nuancing and shading" (1995:99–100). As opposed to single-sited ethnography, in which the researcher is located for an extended period of time in one easily definable place, multi-sited research is "mobile and multiply situated" (1995:102). As such, for many "something of the mystique and reality of conventional fieldwork is lost" (1995:100).

In conducting multi-sited fieldwork, the aim is not to write an all-encompassing account of each of the five museums,[1] but instead trace how each institution engages with the idea of intangible heritage and its safeguarding. Taking forward Marcus's call to "follow the people," "follow the thing," "follow the metaphor," and "follow the plot, story or allegory" (1995:106–109), I follow intangible heritage and trace its different negotiations from the international sphere to the local context of museum practice across the North and the South.

A further characteristic of multi-sited research that is particularly relevant is the idea of comparison. For Marcus, multi-sited research is "a revival of comparative study . . . a research design of juxtapositions in which the global is collapsed into and made an integral part of parallel, related local situations rather than something monolithic or external to them" (1995:102). As such, conducting multi-sited research allows for the examination of the global concept of intangible heritage in different museological settings and narratives. This would, in a sense, provide further methodological tools for building on the idea of "comparative museology" as "the systematic study and comparison of museological forms and behaviour in diverse cultural settings" (Kreps 2003:4).

MUSEUM LOCALITIES

Rather than prioritising a West versus non-West museological divide, this book explores the idea of the twenty-first-century museum as an institution that grapples with multiple constituencies and engages with calls for a reinvented museology. The five organisations I studied in Europe, North America, and the Pacific often expressed different museological and disciplinary traditions. As was stressed in interviews at the quai Branly, each museum is "a culture in itself," entangled in different historical, political, and social webs. It is those webs that provide parallel vantage points for thinking about intangible heritage both as global narrative and as local tool.

The five museums are defined by different cultural, political, and social contexts. Yet one common characteristic is that they are all embedded in the colonial project and in the rise of anthropology as an academic field of study in the late nineteenth and early twentieth centuries (Stocking 1985; Ames 1992, 2006; Thomas 1994). As a consequence, they care for similar types of collections that belong to the broad category of ethnographic artefacts.[2] In a sense they could be described as museums of ethnographic collections, which traditionally fall under the disciplinary remit of anthropology and, as was stressed in one of my interviews in Paris, are "in the business of representing other cultures" (see also Ames 1992; Shelton 2000; de l'Etoile 2007a). During fieldwork, however, it became evident that the label "ethnographic" is increasingly contested. On the one hand, as stressed by informants in the USA and New Zealand, it reinforces colonial stereotypes, rooted in the dichotomy between the self and the other (Fabian 1983), as well as the objectification and essentialisation of the cultures on display. Moreover, as was argued in Paris, it equates the museum with a particular discipline, and as a consequence it is often didactic and monodimensional in its narrative.

Chapter 3 for example examines the controversies surrounding the National Museum of New Zealand Te Papa Tongarewa (Te Papa). Opened in 1998 on the Wellington Waterfront, the museum is celebrated as an embodiment of the country's bicultural partnership between Indigenous Maori and subsequent European settlers (*Pakeha*). Te Papa features prominently in the museological literature (see Henare 2004, 2005; Williams 2005; Message 2006) as a museum that prioritises the narration of stories over the display of artefacts. However, the museum's new inclusivity of Maori traditions and beliefs has not been uncontested. Building on the fieldwork I conducted in New Zealand in 2007, this chapter examines how the partnership between the museum and the diverse ethnic communities of New Zealand informs local understandings of intangible heritage and provides a space to examine the articulations of a bicultural museology.

In chapter 4 the analysis shifts to the Vanuatu Cultural Centre (VCC) in Port Vila, the capital of the Melanesian island state of Vanuatu. This is an institution that has been transformed from a small museum founded by colonial officials in the 1950s into a national cultural establishment, following the country's independence in 1980. Today it administers not only typical museum practices such as collections care and exhibitions, but also international research and community development (Bolton 2003, 2006, 2007). The VCC's mission to preserve ni-Vanuatu traditional culture and its calls for economic, social, and political development offer a critical perspective for examining local uses and negotiations of intangible heritage. The VCC is unique for choosing to preserve not only material culture but also living cultural expressions, often dubbed as intangible heritage, through grassroots projects of community participation and research. In this sense, the proclamation by UNESCO in 2003 of the *sandroing*, a local practice of writing or drawing on the sand, as a Masterpiece of Intangible Heritage raises further issues about local engagements with the global intangible heritage terminology.

The third museum examined in this study is the National Museum of the American Indian (NMAI). This is a multi-sited museum with three buildings: on the Washington Mall, in Suitland, Maryland, and in New York's lower Manhattan.[3] In preparation since 1989, the NMAI is celebrated today as a living memorial to the Native American cultures of the Western hemisphere that throughout the European colonisation of the Americas were fought, persecuted, and often violently destroyed (West 2000). Being conceived of as a "Native place," the museum was built in accordance with customary beliefs and knowledge systems, and the inaugural exhibitions were planned in partnership with community elders and tribal representatives (Volkert et al. 2004). The idea of founding a "living museum" meant looking beyond nineteenth-century collections of Native artefacts and engaging instead with the contemporary reality of changing tribal identity, celebrating the survival of Indigenous people and the flourishing of contemporary cultures. The aim of this chapter, then, is to explore intangible heritage in the context of Native American politics of recognition (see Taylor 1992) and reflect on the challenges of participatory paradigms.

The final two sites are the Horniman Museum in South London and the musée du quai Branly (MQB) in Paris (see chapters 6 and 7). Although rooted in the same nineteenth-century colonial museology that gave rise to the modern museum—with very similar types of collections like nineteenth- and early twentieth-century African masks, Buddhist sculptures, Native American feathered headdresses, and Melanesian carvings[4]—each of these museums has adopted different strategies regarding the making of exhibitions, the collaboration with local communities, and the interpretation of collections. While the Horniman Museum is largely defined by its history, the vision of its founder, and a strong anthropological lens, the musée du quai Branly is very much based on the erasure of its museological past. What they have in common, however, is the fact that they both acknowledge artefact collections as their first port of call. A central question to explore here is how the Horniman and the MQB engage with intangible heritage in response to the legacies of colonial and collection-centred museology.

The Horniman Museum opened in 1901 as a public museum bequeathed to the people of London, in terms of both site and collections, by tea merchant Frederick J. Horniman (1835–1906). Its main collections are ethnographic[5] and archaeological objects, natural history specimens, and music instruments, as well as living animals in the outdoor animal enclosure. In the last hundred years that it has been open to the public, the museum also served as a public space for the presentation of controversial anthropological theories like evolutionism (Coombes 1994; Shelton 2000). Yet in the last decades and since its centennial inauguration in 2002, the Horniman has ventured into new territories by establishing partnerships with different ethnic and diaspora communities in the UK to realise exhibitions and interpret collections. The tensions between Frederick J. Horniman's gift and the challenges of inclusive museum work emerge as central foci of chapter 6.

The musée du quai Branly opened its doors on Seine's left bank in June 2006. A political project conceived by former French president Jacques Chirac, it became the subject of debate even before its opening primarily because of the decision to present artefacts from Africa, Oceania, the Americas, and to a lesser extent Asia as works of art rather than ethnographically contextualised objects—a decision that resulted in the intensification of the art-artefact debate and the creation of two opposing camps, anthropologists and "aesthetes" (Dupaigne 2006; de l'Etoile 2007a, 2007b). Aiming to break away from traditional museum anthropology and from the discourse of its predecessor, the *Musée de l'Homme*, the MQB has been conceptualised as a "dialogue of cultures," a versatile and multifunctional museum with permanent and temporary exhibitions, public debates, cultural performances, and an open university, all in a state-of-the-art building designed by French architect Jean Nouvel. However, the MQB has also been criticised as firmly rooted in Eurocentric museology with little or no concern for including alternative discourses and voices in its narrative (Clifford 2007; Price 2007, 2010; Alivizatou 2008a; Desvallées 2008). Taking forward issues of participation and cultural preservation, chapter 7 explores how the museum's activities and narratives provide a context for discussing intangible heritage in relation to a new European ethnographic museology.

In presenting the complexities of these five microenvironments, the book examines intangible heritage on the global and local as well as the intellectual and operational levels. Within each museum, understandings of intangible heritage are much informed by institutional thinking and early twenty-first-century social and political concerns with globalisation, multi- and interculturalism, and recognition. Whilst preservation is a key motive defining UNESCO's approach to intangible heritage, other negotiations emerge in local settings reflecting concerns around survival and change. By proposing a framework that goes beyond a global preservation scheme, this book makes a further call for a multidimensional examination of intangible heritage as something that is bound up in the interrelations of tradition, modernity, cultural change, and authenticity.

Chapter 2

Global Preservation and Beyond

> In premodern times, people didn't speak of "identity" and "recognition"—
> not because people didn't have (what we call) identities, or because these
> didn't depend on recognition—but rather because these were then too
> unproblematic to be thematized as such.
>
> —Charles Taylor (1992:35)

In the last decade, UNESCO-driven projects, like the 2003 Convention for the Safeguarding of Intangible Cultural Heritage or the Proclamation of Masterpieces (1997–2005), have expanded the notion of universal heritage, with a significant impact on policies and ideas about tradition and knowledge from the past (Nas 2002; Deacon et al. 2004; Kurin 2004a, 2004b; Brown 2005; Alivizatou 2008a; Smith and Akagawa 2009). UNESCO's activities on intangible heritage cannot be separated from the broader intellectual and normative framework of cultural preservation articulated in the course of the previous centuries (Gruber 1959; Lowenthal 1985, 1998; Smith 2006). A key aim of this chapter is to problematise this global framework of cultural preservation with regards to the transmission of embodied skills and cultural practices. Furthering the examination of intangible heritage in the context of international cultural protection, I introduce the idea of erasure, the creative interplay of heritage destruction and transformation, as a way for exploring alternative paradigms of cultural transmission.

The nineteenth century is widely regarded as the time when the protection and conservation of cultural patrimony emerged as a social, scholarly, and scientific pursuit (Lowenthal 1985; Harvey 2001; Smith 2006). Pierre Nora's study of the *lieux de mémoire*, the official and often state-sanctioned sites of memory, in the form of museums, archives, and commemorative events (1989:11–12) further relates the rise of the modern preservation ethos to the consolidation of nation states, the growth of industry, and the development of science. The earlier Renaissance fascination with the ancient world was expressed in the systematic study of the material culture of the past through the collection of ancient objects and artworks and the excavation of sites. Modern archaeological thought gradually grew out of those nineteenth-century romantic ideas of rediscovering the past and its treasures (see Trigger 2006). At the same time, the destruction of older buildings and ancient monuments caused by processes of industrial development called for the establishment of protection and preservation mechanisms for the cultural patrimonies of Western European nations (Choay 2001; Smith 2006).

Modern preservationism saw the emergence of new types of scholarly activity. Just as early archaeologists had been concerned with the discovery and preservation of ancient objects and sites, nineteenth-century ethnologists and anthropologists were concerned with the discovery, study, and documentation of traditional and tribal communities much within the context of European expansionism and colonialism (see Thomas 1994; Gosden 1999). From the late eighteenth century, romantic ideas around the *Volk*, the peoples and their customs—embodied for instance in the work of Johann Gottfried Herder (1744–1803)—underlined the links between culture, region, and identity. This conception provided an intellectual impetus for the systematic study of human cultures, Indigenous groups, tribal communities around the world, and also of folk peasantry in rural areas of Europe. The need to study and document local traditions, customs, and languages emerged as the moral duty of a new generation of social scientists tasked with the mission to document the human diversity that was bound to disappear in the face of modernity. During the late nineteenth and early twentieth centuries, scholars and amateur ethnologists raced around the world to discover and document human cultures,[1] in a practice that has subsequently been labelled as "salvage ethnography" (see Gruber 1959; Clifford 1988; Penny 2002).

The first institutional efforts to preserve national patrimonies and salvage cultures took shape in the nineteenth century with the establishment of special groups and committees and the adoption of legal measures, like for example the establishment of the French Comité Historique in the 1830s, the adoption of the British Ancient Monuments Act in 1882 (Smith 2006:19), and the foundation of the Ethnological Society of London in 1843 and of the British Folklore Society in 1878. The rationale behind these efforts was that rapid processes of economic development and industrialisation were threatening the material remains of the past or peoples' vernacular culture and traditions, and that it was therefore necessary to preserve them through regulations, study, and scientific examination. Inherent in the above was the understanding that the study and protection of the past—tangible or intangible—would serve the public benefit by creating and safeguarding national symbols and emblems of identity. Whilst these processes of heritage designation initially took shape primarily at the national level in Europe and North

America, by the first decades of the twentieth century issues of heritage preservation were also raised on an international level, mainly because of the consequences of international warfare.

In 1931 the first major international conference on architectural conservation took place in Athens, as a response to the loss and destruction of monuments and sites during the First World War. This resulted in the Athens Charter for the Restoration of Historic Monuments, a document drafted by Le Corbusier (Charles Edouard Jeanneret 1887–1965) that laid the foundation of the international heritage preservation movement (http://www.international.icomos.org). At the heart of the Charter were provisions for a legal framework for the protection of ancient monuments, the introduction of scientific rules and principles in restoration processes, and the establishment of national inventories of monuments and sites (ICOMOS 1931). After the Second World War this movement would culminate with its own distinct ethos in the foundation of the United Nations and its Education, Scientific and Cultural Organisation (UNESCO), an institution that has played a central role in the articulation of cultural preservation globally.

THE ROLE OF UNESCO

UNESCO is a member of the United Nations, and like its mother organisation was founded after the Second World War. Based in Paris, but with offices around the world, it is run by the General Council of its about two hundred member states, whose decision making is facilitated by the organisation's multinational Secretariat. Since its foundation, UNESCO has been concerned with the adoption of legal measures and the implementation of programmes in the areas of education, science, culture, and communication. In principle the largest share from the contributions of its member states has been mostly directed towards developing countries. This chapter focuses on the Cultural Heritage section of UNESCO, founded in the late 1960s. The strict segmentation that exists between the different operational areas facilitates this rather monodimensional examination of the organisation's work.

Following the Second World War and the ensuing destruction and loss of life, international bodies increasingly sought the establishment of legal measures for the prevention of similar atrocities. The protection of cultural patrimony, which was crucial in providing a sense of national and cultural identity and continuity, became a key priority (Conil-Lacoste 1994). In the early 1950s the development of a legal portfolio was initiated with the Convention for the Protection of Cultural Property in the Event of Armed Conflict in 1954 (ICOMOS 1954), a document that recognised the need to set international mechanisms for the protection of built heritage and cultural artefacts during warfare.

In 1970 UNESCO adopted the Convention on the Means of Prohibiting and Preventing the Illicit Import, Export and Transfer of Cultural Property (UNESCO 1970), which addressed the issue of the illegal traffic in moveable cultural property. Two years later the international organisation adopted the Convention Concerning the Protection of the World Cultural and Natural Heritage (UNESCO 1972), which has played a fundamental role in the definition and demarcation of world heritage. It was with this document that the term *heritage* replaced the term *property*, and the idea of *outstanding universal value* was introduced in the global preservation movement.

The 1972 Convention was adopted a few years after the first major UNESCO campaign in the field of heritage preservation regarding the relocation of the Nubian monuments to Abu Simbel in Egypt. Egyptian monumental sculptures were threatened with immersion by the construction of the Aswan High Dam and the creation of Lake Nasser, and relocation was considered at the time as the only way to guarantee their survival. Alarmed by the potential loss of the monuments, UNESCO mobilised the international community, both diplomatic and scientific, towards the protection of the antiquities. Eventually, the successful titanic relocation was instrumental in the foundation of the idea of world heritage (Hassan 2007), a cultural patrimony belonging not only to specific nations, but also to the entire humanity and future generations. The Egyptian campaign indeed led to the foundation of the World Heritage Centre, a UNESCO-based organisation specifically charged with monitoring the preservation of designated universal cultural heritage sites, monuments, and buildings.

It is important to mention here the influence on the World Heritage Convention of the 1964 International Charter for the Restoration and Conservation of Monuments and Sites (Venice Charter). The Venice Charter was written by archaeologists, conservators, and other heritage scientists, and underlined the heritage value of monuments as inherent in "the full richness of their authenticity" (ICOMOS 1964). *Authenticity* was thus one of the keywords of the 1972 Convention (McBryde 1997; Cleere 2001; Munjeri 2004); according to its Operational Guidelines, it could be located in the monument's materials, workmanship, design, and setting (UNESCO 1972). In addition to the different criteria that monuments and sites were obliged to meet in order to be inscribed on the World Heritage List, they also needed to pass the "test of authenticity" (McBryde 1997:94). This was a detailed examination, carried out mainly by international experts, architects, art historians or archaeologists working in partnership with ICOMOS.[2]

Based on this history, it is not surprising that by 2001 more than half of the total inscriptions on the List were found in Europe (Cleere 2001:25)

Jolly 1994; Stanley 1998; Nas 2002; Lindholm 2008:39–51). The transformation of cultural expressions from community rituals to tourist spectacles is often viewed as inauthentic or fake. In a sense, although never mentioned in the official documents, authenticity is very much present in the intangible heritage discourse. Concerns for the undermining of the authenticity of intangible heritage can be read between the lines of the 2003 Convention and the Proclamation (1997–2005). Fears of acculturation, commercialisation, or folklorisation, for example, reveal an institutional will to protect intangible heritage from the threats of modernity, suggesting that the latter will harm original, authentic, and uncontaminated traditions.

This hints at another paradox characterising the UNESCO's approach to intangible heritage: while acknowledging that intangible heritage is living and constantly changing, the normative framework of UNESCO is designed in such a way as to impede its modernity-engendered transformation. In a way, the UNESCO approach implies that tradition and modernity cannot go together, as the latter impairs the authenticity of the first. Similarly, by acknowledging that traditions are rooted in a particular community, that they have not changed over the course of time, and that they are still practiced as they used to, the Proclamation favours a particular type of "authentic" cultural phenomena, described as "marginalised" (Handler in Nas 2002:144) or "preindustrial, folkloric traditions" (Brown 2005:47) as opposed to mass cultural practices.

INTANGIBLE HERITAGE AND THE INVENTION OF TRADITION

The examination of the making of intangible heritage by UNESCO points at different gaps, paradoxes, and controversies. Heritage theorists and practitioners have problematised the wider implications of the entire initiative, with the major source of concern being the institutionalisation of culture and peoples' ways of life. For Barbara Kirshenblatt-Gimblett, for example, intangible heritage is as a "metacultural production." As she explains,

> while persistence in old life ways may not be economically viable and may well be inconsistent with economic development and with national ideologies, the valorization of those life ways as heritage (and integration of heritage into economies of cultural tourism) is economically viable, consistent with economic development theory, and can be brought into line with national ideologies of cultural uniqueness and modernity. [Kirshenblatt-Gimblett 2004:61]

De Jong's analysis of the Kankurang reveals similar concerns. Governmental and international involvement can have a radical impact on how local communities and practitioners perceive and engage with tradition. Once regarded as "degenerated," only to be subsequently celebrated as national heritage and heritage of humanity, local traditions become entangled in various layers of meaning often serving different motives (see Churchill 2006). This points to the older debate about the invention of tradition (Hobsbawm and Ranger 1983), mobilised here with reference to postcolonial politics of recognition. Marshall Sahlins, for example, observes:

> All of a sudden, everyone got "culture." Australian Aboriginals, Inuit, Easter Islanders, Chambri, Ainu, Bushmen, Kayapo, Tibetans, Ojibway: even peoples whose ways of life were left for dead or dying a few decades ago now demand an indigenous space in a modernizing world under the banner of their "culture." [1999:401]

Examined from this angle, intangible heritage becomes a potent political tool, alternatively viewed as "an ideological smokescreen of more fundamental interests, principally power and greed" (Sahlins 1999:403). In other words, as identity is increasingly defended as a "scarce resource" (Harrison 1999), local groups and communities use it to affirm their place in the international diplomatic arena (Bowen 2000; Kuper 2003; Niezen 2003; Brown 2005). In this sense, by making special reference to "Indigenous communities," the 2003 Convention proves to be a sister document not only to the 1972 Convention, but also to the different international conventions, declarations, and statements regarding cultural diversity (UNESCO 2001, 2005), biological diversity (UNEP 1992), and the rights of Indigenous people (UN 2007). As Michael Rowlands has observed, "the contrast between rainforest conservation, indigeneity, and the transmission of grievance could not be greater, but at another more abstract level, these shade into each other as part of the struggle for existence in the twenty-first century" (2004:223).

The "struggle for existence" and the mobilisation of "culture" as tools for asserting difference and power have long been the subject of critical investigation (see for example Thomas 1997; Brown 1998; Kuper 2003; Lindholm 2008). In a paper entitled "The Making of the Maori: Culture Invention and Its Logic," Alan Hanson (1989) analyses the construction of "Maoriness" in the course of the twentieth century. Based on the assumption that "traditional culture is increasingly recognized as an invention constructed for contemporary purposes," he explores how scholars, government officials, and members of the Maori community have reinvented the idea of the Maori people "to maintain their cultural distinctiveness and to assume a more powerful position in society" (1989:890–891). Revisiting early twentieth-century discussions about the Aryan origins of the Maori, and questioning the late twentieth-century Maori revivalism expressed, for example, in the surge of spirituality accompanying the international exhibition Te Maori (see chapter 3), he seems to suggest that "distortions have been accepted by Maori as authentic to their heritage" in order to serve political agendas (1989:897).

Along similar lines, anthropologists have examined the revival of pre-colonial culture, or *kastom*,[5] in postcolonial Melanesia. In a special issue of the journal *Mankind*, entitled "Reinventing Traditional Culture: The Politics of Kastom in Island Melanesia" (Keesing and Tonkinson 1982), a group of anthropologists problematised the political and ideological use of the term. For example, Tonkinson, writing about Vanuatu, noted how kastom emerged "as a non-European 'grassroots' force exemplifying 'the Melanesian way' as opposed to the 'white man's way'" (1982b:306). In this process it could also "be used internationally to assert a measure of independence and autonomy for a small country in a world dominated by superpowers" (1982b:314).

Reflecting on the development of intangible heritage as a global political tool, Richard Handler has questioned the transformation of cultural practices brought about by preservation measures and the impact of such measures on local recipients (in Nas 2002). Although planned in order to benefit local communities, documentation programmes, inventories, and lists are often confined within a technical framework and moved by political concerns. This suggests that they are frequently entangled in political controversies powered by cultural bureaucrats rather than actual practitioners.

A further problematic issue is the idea of exclusion. Intangible heritage as envisioned by UNESCO seems to include a set of inoffensive cultural phenomena that act as markers of a national or regional identity resisting global forces. For Handler, "the list favors folkloric or marginalised expressions" (in Nas 2002:144), suggesting that contested and contemporary popular cultural expressions or ways of life are not part of the celebrated living heritage of humanity. In addition to leaving out popular, global, and hybrid culture, the intangible heritage discourse creates a problematic relationship between a dominant national and a more marginalised minority heritage. The traditions of religious, ethnic, or cultural minorities are often left out of the official national narrative. As Richard Kurin remarked, "culture defined and selected by national governments may not be the best basis for deliberative and compassionate consideration" (in Nas 2002:145). The involvement of the state in the construction of national narratives turns intangible heritage into an ethnocentric and unproblematic celebration.

But the most controversial point regarding the 2003 Convention is the idea of "safeguarding." For many critics, international and national governmental programmes like archives, lists, databases, and inventories are "oddly reminiscent of early anthropology, which was driven by the conviction that primitive cultures should be documented in their entirety—from basketry techniques and healing arts to kinship systems and religious beliefs—because their extinction was inevitable" (Brown 2005:48).

Although today (and in the context of cultural revival further discussed in chapters 3, 4, and 5) those early anthropological collections are proving to be of great value to the descendants of the peoples studied (see Abil in Speiser 1996[1923]; Herle 2003; Lenz 2004), the methods and techniques employed then and now reveal a tendency towards the objectification, segmentation, and eventual simplification of cultures and ways of life. In this sense, critics talk of cultural decontextualisation, alienation (Nas 2002:139), and fears of "fossilisation" (Brown 2005:54). For many, the bureaucratisation of culture as national intangible heritage will alienate practitioners and eventually transform peoples' lifeways into a sanitised and well-protected reflection of what they used to be (de Jong 2007).

Peter Nas wrote about his experience as reviewer of the candidatures for the first Proclamation of Masterpieces in 2001 in the journal *Current Anthropology* (Nas 2002). After explaining the programme and analysing its contradictions and paradoxes, he argued that the preservation of expressions of intangible heritage could extend beyond the level of national politics and act as inspiration for the development of new identities. For him, "these valuable cultural complexes may play a dominant role in the constitution of a simultaneously globalized and localized world" (2003:143).

As Kirshenblatt-Gimblett has observed, "metacultural productions," lists, masterpieces, and cultural performances are a key part of modern cultural economies (2004:61). What is interesting, then, is to move the debate beyond the ideas of authenticity and endangerment inherent in the "heritagisation" of cultural practices and ways of life, and focus instead on how intangible heritage as a "metacultural" product shapes and expresses contemporary identities in a world where local and global, modern and traditional constituencies are increasingly intertwined. This invites a more flexible and complex approach to intangible heritage, to which I now turn.

INTANGIBLE HERITAGE AND ERASURE

Concerns about cultural authenticity have been at the core of international heritage preservation from the early twentieth century. The development of a professional approach to the conservation and care of the material relics, founded on global scientific principles, set out criteria and guidelines for the valorisation of heritage. These were mostly embodied in the 1964 Venice Charter and the 1972 World Heritage Convention, which aimed to protect and define heritage on a global scale. The age of a monument or a building, the materials used for its construction, the preservation of the traditional setting, and the clear separation between the authentic fabric and the subsequent restorations were important principles that needed to be taken into consideration and respected in modern preservation (ICOMOS 1964). Underlying this approach was a conception of cultural authenticity whereby the true essence and value of monuments, buildings, and artefacts, and the reasons for which they needed to be protected, were primarily bound up with the original fabric, materials, and production techniques, rather than with their use, function, or symbolic meanings. For Laurajane Smith these scientific principles laid the foundation of an "authorised heritage discourse" (2006). Whilst rooted in nineteenth-century ideas of cultural preservation, this authorised discourse has dominated professional understandings of heritage for the largest part of the twentieth century, often overriding more subtle, personal, and subaltern engagement with the past (Butler 2006; Smith 2006).

The above arguments draw on a larger body of critical thinking about the construction of heritage in the twentieth century. Denis Byrne, for example, has problematised the Western-centric and top-down ways in which cultural heritage has been valued and managed internationally, often ignoring local contexts and traditional practices (1991, 1995). Investigating the preservation of Buddhist *stupas* (reliquaries) in Thai monasteries against the backdrop of local religious demands for parts of the monument, he raised the issue of the symbolic meanings and values attached to buildings and sites by local people and religious practitioners (Byrne 1995). If the stupa is not allowed to decay and parts of it to be removed by worshippers and believers, does it lose part of its symbolic meaning and use as an expression of Buddhist heritage? Does the scientific commitment to the preservation of the original and authentic material distort the meanings of a site and alienate local communities and practitioners?

The issue of scientific preservation versus local engagements with cultural heritage becomes particularly poignant in cases in which top-down scientific approaches to cultural preservation are imposed on disenfranchised or minority groups. A controversial case, for example, was the debate in the 1980s surrounding the repainting of Australian Aboriginal rock art in the Kimberley district (Bowdler 1988; Mowaljarlai et al. 1988), and the question of whether descendant communities should be allowed to repaint and retouch the images or whether that would threaten the integrity of the site. For some archaeologists and other scientists, the repainting of the images would destroy important information about past painting practices and decrease the historical and aesthetic values of the old paintings. Yet banning the repainting of the images could lead to the discontinuation of Aboriginal customary practices related to ongoing beliefs and cultural traditions. Living traditions that had survived the European colonisation of Australia would be placed under control and possibly banned.

The tension between the preservation of sites and other alternative and creative uses has been at the core of a new tradition of critical heritage studies (Butler 2007; de Jong and Rowlands 2007). Cornelius Holtorf notes for example the transformative powers of heritage preservation and destruction, arguing that "a certain degree of heritage destruction and loss is not only unavoidable, but can indeed be desirable in order to accommodate fairly as many genuine claims to that heritage as possible" (2006:106). From the dismantling and rebuilding of the Ise Jingu temple in Japan to the "looting" of Buddhist stupas by believers in Thailand and the dismemberment of pieces of the Berlin Wall, Holtorf explores how the destruction of heritage creates alternative ways for relating to the past that often conflict directly with the heritage preservation ethos. Ideas and principles that have become ingrained in modern archaeological and conservation practice, such as the authenticity of heritage, its endangerment, and the benefit of future generations express the values of a scientific community at the expense of other perspectives (Holtorf 2001). It is those other perspectives and engagements with the ancient past and its material relics that a recent critical turn towards "archaeological ethnographies" has striven to uncover (Hamilakis and Anagnostopoulos 2009).

Examining the preservation of objects, sites, and practices from an anthropological perspective raises further questions regarding the dynamics between preservation and destruction. At the core of modern museum work is the safeguarding of collections for future generations (ICOM 2007). Yet in researching the meanings and values associated with the destruction of objects as part of wider social and cultural processes, theorists and researchers have questioned the dominance of modern museological principles (Kreps 2003). Commenting on the possibility of a "new Asian museum" that makes a rupture from Western museum practice, Rustom Bharucha mobilises the "politics of erasure" as a metaphor for "pushing the boundaries of imagination" and effecting "mutations of specific practices" (2000:17–18). For him, "museums need to confront the insularity of their implicit non-trespassing zones, which have denied vast sections of the population, particularly from the minority and immigrant sectors, not merely access to the museum, but the right to interrogate its assumed privileges and reading of history" (2000:19). Bharucha questions the Euro-American museum with its reliance on "the periodisation, classification, and categorisation of its artefacts," and projects the "new Asian museum" as dismantling a "factitious past by exploring new imaginaries" and drawing on ecological principles. These principles relate to erasure, renewal, and impermanence, which ultimately are a "resistance to conservation and commodification" (2000:15–16).

Bharucha offers two examples of "pre-modern" performances that rely on ideas of erasure, renewal, and impermanence. *Kolam* are traditional floor drawings/prayers made by women in South India, and their "entire point lies in the *erasure* of the floor-drawing after it has been completed, following hours of meticulous work" (2000:16). Similarly, he describes the traditional clay modelling of Hindu deities *Durga*, *Kali*, and *Lakshmi* during the *Pujas* in Calcutta. Here too, the figures of goddesses are carefully designed, celebrated with fervour, and worshipped publicly for several days, only to be "unceremoniously tossed into the muddy waters of the Hooghly River" (2000:16) after the celebrations are over. Interestingly, the impermanence of the kolam and the immersion of the figures of the goddesses in the river are acts of erasure that ultimately reveal that the past is alive and recreated in cyclical acts of destruction, renewal, and impermanence.

Subversive acts of cultural preservation via destruction also surround the making and destruction of another set of objects, the funerary effigies from New Ireland in the Western Pacific known as *malanggan*. In her examination of these effigies and of the ceremonies that accompany their use, Susanne Kuechler explains how malanggan are produced, performed, and eventually disposed of by being destroyed, abandoned in the forest, or sold in the art market (2002:1–4). What her analysis reveals is that malanggan do not preserve memories "by virtue of their durability" but rather they "effect remembering in an active and continuously emerging sense as they disappear from view" (2002:7). As she notes, "what appears to matter most is not the circulation of an object, but the recollection of an image" (2002:3).

Kuechler's analysis of malanggan brings to the fore the idea of a "polity of images" (2002:2) as a site of cultural transmission. The power of the image as intellectual property reveals the dynamics at play between the materiality of the artefacts and their performative functions. Once performed and ritually sacrificed, the effigy is disposed of, but "the death of the object leaves behind a named and remembered image . . . recalled from time to time to re-direct ancestral power to the land of the living" (2002:2). Remembering is not inscribed in the materiality of malanggan, but is effected through the images left behind after the objects disappear. Cultural transmission is, thus, enacted not via the conservation of malanggan, but through their destruction. Their value does not lie in the authenticity of the material, but rather in the knowledge, information, or images that are inherent in their materiality and ultimately reside in human thought and memory. As such, malanggan collected and displayed today in museums in Europe and North America are "empty, hollow remains of objects of sacrifice" (Kuechler 2002:8). Their creators chose to get rid of them, since the images left behind after their performance would perpetuate their production.

What emerges is a distinction between heritage as form, embodied in the preservation of objects, buildings, and sites, and heritage as performance or process, embodied in the transmission of broader cultural practices and beliefs. Yet the creative potential of destruction and renewal can be considered in relation not only to physical objects and sites, but also to intangible culture. According to the global movement of heritage preservation, modern processes of economic and technological development threaten the viability of intangible heritage (UNESCO 2003), as local and traditional practices embedded in a sense of place and community are transformed, lose their meanings, and eventually disappear. Destruction here is not part, but rather a threat to heritage as process. But is it?

The creative destruction thesis, which has been part of economic and sociological thought since the writings of Karl Marx, offers an interesting vantage point for considering this question. Reflecting on the impact of capitalism and modernity on markets, labour, and production, creative destruction suggests that growth, innovation, and development often require the destruction of previous and established modes of production (Schumpeter 2010[1942]). Transplanting these ideas in the field of globalisation and culture, economist Tyler Cowen (2002) explores how processes of cross-cultural exchange, the trade of goods and ideas, and the movements of peoples impact on local cultures and practices. Using food, dance, textiles, music, and crafts as examples of cultural creativity, Cowen maintains that "cross-cultural exchange, while it will alter and disrupt each society it touches, will support innovation and creative human energies" (2002:17). Cowen does not always acknowledge the unequal North-South power relations or the disparities between local communities and colonial settlers; nevertheless, his perspective interestingly illustrates how cultural practices flourish and grow through seemingly devastating processes. Amongst other examples, he discusses Navajo weaving as an Indigenous practice that developed through contact with settlers (2002:43–46). The conquest and colonisation of the Americas in the fifteenth and sixteenth centuries had detrimental consequences on Native cultures (Todorov 1999; see also chapter 5 below for its contemporary articulation); yet it also brought different peoples and traditions together and introduced practices that led to innovative creative outputs, like the Navajo rugs. Fabrics and materials for the making of these rugs came from the domestication of sheep, a practice introduced by the Spanish, and various patterns and motifs were influenced by European and settler weaving (Cowen 2002:44; Brown 2004). Cowen questions the notion of pure and authentic traditions and explores how synthesis and renewal are a key part of cultural vitality: in this sense, globalisation is not a threat to cultural distinctiveness, but rather an opportunity for cross-cultural innovation and fertilisation (see also Nederveen-Pieterse 2004).

INTANGIBLE HERITAGE: PRESERVATION OR TRANSFORMATION?

The creative destruction thesis raises interesting questions about the safeguarding of intangible heritage. Inherent in the state-sanctioned preservation of peoples' traditions and ways of life are concerns not only about their fossilisation in space and time, but also about their manipulation for dubious, often political, motivations. On the contrary, ideas of impermanence and erasure suggest that the continuity and vitality of practices and ceremonies can take place outside the context of formal preservationism and through more fluid and unfixed processes. As discussed above, UNESCO has developed a mostly conservationist approach to both tangible and intangible heritage, often treating the past as a pure entity that must be kept safe from the threats of deterioration (in the case of tangible heritage) or globalisation (in the case of intangible heritage). Yet the creative potential of destruction and transformation emerges as a possible alternative framework for negotiating ideas of identity and contemporary engagements with the past. Based on these assumptions, the next chapters drill into the practice of five museums and heritage organisations across the North and South in order to further investigate how the global narrative of intangible heritage is translated in their local complexities and what this suggests not only about the meanings of intangible heritage, but also about the roles of these institutions.

Chapter 3

From Artefacts to Communities: Participation and Contestation at Te Papa Tongarewa

> In terms of Maori identity, there is a cultural renaissance and revitalisation. Maori *taonga* constitute a large part of our identity and this begs the question: Can we actively assist in that recovery and renaissance?
>
> —Arapata Hakiwai, director, Matauranga Maori, Te Papa

The previous chapter introduced the themes of erasure, impermanence, and transformation as an alternative framework for thinking about intangible heritage. In what follows I examine how this global heritage narrative is further interpreted in local contexts of contemporary museum practice. Over the last centuries museums have functioned as major preservation institutions, treasure houses, and archives of material culture. In recent years, however, they have been increasingly seen as social spaces of civic engagement and public benefit—a movement that has been related to the shift of museological interest from collections to a more active engagement with the public. Building on the dynamic interconnections between preservation and erasure, the following chapters explore how intangible heritage is articulated in fundamental museum activities, including the care of collections, exhibitions, and programmes as well as forms of community engagement.

My fieldwork takes off in Wellington and the National Museum of New Zealand Te Papa Tongarewa (Te Papa). Both English and Maori words make up the name of New Zealand's national museum, a manifestation of the institution's bicultural identity (O'Regan 1997; Williams 2005; Message 2006; McCarthy 2007). Throughout this chapter, emphasis is placed on the way biculturalism is expressed in the museum, and how this provides a context for local negotiations of intangible heritage. Rooted in the signing of New Zealand's founding document, the Treaty of Waitangi,[1] biculturalism informs everything in the museum: from

Intangible Heritage and the Museum: New Perspectives on Cultural Preservation by Marilena Alivizatou, 49–75. ©2012 Left Coast Press, Inc. All rights reserved.

the planning of exhibitions and the management of the institution to employment opportunities. Conducting research at Te Papa meant therefore critically examining the ways biculturalism is reflected in its practice.

Since it opened on the Wellington Waterfront in 1998, Te Papa has been one of the most popular museum destinations in the Pacific. It has also been the subject of debate. Its popularity with the wider public is often attributed to the fun-fair, leisure-centre (Henare 2004:61) and shopping-complex (Message 2006) characteristics of its architecture. But for many authors the museum's adoption of Maori knowledge and tradition (Williams 2005) and the purported trivialisation of settler European or Pakeha history (Brown 2002; Goldsmith 2003; Henare 2004) have been important sources of controversy.

As the country's major national museum, Te Papa is a charged space of national mythmaking. By celebrating moments of national unity and consolidation, such as the Treaty of Waitangi, and often omitting darker sides of the country's history, its narrative aims to foster pride in bicultural identity and a collective sense of belonging (Figure 3.1).

Moreover, by inviting different New Zealand communities, Maori tribes (*iwi*), and European and Asian groups to take active part in museum work, Te Papa firmly establishes its place as a postcolonial museum in a country with a complex colonial past and much divided present (Tuhiwai Smith 1999). This invites a closer examination of the politics of recognition and representation that are at its heart.

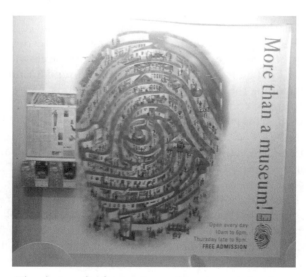

Figure 3.1: The choice of a fingerprint as the museum's logo conveys the idea that Te Papa symbolises the identity of New Zealand.

Te Papa's biculturalism, the fact that (in theory at least) it is run according to both Maori and European cultural principles, protocols, and understandings significantly challenges traditional museum work and influences local approaches to intangible heritage. Te Papa is different not only because apart from a chief executive it is also run by a Maori *kaihautu* (literally captain of the canoe), or because it houses the country's most active *marae* (Maori meeting place), or because every two years it hosts a different resident iwi with two *kaumatua* (elders) as Maori protocol advisors. The museum is quite distinct in the sense that it aims to tell stories rather than only showcase collections, and in so doing invites multiple perspectives, readings, and understandings of the national past, heritage, and tradition.

FROM THE COLONIAL MUSEUM TO TE PAPA TONGAREWA

Te Papa was established in 1992 with the Museum of New Zealand Te Papa Tongarewa Act of Parliament. Similar to the case of the National Museum of American Indian (see chapter 5) and the musée du quai Branly (chapter 7), this Act called for the creation of a new museum following the dissolution of the older National Art Gallery and of the National Museum (which would be incorporated in the new institution). Te Papa, therefore, is the culmination of a long history of displaying art and culture in New Zealand's capital that commenced in 1865 with the foundation of the Colonial, subsequently called Dominion and finally National Museum.

Officially, Te Papa was established as "a forum for the nation to present, explore, and preserve the heritage of its cultures and knowledge of the natural environment in order to better understand and treasure the past, enrich the present, and meet the challenges of the future" (New Zealand Government 1992). Its exhibitions, research programmes, and activities are explicitly founded on three concepts: "Papatuanuku—the earth on which we all live; Tangata Whenua—those who belong to the land by right of first discovery; Tangata Tiriti—those who belong to the land by right of the Treaty of Waitangi" (National Museum of New Zealand Te Papa Tongarewa 2006:6). On the one hand, therefore, the museum acknowledges and celebrates the plurality of New Zealand cultures, and on the other it underlines the strong bonds between people (both *tangata whenua* and *tangata tiriti*) and the land.[2]

In a study commissioned by the National Services of the National Museum of New Zealand and the Museum Association of New Zealand prior to the opening of Te Papa, museum researcher Gerard O'Regan (1997) has examined through surveys and interviews with New Zealand curators and museum professionals the challenges raised by the bicultural agenda for national and local museums. Although he acknowledges the strong presence of biculturalism in Te Papa, he also admits that "the museum sector has not attained a common understanding of what 'biculturalism' means within the museum environment, despite an often strong philosophical commitment to the principle" (1997:8). This apparent difficulty to grasp what biculturalism means emerged also in discussions I had with Te Papa staff and has been commented by several museum critics (Jolly 2001; Brown 2002; Goldsmith 2003; Henare 2004; Williams 2005; Message 2006).

Yet Te Papa's bicultural ethos, despite its often vague connotations, hints at an important break with past New Zealand museology in that it invites the active participation of different communities and primarily that of Maori tribes. For example, O'Regan notes:

> If a museum is to take proper account of *matauranga* (traditional knowledge) Maori, the ramifications go right across the organisation—collection and acquisitions policies, the content of exhibitions and other programmes, the role of the museum in the community, its niche within the cultural sector, its research agendas, and ultimately its staffing structure, especially the skills, competencies and inter-staff responsibilities within it. [1997:93]

This has been an important step forward for New Zealand museology, which previously had by and large followed Western paradigms of collections management and curation. For example, Conal McCarthy (2007) observes how the first national museums in New Zealand, following the tradition of British museums like the Pitt Rivers Museum in Oxford or the Horniman Museum in London (see chapter 7), were an effort on the part of European settlers to understand, classify, and possess the new land and its peoples. Maori artefacts were labelled as "curios" or "ethnographic specimens" within the context of the Colonial and later Dominion Museum, and were often presented in trophy-like displays to be viewed predominantly by European New Zealanders. As McCarthy explains, there was little Maori visitation, let alone participation in museum work (2007).

However, the political and economic unrest of the 1970s that followed decolonisation and the weakening of the links between New Zealand and Britain (Belich 2001) triggered a massive Maori mobilisation in different spheres of public life (Durie 1998). Maori rallied for political and economic rights and land reclamations, and in 1975 the Waitangi Tribunal was established to address grievances and past injustices. From a Native minority often described as a "dying race" (King 1985; Thomas 1999), Maori people emerged as key players in national politics, and this political consolidation was a key factor in the revival of Maori traditions and language (see Durie 1998:52–84).

A major locus for the celebration of Maori renaissance was the exhibition Te Maori: Indigenous Art from New Zealand Collections, which was prepared in Wellington, toured major U.S. cities in 1984, and was later presented in museums around New Zealand (Hanson 1989; Kaeppler 1994; Thomas 1994; Brown 2002; Hakiwai 2005; Henare 2005; McCarthy 2007; Tapsell 2011). Te Maori was the first travelling exhibition of Maori material culture to take place in prestigious museums of the Western world like the Metropolitan Museum of Art in New York, with a great impact on the appreciation of Maori art and culture. McCarthy describes it as "groundbreaking" (2007:135) and as a turning point in the relations between Maori and museums, underlining their "enthusiastic involvement in the ceremonies accompanying the exhibition" (2007:138). Similarly, in an interview with me Arapata Hakiwai, director for Matauranga Maori at the Te Papa, described the exhibition as a historical moment in the history of New Zealand and a turning point in the relationship between Maori and Pakeha.

Not surprisingly, the exhibition was met with significant scepticism by scholars engaged in the "invention of tradition" debates. Thomas, for example, argued that the displays put forward "a radical aesthetic decontextualisation that excludes non-traditional contexts of production, colonial processes and European influences of all kinds" (1994:184), ultimately idealising a lost past and marginalising contemporary Maori. In a paper that provoked much debate in New Zealand (see chapter 2), Hanson noted that the exhibition suggested that "Maori people have access to primal sources of power long lost by more rational cultures" (1989:896), and favoured a romanticised image of Maori in order to serve political agendas. Such criticisms sparked rows in New Zealand among academics, members of Maori communities, and the press, as it was felt that the legitimacy of Maori over their past and the authenticity of their contemporary culture had been questioned (see Thomas 1997:8–11; Henare 2005:205–209).

Despite its success and popularity both in New Zealand and abroad, the exhibition was met with further criticism by Maori groups. Many iwi, claiming the cultural or spiritual ownership of artefacts, were sceptical about their being displayed outside New Zealand and incorporated in Western museological discourse. Even the authority of Sidney Moko Mead, the Maori scholar who took part in the organisation of the exhibition, was significantly questioned by unconvinced Maori (Kaeppler 1994:28). These debates on the one hand revealed the tension surrounding the ownership and appropriation of Maori artefacts; on the other, they demonstrated a fundamental re-conceptualisation of Maori material culture, which since the exhibition has been widely regarded not as a typical museum collection, but as *taonga*,[3] treasured and living objects. More importantly, as O'Regan remarked, "since Te Maori it has no longer been acceptable to embark on presentation of things Maori without the appropriate approval, support and involvement of Maori people" (1997:6).

Maori participation is strong in the museum with labels in Te Reo (language) Maori, iwi first voice interpretation, an active marae, community based projects, and Maori staff. Interestingly, however, Te Papa does not invite only Maori participation, but also the involvement of the wider New Zealand community. As Stephanie Gibson, history curator, observed in the course of an interview, the influence of the new museology and the social history approach has transformed Te Papa into a story-driven museum. The museum indeed often prioritises the narrative over the display of artefacts, something that is not unchallenged. According to some of its critics, in shifting attention away from its collections Te Papa's narrative approach has "actively undermined the very purpose for which museums were founded in the first place—the gathering and analysis of artifactual knowledge, and its preservation for future generations" (Henare 2004:59).

Drawing on these debates, in the rest of this chapter I will examine in more detail how understandings of intangible heritage emerge in the context of artefactual knowledge and community participation.

TE PAPA: THE MUSEOLOGICAL NARRATIVE

Once on the Wellington waterfront, missing the Te Papa is difficult (Figure 3.2). The museum occupies a large edifice standing between the sea and Cable Street, a symbolic and contested location that joins the natural environment to the city and was the subject of land reclamation by local iwi (see Jolly 2001:442).

The building, the north side of which evokes a ship's prow, faces the Wellington harbour and is surrounded on one side by the Bush City—an outdoor space featuring Native trees, plants, stones, and minerals—and on the other by the museum's car park. In terms of its architecture, Te Papa was built on the model of a shopping mall complex, something that for many hints at the market- and consumer-oriented philosophy of the museum (Message 2006:169). Despite critiques, the museum has been very popular with New Zealanders and foreign visitors (McCarthy 2007).

During my research Te Papa's exhibits were presented over six levels. Level one was the main entrance to the museum, with the museum store, cloakroom, restaurant, and the escalator that leads to level two. Level two featured a large open space, the Wellington Foyer, and the main information desk. This led to the natural history exhibits on the same level and to several virtual reality attractions that were particularly popular with children, but have been criticised by techno-sceptics who feared the museum would become a theme park (Goldsmith 2003).

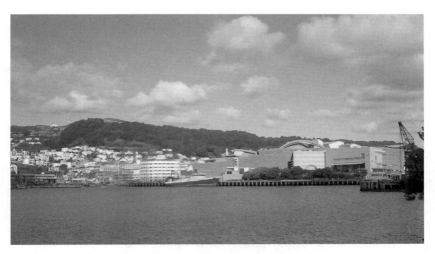

Figure 3.2: View of the Wellington Waterfront with Te Papa.

Level three presented the exhibition Blood, Earth, Fire, which explored the human impact on the New Zealand environment and was regarded as one of the bicultural exhibitions of Te Papa.[4] The heart of the museum beat on the fourth level, in Rongomaraeroa, Te Papa's marae, and the exhibitions that are dedicated to the peoples of New Zealand, Maori, Pacific islanders, European settlers, and other migrant communities. Finally, levels five and six featured the art exhibits of Te Papa, Toi Te Papa (Art of the Nation), previously part of the National Gallery collections.

Te Papa with its popular, virtual attractions, dramatic scenography, emphasis on telling stories, and reflexive historical interpretations challenges old museologies. During fieldwork, it also became evident that standard European scholarly categorisations of natural history, ethnography, history, and art were interpreted through the lens of Maori traditional knowledge, or matauranga (O'Regan 1997; Durie 1998; Oliver 2004), and custom, or tikanga, creating a mixed interpretative framework at the interface of modern science and Indigenous tradition.

The Marae

At the heart of the museum is Rongomaraeroa—the museum's marae, or Maori customary meeting place, on level four. Te Ara a Hine (pathway of women), the ascending pathway leading to Te Papa's marae, features artworks by contemporary Maori women artists and explains in contextual information the marae protocol, introducing important Maori ideas such as *karanga* (ceremonial call), *tikanga* (custom), *karakia* (blessing ceremony), and *whakapapa* (genealogy). It thus provides visitors going into the space with a sort of a performative script of how to behave and what to expect in the marae.

Rongomaraeroa is unlike any traditional marae in terms both of its appearance and of what takes place in it, for which reason it is described as postmodern (Williams 2005). Te Hono ki Hawaiki (return to Hawaiki[5]), the multicoloured *wharenui* (meeting house) that dominates the site, features contemporary carvings by Maori carver Cliff Whiting, representing traditional creation legends along with settler figures (Figure 3.3). A panel at the entrance to the marae explains the function of the space. In an inclusive tone, it states:

> The marae is the very heart of the Maori world. It is where we meet to welcome and celebrate the living, mourn and farewell the dead, to learn where we are coming from and to debate where we are going. On the museum's marae all iwi have the chance to host others and to honour their taonga. It is a marae for all the people of New Zealand.

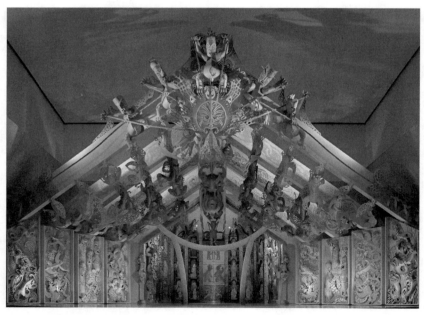

Figure 3.3: The wharenui (meeting house) Te Hono ki Hawaiki is at the heart of Rongomaraeroa, Te Papa's marae. (Photograph by Norman Heke, Museum of New Zealand Te Papa Tongarewa, MA_I.007526.)

In front of the meeting house and facing the Wellington harbour is the *waharoa*, or gateway, carrying different ancestral carved figures. The introductory panel reads: "Our waharoa pays tribute to the great navigator Kupe and the many ocean-going people who followed him to Aotearoa. It also acknowledges Abel Tasman and James Cook and the great migration which came in their wake. The aeroplane on the outside of the waharoa welcomes those people who continue to arrive in this country."

The coexistence of Maori and European ancestral figures in Rongomaraeroa's carvings breaks away from traditional marae canons to create a contemporary meeting space that demonstrates Te Papa's bicultural commitment to cross-cultural dialogue. Also, the use of pronouns "we" and "our" reveals the inclusive spirit of the museum. Here, it is not a detached curatorial voice that speaks about Indigenous cultures, but a museum made up of a plurality of Maori and Pakeha communities.

Occupying a prominent place in the marae is a large piece of *pounamu*, the Maori word for greenstone, lying in a water pond. The pounamu is one of the distinctive minerals of New Zealand that have been used by Maori for making special weapons and jewellery. Many Maori taonga are made out of it, and the mineral is considered a special attribute of Maori peoples and New Zealand. The impressive piece of unprocessed pounamu is not presented as a static museum display, but rather as incomplete and in flux. People in the marae are asked to take grains of sand from the pond and rub it against the pounamu, so that the polished stone can reveal its green colour. Through its active transformation, the piece of pounamu challenges the fixity of museum artefacts and conveys messages of impermanence and change.

Rongomaraeroa is a complex space, crossed by different and competing discourses. The Maori tradition of the marae, with all the accompanying practices and protocols, has been reappropriated by Te Papa to serve its reconciliatory, bicultural remit, often at the expense of more contested issues such as Maori self-determination and historical grievances (Tapsell 1998; Williams 2005). In this sense, as Kylie Message remarks, Rongomaraeroa seems to "embody the feel-good Treaty aspirations of New Zealand" (2006:189), but significantly ignores controversial issues with which the country is faced. Along similar lines, Paul Williams claims that with its reappropriation of the idea of the marae, Te Papa undermines Maori traditions. For him Rongomaraeroa is a "customary non-space" (2005:85) where traditional Maori protocol is not respected, as the consumption of food and alcohol are allowed, men and women have equal rights, and visitors are not asked to remove their footwear.

In my discussions with them, members of Te Papa's bicultural team significantly challenged these concerns with the authenticity of what Maori tradition is, and how it should be treated. According to Turei Reedy and Lucy Arthur, who worked for the museum's bicultural team, "this is a narrow view of what a marae is," "as if we are not allowed to change and we need to stay the way we were so as to maintain our integrity." During my research I observed Te Papa's marae being used as a space for ceremonial practices as well as contemporary performances. Resident iwi use the marae for *powhiri* (welcoming ceremonies), *hui* (meetings), *kapa haka* (dances and performances), and museum staff use it for *waiata* (songs) practice and also for more contemporary activities, such as concerts of classical music or educational workshops. Therefore Rongomaraeroa is not only a Maori meeting place for the preservation of Maori traditions, but also a space where contemporary identities are acted out.

Mana Whenua

The marae lies in proximity to the main Maori exhibition space, Mana Whenua (the power/ prestige of the land). This exhibition features some of the most treasured Maori taonga, like the 1864 wharenui Te Hau ki Turanga and the 1897 *pataka* (raised storehouse) Te Takinga. Entering Mana Whenua from the marae entrance, one is immediately struck by the change in the atmosphere and overall environment. While the marae with the brightly coloured contemporary meeting house is bathed in sunlight, the lighting in Mana Whenua is sombre, and dark colours—green, black, and blue—dominate the entire exhibition creating an atmosphere of deep spirituality and respect for tangata whenua (the people of the land).

Maori tradition and cultural revival are fundamental concepts of the exhibition, which revolves around key taonga and their connection to iwi. The exhibition's highlight is Te Hau ki Turanga. Its placement at the top of a staircase in the middle of the exhibition underlines its historical importance, while discrete spotlights both outside and inside the house reveal its renowned carvings. Unlike Te Hono ki Hawaiki, visitors to Te Hau ki Turanga are asked to remove their footwear. The label next to it reads:

> Greetings to all our visitors! We, the Rongowhakaata people of the Gisborne district, welcome you to our great house . . . Our love for our ancestors and their heritage keeps alive our interest and involvement in this house. Today, Te Hau ki Turanga symbolises the proud identity of Rongowhakaata, our contribution to the nation and our commitment to a bicultural partnership with Te Papa Tongarewa, the Museum of New Zealand.

Next to Te Hau ki Tiranga stands Te Takinga, the suspending storehouse adorned with feathers. Here is the Ngati Pikiao that greet visitors in the same tone: "Welcome visitors to this magnificent storehouse called Te Tikanga, part of the proud heritage of Ngati Pikiao, one of the Arawa tribes of Rotorua. We see this unusually large and elaborate pataka as evidence of our mana in Te Papa Tongarewa, the Museum of New Zealand." Rather than a detached curatorial voice, it is Maori iwi who welcome visitors and declare their presence by sharing their proud heritage with Te Papa and the rest of the world. The discourse of partnership, but also the power and authority embodied in the word *mana*, is particularly strong, with no direct reference to the ownership disputes between the museum and iwi that were subsequently stressed in my discussions with Te Papa staff.

At the other end of the exhibitions stands the Moriori[6] display case, presenting a series of adzes and hooks. The presence of the Moriori is made clear in the introductory label:

> Our Moriori traditions state that our earliest karapuna or ancestors sprang from the earth, while other karapuna migrated directly from Hawaiki. We are a distinct people with our own culture from the same rootstock as Maori, but have lived in our own islands for over six hundred years. Long ago, Moriori chiefs laid down a covenant for peace, prohibiting the killing of people. On distant Rekohu, pounded by turbulent seas, we have held steadfast through invasion and disaster and today we share our story.

Traditional beliefs and historical events are interwoven to represent and legitimise contemporary Moriori perspectives. As a museum host observed, however, the controversies and painful memories of the 1830s clashes between Moriori and Maori are silenced, hinting at the powerful relationship between remembering and forgetting.

A major aspect of Mana Whenua is the presentation of cultural revivalist projects. These include the display of Te Aurere Iti, the model of a *waka* or canoe that was made in 1992 based on traditional fabrication methods and sailed from Hawaii to Rapa Nui (Easter Island) and New Zealand. The label nearby reconfirms Maori spirituality by stating that "as the waka retraces ancient migration routes, the crew begin to feel the presence of atua (gods) in the sea, in the storms, even in the timber of the vessel itself." The label also explains that "Te Aurere Iti can inspire present and future generations of Maori to examine their origins and identity."

Along similar lines, Makotukutuku is a *wharepuni* or storehouse that was made by members of Ngati Hinewaka in the late 1990s based on archaeological findings in the Makotukutuku Valley. In an interview, curator Awhina Tamarapa described the conflicts raised during the reconstruction of the house between iwi members and archaeologists, which revealed the different approaches of academic scholarship and traditional knowledge. Matauranga Maori does not always agree with academic perspectives, and their relationship in the context of inclusive museology has been a subject of critical reflection. Should the house be built according to the traditions, memories, and opinions of the community, or the archaeological record?

Another interesting aspect of the museological narrative of Mana Whenua is the presentation of traditional musical instruments made and donated to Te Papa by Maori instrument maker and player Hau Manu. These instruments, their sounds, and related performances are regarded as taonga and respected as such, even though they are not historical objects but have been created only recently. A multimedia installation enables visitors to listen to their sounds. Accompanying labels explain contemporary efforts to revive the skills and tradition associated with these instruments: for example, one of them states that "Formerly such music played a part in the rituals of everyday life—healing, making things grow, fishing and hunting. It would greet the newborn and farewell the dying. Now the voices of these instruments are heard wherever we make music—breathing the spirit of our ancestors into today's world."

Unlike the collections of musical instruments in the Horniman and the quai Branly, here Maori instruments are living objects, used to perform in special events throughout the year.

Living tradition, pride in identity, and knowledge inherited from the ancestors are basic concepts behind Mana Whenua. Iwi are the authors of the museum narrative and their self-representational discourse, inspired by tradition, confirms their strong presence, hopes, and aspirations for the future. The first voice interpretation also hints at the collaboration between iwi and the museum, legitimising the presence of Maori taonga in Te Papa and also reconnecting iwi with their heritage. As such the exhibition becomes a space where tribal communities affirm their living bonds with tradition and consolidate their presence in the museum narrative.

Iwi Exhibition—Mo Tatou: Ngai Tahu Whanui

Next to Mana Whenua is a space for short-term exhibitions co-curated by iwi in collaboration with Te Papa in which Maori communities are given the space to present their cultures, traditions, and contemporary ways of life. At the time of my research, Ngai Tahu was the resident iwi.[7] Megan Tamati-Quennell, curator for Contemporary Maori, Indigenous Art, and of the Ngai Tahu exhibition, worked with an iwi steering group of tribal members, encouraging their respective communities to present aspects of tribal history, beliefs, achievements, and vision for the future. She explained, "I wanted to make sure that it was not a classical social history narrative, 'who we are,' 'what we are'; I wanted to use a different curatorial model. I wanted to talk about us as a people historically, but also in modernity and ensure our present was acknowledged and seen as important, that there was not only a focus on our past." Rather than offering a single narrative, the exhibition was centred on four main ideas: culture, tenacity, sustainability, and innovation. These ideas were positioned as cultural characteristics of the tribe both in the past and in the present, and also worked as organising principles for the exhibition. Historic taonga and contemporary artworks were clustered around these themes to speak about Ngai Tahu.

The exhibition presented the people as the backbone of the tribe and handed over a whole section to the *hapu* (subtribes) to select treasured taonga. Members of the tribe provided a short statement that was used as wall text with the taonga to represent their communities and highlight their uniqueness within the larger tribe. Contemporary artworks were presented alongside taonga to highlight the cultural dynamism of the tribe and evoke the relationship between customary and contemporary, present and past.

Other aspects of Ngai Tahu's history were addressed, including an emphasis on the connection of people and place. Maori knowledge systems and concepts formed the anchors for the exhibition: this included using *pepeha* (tribal sayings) to present oral mapping and naming of landscape, and *whakapapa* (genealogy) to reinforce a sense of belonging and the tribe's ties to land and place. The exhibition also paid tribute to the historical moments that changed the tribe, the political struggles including the settlement of Te Kereme, their land claim; grievances that highlighted breaches of the Treaty of Waitangi; and the Crown apology that formed part of the claim settlement. The exhibition was also accompanied by an audiovisual explaining the claim history and claim settlement. Overall, Ngai Tahu emerge as a vibrant and dynamic tribe with strong roots in tradition, but well informed and engaged in contemporary economic, political, and cultural affairs.

A key theme of the exhibition that was also confirmed by the Ngai Tahu kaumatua Maruhaeremuri Sterling is that iwi members respect and maintain cultural traditions and knowledge in ways that enable them to preserve tribal identities in a changing world. As such, iwi-run Kaikoura whale watching and pounamu jewellery businesses are presented as a modern way for maintaining and reviving traditions, stressing the dynamic interaction between Maori and the natural environment as well as between modern and traditional ways of life and beliefs.

Mana Whenua and the iwi exhibitions gallery are the two main spaces for the presentation of tangata whenua (the people of the land). At the end of these displays stands the historic *waka taua* (war canoe) Teremoe. Teremoe is dimly lit and adorned with white feathers, while a hidden installation recreates sounds of waves. Information is provided about its history, the battles it took part in, and how it came to be in Te Papa. Facing Teremoe, at the opposite site of the void cutting through Te Papa, is a European New Zealanders icon, the Britten race bike, introducing the tangata tiriti displays. Facing each other, the historical war canoe and the modern race bike provide an interesting point of reference to Te Papa's biculturalism. The selection of a cherished taonga, an old war canoe, for the Maori and of a racing bike for the Pakeha hints at what each party brings into the bicultural partnership—tradition and innovation—and how these stand for the two faces of the museum's biculturalism.

Signs of a Nation: Nga Tohu Kotahitanga

Standing between the two, as if bringing together tangata whenua and tangata tiriti, is the exhibition Signs of a Nation, which presents the 1840 Treaty of Waitangi as the embodiment of the country's biculturalism. This exhibition, featuring the magnified copy of the almost destroyed original treaty document in both English and Te Reo Maori, is a reflexive commentary on the country's biculturalism and the Maori-Pakeha relationship. Surrounding the treaty are talking poles that present peoples' opinions, doubts, and questions on the document and its implications. The public is invited to sit, read the two versions of the treaty, and reflect on its legacy, impacts, and the different controversies that have resulted from its ambiguities. This is a space for contemplation. There are no auratic objects—only historical information and peoples' voices and opinions. The narrative takes precedence over the objects, voicing the concerns of contemporary New Zealanders.

Just above, on the mezzanine, the exhibition Poringi: The Ongoing Story of Treaty Partnership examines in a critical manner the consequences of the treaty and the evolving relations between Maori and Pakeha. For example, it questions the role of missionaries in converting Maori to Christianity and introducing diseases, or the revival of Maori language. Moreover, it addresses contemporary issues related to the treaty and the establishment of the Waitangi Tribunal. It even touches upon heritage property issues affecting Te Papa itself and the items in its possession. One of the labels reads: "Te Hau ki Turanga the wharenui (meeting house) in Mana Whenua, is alleged to have been confiscated by Crown officials in 1867. Its display in Te Papa is subject to agreement with Rongowhakaata, but their loss of the wharenui is part of a wider claim that Rongowhakaata are bringing against the Crown."

This exhibition is more political and self-critical compared to Mana Whenua, something that can be attributed to its strong, discursive narrative. Through a combination of historical information, photographic material, and multiple personal narratives, Poringi transcends the visual contemplation of collections to address more contested issues of cultural continuity and belonging. Its location in a rather isolated mezzanine, however, makes it easy to miss.

Tangata Tiriti Exhibitions

The celebratory tone of the Maori exhibitions raises questions about how the other party to the bicultural agreement, the post-Treaty settlers[8] in their great diversity, would fit into Te Papa's bicultural discourse. This is ventured in five exhibitions.[9]

The exhibition Passports traces the migratory journeys from Britain and the rest of the world to New Zealand in the late nineteenth and twentieth centuries. The stories of different individuals who came to New Zealand in pursuit of a better life are narrated through oral history videos and sound recordings. Souvenirs, mementoes, and other items of personal rather than collective or aesthetic value, such as coffee cups, prayer books, and toys metonymically represent the people who carried them to New Zealand. The exhibition is not about the artistic or political achievements of the settlers, but about their passage to New Zealand and the challenges they faced in starting a new life. The personal narratives and individual stories of migration present collections in a new light.

Along similar lines, the community gallery every two years gives the floor to the presentation of the histories of various national or ethnic communities that made their homes in New Zealand. At the time of my research the community gallery presented the Italians in New Zealand and their migrations following the Second World War. Much like the Ngai Tahu exhibition, community representatives collaborated with Te Papa curators for the making of Qui Tutto Bene. In our discussions, Stephanie Gibson, history curator, highlighted the challenges of the partnership between museum and communities. While ethnic communities are in a sense segregated from the bicultural partners, Gibson noted that the community exhibition space provides ethnic groups with their own place to express identity.

Pacific nations and their relationship with New Zealand through migration and exchange was the focus of the exhibition Mana Pasifika, a permanent exhibition which closed in 2007 and was replaced with a new exhibition. Contrary to the tradition-focused Mana Whenua, the museological approach chosen here combined elements of traditional and contemporary Pacific culture. Sacred objects for handling the flesh of slain enemies introduced the theme of cannibalism in Fiji, whereas music practices in Hawaii were represented by the display of ukuleles.

Contemporary artworks like *Pisupo lua afe*, the corned beef tin cow by Michel Tuffery, were also part of the museological discourse of Mana Pasifika. What was striking, however, regarding Mana Whenua and Mana Pasifika is that while the first emphasises Maori tradition through the display of historical taonga, the latter prioritised contemporary Pacific Islanders living in New Zealand rather than the historical ties between New Zealand and the rest of the Pacific Islands.

Next to Mana Pasifika until the summer of 2007 was the display On the Sheep's Back, which explored the bonds between New Zealanders and sheep farming by employing oral histories and personal testimonies. The exhibition highlighted the connections between Pakeha and the land and how stock raising became part of the New Zealand national psyche. As opposed to the spiritual links between Maori and the land that characterised the Maori displays, the bonds that connect Pakeha New Zealanders to the land seemed to be related to more mundane activities.

Facing Mana Whenua is the permanent exhibition Made in New Zealand. This presents Maori and Pakeha material culture in an interpretative framework that stresses bicultural exchanges and influences. It features in a chronological order different objects, including paintings, drawings, feathered cloaks, *hei tiki*, the Maori *Madonna and Child*, and Brian O'Connor's *Paua* surfboard. The emphasis, through the sequence and juxtaposition of objects, is on material culture. Yet the curatorial voice is strong and critical of Pakeha perceptions of Maori culture, like the commercial exploitation of Maori iconography on cigarette packages, or the appropriation of Maori symbols by Air New Zealand. For example, the label next to Charles Goldie's 1903 portrait of Maori elder Ina Te Papatahi reads: "The erroneous belief that Maori were a dying race and that settlers had only to 'smooth their pillow' had some currency at the time. Whether Goldie himself believed this is not clear. What is clear is that his fame would soon be 'smoothed' by the arrival of modern ideas about art." Notwithstanding such critical statements, however, the overall discourse focuses on bicultural exchange, innovation, and tradition, something which is in line with Te Papa's reconciliatory and politically correct approach.

Nature and Culture

Levels two and three feature the natural history displays, which examine the environmental richness and diversity of New Zealand and underline the close bonds between culture and nature. The exhibition Awesome Forces explains the geological phenomena that led to the creation of the North and South Islands of New Zealand, introducing the scientific interpretation of the seismic activity that led to the emergence of the islands. A virtual reality installation also emulates the experience of an earthquake. Next to this, in the Papatuanuku theatre, Maori legends and beliefs about the creation of New Zealand are presented in a sound and light show.[10] Unlike traditional natural history exhibitions that tend to present primarily academic, geological, or zoological perspectives, science and matauranga are presented as equally important narratives.

Next to Awesome Forces stands the exhibition From Mountains to Sea, which is about New Zealand wildlife. It features a model of a *moa*, the gigantic flightless bird that was hunted to extinction by Maori, as well as a display of marine animal skeletal remains. Dark lighting, reconstructed trees, and sounds of the bush create an immersive environment. This space leads to the Bush City, the outdoor bush of Te Papa comprised of plants and trees. A winding path goes into the bush, over a swinging bridge, and through caves that present true to life replicas of stalactites, animal fossils, and glowworms to create the feeling of being in nature.

The natural environment and how humans have transformed it is the focus of the exhibition Blood, Earth, Fire on level three. Roma Potiki, concept developer at Te Papa, showed me around the exhibition and underlined how it had been informed by Maori traditional knowledge. The exhibition is concerned with the destructive impact of humans on the New Zealand ecosystem, such as farming and the introduction of foreign species like cats, dogs, and rats. Maori perspectives on the land are particularly strong, underlining again the powerful bond between nature and Native culture.

The first room of the exhibition, immersed in a dark and mystic atmosphere, presents Maori beliefs on the sacredness of the land, focusing on the notion of *whenua*, which means both land and placenta. Important taonga are presented, like a *rakau whakapapa* (genealogy stick with notches that stand for previous generations), *tauihi* (canoe prow), adzes, and an *ipu whenua* (afterbirth container). As Roma Potiki explained to me, the planning team wanted to create an immersive environment to emphasise the spiritual connections with the sacredness of the land.

In a secluded area of the exhibition, a Maori lament is digitally performed to express the feelings of loss and sorrow over the extinction of the *huia*, the Native New Zealand bird whose feathers used to be worn by the Maori elite. This section contrasts greatly with the nearby audiovisual installation, which displays images from a camera placed on a sheep's head to represent Pakeha farming practices as their bond to the land.[11] Further down the exhibition, and again in great contrast to the sheep installation, an interactive display presents the Maori lunar calendar as a symbol of Native sustainable interaction with nature.

A short film entitled *My Place* is presented in a small theatre at the end of the exhibition space, featuring interviews with New Zealanders and examining their relationship to the land: landowners, artists, and youth from the North and South Islands talk about their personal stories and narrate how they found a place to express their identities. Interestingly, the film circumvents the Maori and Pakeha distinction, and all interviewees are presented as tangata whenua.

Taken as a whole, Te Papa's narrative is based on a mixed discourse of art, science, and social and oral history. Maori, Pakeha, and natural history collections and their multidimensional interpretation shape the museum's bicultural identity. Exhibitions are often immersive with special lighting, virtual displays, music, song, and video, and a strong emphasis is placed on the people of New Zealand rather than solely on material culture. This creates a strong multivocal narrative: oral history, traditional knowledge, historical documents, and scientific interpretations provide different approaches to the country's cultural, artistic, and natural heritage.

But what sets Te Papa apart from other multivocal museological approaches is the strong presence of matauranga Maori not only in the Maori exhibitions, but throughout the museum. Te Papa's biculturalism is thus expressed in efforts to give equal importance to both Western and Maori perspectives. As such, the reappropriation of traditional knowledge reveals further negotiations of traditional beliefs in a contemporary museum context. This also emerges in the museum's performative spaces like the marae and in symbolically charged exhibitions like Mana Whenua: spaces that are important not only in terms of their physical or aesthetic dimensions, but also because they invite participation and the expression of contemporary identities.

Intangible Heritage at Te Papa: Locating Biculturalism

The museum's biculturalism and the revival of traditional knowledge provided a central framework for discussing intangible heritage during my fieldwork. Turei Reedy and Lucy Arthur worked for the museum's bicultural team and explained the importance of communicating biculturalism across both intellectual and practical levels. As Lucy Arthur argued:

> When the museum was conceived as a bicultural institution in the early 1990s, that was a very new way of looking at museums in New Zealand. But having this foundation . . . does not really mean that everyone in the museum knows what biculturalism is. You can't just say I work in the café, I should not worry about that. Biculturalism affects all members of staff.

For Te Papa's late chief executive Seddon Bennington, the museum's bicultural identity is expressed in that "we recognise the great importance and significance of reflecting the partnership with Maori, as something that we do internally and this affects all our staff. But also this is related to our public role; it is something that is a real strength and value that we can add to what Te Papa does."

In our conversations, Megan Tamati-Quennell, curator for Maori and Indigenous Art, compared Te Papa to the earlier Dominion Museum, which she described as a "scary place" that was "intellectually intimidating" and rarely visited by Maori. Karl Johnstone, matauranga Maori researcher and concept leader for various exhibitions, among which the temporary exhibition Whales, commented "biculturalism is not cognitive; it is not about the way you think; it is not about the way you process; it is about values and philosophy and changing values and philosophies is a lot harder than changing mindsets." For him, Te Papa's main difference compared to its ancestors is that it is "build around trust." His comments become more relevant with regard to the concept of *mana taonga*, two words that were repeated several times in my discussions with the Te Papa staff. As Arapata Hakiwai stressed, mana taonga, the power and agency of the historic treasures, suggests the reconnection of historic Maori collections with tribes and subtribes in an active and reciprocal process of trust and recognition. In this process the cultural ownership of the taonga remains with the iwi and Te Papa's role is that of a caretaker.

The bicultural management framework actively seeks the engagement of Maori. The museum is run by the chief executive and the kaihautu, a Maori leader ensuring that Te Papa operates in accordance with Maori cultural practices. At the time of my research, Te Taru White, Te Papa's kaihautu, had just resigned, something that for many hinted at the underlying problems of the bicultural partnership. Traditional cultural practices are also maintained and kept by Te Papa's kaumatua, two Maori elders that consult the museum on issues of appropriate practice regarding the taonga and the role of the museum towards other iwi. These elders are nominated by Te Papa's resident iwi, who changes every two years. While at Te Papa, Maruhaeremuri Sterling, one of the two Ngai Tahu kaumatua, was involved in the conduct of prayers, karakia (blessings), and powhiri (welcoming ceremonies in the marae). For her, becoming a Te Papa kaumatua was a way to honour her tribe and ancestors and to educate younger generations about Maori culture. Although she represented the public face of Te Papa, she had little input in management issues.

While the peopling of Te Papa with staff adhering to the bicultural ethos and the cultivation of trust seem to operate on an institutional level,

Hakiwai acknowledged that many sceptical or dissatisfied iwi still claim their taonga back. Talking about a recent case against Te Papa at the Waitangi Tribunal, he told me: "I am a proactive supporter and advocate of repatriation for the right reasons. I think that there are a lot of taonga in this museum that can go home and that they should go home and in due course will go home." It seems therefore that Te Papa's attempts to convince Maori to trust it with their taonga have not persuaded all iwi, who are still suspicious of the idea of the museum as a "home" for their cultural and spiritual treasures. The repatriation of taonga and the relationship between Te Papa and iwi was also discussed by Aaron Brown, a member of the repatriation team who was concerned with the repatriation of skeletal remains and *toi moko* (tattooed heads) from New Zealand and overseas museums to iwi. Regarding collaborations with iwi, he acknowledged that "ultimately iwi drive the project through their engagement with the museum . . . once the remains go back to iwi, it is a non-conditional return." In the context of a postcolonial politics of recognition and reconciliation, Maori claims feature prominently and are respected deeply as the first party to the bicultural partnership.

Participation

The collaboration with iwi as Te Papa's fundamental museological principle emerged as one of the main characteristics of the Maori exhibitions. For Awhina Tamarapa, who was a member of the organising team of Mana Whenua, one of the most rewarding moments in preparing the exhibition was the collaboration with Ngati Hinewaka for the building of the storehouse currently displayed in the exhibition, which was based on archaeological finds and the revival of traditional skills. For her, being a curator at Te Papa is "being a conduit between the taonga and the people." In a similar tone, Hakiwai acknowledged that "taonga are very important, but to make them live, we need to bring the people in the museum." Both Awhina Tamarapa and Arapata Hakiwai acknowledge the importance of reconnecting people with objects as central principles directing their work rather than "leaving our taonga lying in the dark storeroom."

For Karl Johnstone, "indigenising the museum" could not be achieved only with the aesthetic presentation of taonga, but needed the inclusion of "Indigenous worldviews" in the museum narrative. Referring to the example of the Whales exhibition, he explained that his intention as a concept leader was to marry the scientific approach that had dominated the understanding of the natural world with matauranga Maori, the Native knowledge concerning the development of the world. Similarly, Roma Potiki spoke extensively with me about the efforts to combine both Maori and Pakeha perspectives on the land in the narrative of the Blood, Earth,

Fire exhibition: the inclusion of the Maori lunar calendar emphasised an alternative Maori approach to the understanding of time and nature.

While such efforts have been praised and acknowledged as important factors in honouring the bicultural partnership and engaging Maori audiences, several concerns have been raised regarding "indigenised" and "postcolonial" museological approaches that combine traditional knowledge and self-representation. Megan Tamati-Quennell, who curated the Ngai Tahu exhibition, remarked:

> It is all about how you want to represent yourself. The exhibition was a representation of our history and culture as we understand it today. We (myself and the Iwi Steering Group) decided against focusing on our history of pre-European tribal warfare including the Kai Huaka feud which was a battle which in English translates as "eat relations"; we did not talk about the severe impact of colonisation on the tribe apart from the focus on Te Kereme—our land grievance claim and claim settlement. Instead we wanted to present our people as the backbone of the tribe and talk about the unique aspects of culture—specific to us, unique within Maori and within the world; of our achievements, of us as a tribe with strong cultural anchors but of our future aspirations, where we are looking to in the future.

Talking about the dynamics between Maori knowledge and academic scholarship, Awhina Tamarapa recalled:

> When we were working with Ngati Hinewaka to build the *whare* upstairs [in Mana Whenua], the archaeologists had one theory about how the house was constructed and the people had another theory. So, it was traditional knowledge versus science. In the end the people won, because it was their house. They said thank you very much about your theories, but we want to do it our way.

Te Papa's effort to actively engage iwi and prioritise Maori tikanga/ matauranga has established new representational strategies that hint at the politicisation of the museum discourse and the challenges of reconciling traditional and academic knowledge. "I guess to me where we are at the moment is getting those people involved. If it is coming from their perspective and if this is what they want to say about themselves, I think this has a merit of its own. Besides, they are making it clear that this is their voice. This is valid," remarked Lucy Arthur. Along the same lines, Turei Reedy observed that "there was a very long history of having no voice that I think that the step toward letting tribal people speak is quite huge."

The politics of recognition and representation have transformed museums into meeting points of different intersubjectivities. In this sense, there is not one museum truth, but different discourses that often compete or clash, demonstrating the complexities of participatory work.

Contesting Biculturalism

So far, biculturalism has been examined from the perspective of Maori participation. An examination into the second party of the treaty, however, raises a series of problems with which Te Papa staff are faced. "When a Pacific islander comes to New Zealand today, he or she would be classified as tangata tiriti. However, their genealogy, their *whakapapa*, places them in the first category, tangata whenua," Karl Johnstone explained to me commenting on the vague areas of biculturalism. It seems that for many the bicultural framework operates on a conceptual level, but has little relevance to contemporary New Zealand. My discussions with the staff of the Ministry of Internal Affairs off the busy Lampton Quay in Wellington pointed out that New Zealand public policy has always been influenced by immigration policy. Since the mid-1990s, the country has become an immigration destination not only from Europe, but also from East and South Asia and the Pacific Islands. This has created a huge diversity of ethnic groups in New Zealand, of which the Maori are just a part. The bicultural framework cannot respond to these demographic changes, and a new intercultural framework is needed to prioritise cultural exchange and fluidity rather than build walls separating groups.

As Turei Reedy observed, Te Papa needs to "break down the hard lines between the exhibitions" and instead "focus for example on the stories that link up Maori and Pacific." Adding to that, Lucy Arthur observed that for many people "New Zealand does not feel to belong to the South Pacific nor it has links to other countries like Samoa or Fiji." In my discussion with Kolokesa Mahina-Tuai and Sean Mallon, curators for Pacific Cultures, these issues emerged quite strongly as fundamental directions to be adopted for the exhibition Tangata o le Moana (People of the Sea) that would replace Mana Pasifika. As Kolokesa Mahina-Tuai explained, the new exhibition would ask questions about the place of New Zealand in the Pacific and about how Pacific islanders fit into the bicultural framework. The new exhibition would show the one thousand year history of Pacific people in the country, but it would also address more contemporary issues showing the vibrancy of Pacific cultures in New Zealand today, like the Pacific Arts Festival and the links with Maori.

Ten years after Te Papa's opening, biculturalism is under revision towards a more inclusive intercultural framework. For Stephanie Gibson this is of primary importance. While working at Te Papa, she collaborated with representatives from different groups, including the Indian, Italian, and Scottish communities, for the curation of the temporary exhibitions. However, she remains sceptical as to the bicultural model, which she finds "old-fashioned" in the sense that it creates a museological discourse that "others" and "separates" people in distinct communities. Nevertheless, she acknowledged that "even though we 'other' communities, they do get an incredible voice, a national platform for two years, their own space." The challenge for her in this respect is to "face the dark side of history," and not just make an uncritical exhibition based on stereotypical representations of communities.

Understandings of Intangible Heritage

Erana Hemmingsen worked as senior programme developer of the education team. She is a member of Ngai Tuhoe, an iwi on the East side of the North Island that as she acknowledged has been relatively isolated from the rest of New Zealand and whose members uphold traditional beliefs and quite often become teachers of Te Reo Maori. She extensively talked with me about Maori beliefs and knowledge systems and how these are communicated in the museum. Early on in our conversation she explained that "we are an oral people," adding, "For me this is intangible heritage . . . something that you cannot touch, but is passed on from one generation to the next. Before the Europeans came, our meeting houses were our books; the carvings and the panels tell the stories of our tribes; most of it is maintained in the old songs that we sing."

In her work, she applies the Maori perspective and knowledge to the museum's educational programmes and exhibitions: "There are different gods which are responsible for different things. For example, the god of earthquakes is Rua Moko, who is the unborn child of mother earth, Papatuanuku, and every time he moves inside her, we have earthquakes. So, we add our Maori programme to the scientific aspects of the educational programmes."

Further along our talk she observed:

> What Maori people are good at is storytelling and our elders are very good orators. In this way information and knowledge are passed on. So for me, intangible heritage is talking to the old people. I don't go to the library to find a book about my people, because these are predominantly European. I go to the old people and talk to them in their own language.

In a similar tone Lucy Arthur argued that "Maori culture is an oral culture. A lot of their knowledge and history is contained within spoken words, *waiata*, and oral traditions. It is very important for the museum to recognise this in its exhibitions and the way it does things." The idea that intangible heritage emerges from knowledge that is passed from previous generations came up repeatedly during my fieldwork. For example, Awhina Tamarapa noted that

> the tangible is what you can see and touch, but intangible heritage is a culture's spirituality, values, philosophy, cosmology . . . and it is this part that I enjoy in my work: dealing with that aspect; helping people discover who they are by showing to them things that they can connect to and their history. This is why I think that the house building with the Ngati Hinewaka is all about intangible heritage; it is all about reclaiming and passing on knowledge.

"For Maori, taonga is a big part of our identity," acknowledged Arapata Hakiwai. "With colonisation, we had forgotten the older ways of doing things, but our traditions and stories are embedded in our taonga here at Te Papa" underlined Awhina Tamarapa. Similarly, when Megan Tamati-Quennell was preparing the Ngai Tahu exhibition she acknowledged that "the matauranga associated with many of our taonga was not lying within the tribe, but outside with ethnologists and anthropologists . . . So, reclaiming matauranga was really important. We were reclaiming our tradition." Maori taonga provide therefore a context for reconnecting with the past and negotiating identities in the present.

Similarly, Awhina Tamarapa observed that reclaiming tradition was a healing process of "reclaiming identity." As such, taonga are not only regarded as works of art inherited from previous generations, but as a vital source of coping with loss and reaffirming Maori consciousness. The *wairua* (spirit) and the *mauri* (life force) of the taonga, the stories and knowledge carved on the wood, emerge as defining elements of Maori identity; as such, taonga are not dead museum pieces, but living and sacred objects that transmit Maori culture and need to be recognised as such by the museum. The active involvement of the Rongowhakaata in the installation of Te Hau Ki Turanga and the performance of the musical instruments on display in Mana Whenua underline the respect with which taonga are treated as symbols of a cherished past and ongoing tradition.

But cultural preservation is not only related to the care of material taonga. In the last years the museum has hosted Te Paerangi, a national programme targeted at local museums, iwi, and other organisations to raise awareness and engage communities in heritage issues. Rhonda Paku, who is manager for iwi development in that team, stressed the need to empower communities to reclaim and pass on knowledge on taonga and cultural history. She thus discussed various ways in which this is pursued, often with the use of digital technologies. One example was an electronic resource produced by Te Aitanga-a-Hauti tribe from Tolaga Bay about taonga held at Te Papa and in overseas institutions.[12]

It contained not only information about the artefacts, but also recordings of songs, images, and personal stories retrieved and gathered by the community. Initiatives like this constitute bottom-up approaches in heritage preservation and identity reclamation. Through this project, the iwi was transformed into an active agent of heritage advocacy seeking recognition on national and international levels.

Performing Identity

The enactment of community participation in the museum was a central topic in my discussions with Te Papa staff. The importance of the space of the marae in this respect was repeatedly stressed. For example, Lucy Arthur observed: "On the one hand, the marae is an exhibition space, but on the other, it is the bicultural heart of the museum as a real working marae. It enables traditions to be heard in a real way. The resident iwi is able to share its culture in the marae, sing their waiata and perform their dances." "The marae breaks down the traditional notion of the museum" maintained Karl Johnstone, while for Arapata Hawaiki "the beauty of this museum is that we hear the sound of songs, waiata, people greeting and singing to their ancestors in the marae, but also in the exhibitions . . . we don't want a silent museum."

Eric Ngan, the events manager, headed the team that makes sure that Te Papa is never silent. From the celebrations for the Matariki, the festival for the Maori New Year, to the organisation of floor talks, public lectures, and activities, he oversaw more than four hundred events annually. "It may seem sacrilegious to some curators," he argued, "but I personally see the museum as a large performance space. All I see is those large spaces at the Waterfront and I want to transform them into spaces for performances."

The Matariki, which according to Ngan is "developing as Te Papa's signature event," is celebrated once a year in June when Matariki (the Pleiades) appear on the New Zealand sky. The celebrations for Matariki at Te Papa include a variety of activities for adults, families, and children combining elements of the traditional and contemporary. For example, in 2006 when the festival's theme was "innovation," Te Papa hosted a series of lectures emphasising the survival and adaptation of Maori and Pacific cultures in the twenty-first century.[13]

Similarly, the performances that took place in the marae during the 2007 Matariki Festival included traditional kapa haka and *poi* dances, but also contemporary hip-hop by Maori, Pakeha, and Pacific bands.[14] Elements of the traditional, the modern, and the postmodern coexist and create a mixed contemporary living heritage, much like contemporary New Zealand. "There is a special understanding of biculturalism," Eric

Ngan explained to me, "because we are well aware that we live in a very multicultural society. For example, I am of Chinese ancestry and have to create a product that speaks to all the different people in New Zealand." For him, the challenge now is to "extend the events programmes outside the museum into the different communities and also to expand online." In the context of live performance, intangible heritage seems therefore to be mostly associated with the vitality of contemporary culture, rather than with carefully preserved traditional practices and cultural expressions.

Story-Driven Exhibitions

Te Papa staff further discussed intangible heritage in relation to exhibition development. For Karl Johnstone, intangible heritage is "absolutely fundamental" as a way for balancing out the fact that "Te Papa can be very object-centred." He thus claimed that "objects are reference points to culture, people, stories, ceremonies and events," and that "a taonga is not a material object necessarily. It is anything people ascribe value to: a song is as much a taonga as carvings." As such, he added that "what intangible heritage does is that it recognises that intangible culture is as important as artefacts." For him, "This is a great opportunity from a museological perspective in exhibition development, because you develop an exhibition by trying to say a story. The story as a starting point is the most important thing since you can fill it out with tangible and less tangible aspects; you are not starting with an object."

In a similar context, talking about her work in the community exhibition space for the preparation of the Indian, Italian, and Scots temporary exhibitions, but also of Passports, Stephanie Gibson acknowledged that "for me intangible heritage is the low level stuff: the interviews I do with people in the communities, the oral histories, the cultural events and the participation of people on a day to day basis." For her, the human dimension was one of the key areas of concern embodied in "community stories and peoples' memories." "We are a story-driven museum," she underlined. "This museum is driven by narrative and the narrative that we go for is the personal voice. This is a voice-driven museum, not so much an object, or curator-driven institution. The goal was to bring in the New Zealand audience as a whole, which is something that has been achieved."

However, she also expressed some reservations about the issue of collaboration with communities. As she acknowledged, "at the end of the day, it was not co-curating, we were calling the shots; co-curating would be a bit of a dream."[15] As will be discussed in chapter 5, similar issues about the power dynamics of participatory museology have also emerged in the context of the National Museum of the American Indian.

THE CHANGING FACE OF TRADITION

Reflecting ongoing debates on recognition, reconciliation, and unity, Te Papa has been conceptualised as a "forum" for discussing and revising a divided and turbulent national past, a theme that is still perpetuated in the ethnically divided exhibitions on level four. In this sense intangible heritage is tied up with Te Papa's efforts to humanise and indigenise the museum and serve its vision of a national space of dialogue.

The acknowledgement and inclusion of Maori culture and tradition in the official museum narrative has informed local understandings of intangible heritage. Matauranga Maori, embodied in Maori oral history, creation myths, and cosmologies; the spiritual importance of the land; tikanga; Maori customs, protocols, and celebrations; and the symbolical space of the marae constitute a key framework for interpreting intangible heritage as the living legacy inherited from the ancestors and revived and reinterpreted by contemporary generations. The revival of traditional knowledge and skills in the contemporary context of the Makotukutuku house, Te Aurere Iti canoe, Maori music instruments, and kapa haka shows that heritage is not negotiated in terms of endangered traditions that need to be safeguarded from globalisation, but as the active reclamation of a past that had been sleeping and is now waking up.

In the context of the politics of representation, this also affirms a strong Maori presence that has dynamically faced the trials of colonisation and emerged stronger. Through ideas of revival, reconnection, and performance, intangible heritage is not fixed and static, but an expression of ever changing identities rooted in a proud tradition, but also in flux and open to reinterpretation. Nylon might have replaced natural fibres in Maori kapa haka, but in this process people are engaging in new and contemporary ways with cultural traditions. Departing from the official construction of intangible heritage within the preservationist context of global heritage, the examination of its negotiations in Te Papa has revealed alternative paths. Here, themes of reviving rather than documenting tradition are particularly strong. Moreover, the idea of mana taonga, of historic treasures as living ancestors intimately connected with present generations, provides a new context for thinking about the tangible and intangible relationship.

In the next chapter, these issues are further explored in a different organisation in the Pacific, the Vanuatu Cultural Centre (VCC). Celebrated as an exemplary "Indigenous museum," the VCC provides an alternative museological model. It is in this context that intangible heritage becomes a tool for bringing forward local concerns on *kastom* preservation and sustainable development.

Chapter 4

At the Interface of *Kastom* and Development: The Case of the Vanuatu Cultural Centre

The Vanuatu Cultural Centre is unique in the world. It is not only about the things you see in the museum, but about the life that people live.

—Jean Tarisesei, Head of the Women's Cultural Project, Vanuatu Cultural Centre

Cultural revival and traditional knowledge, the empowerment of local communities and the animation of museum collections provided a first context for discussing intangible heritage within Te Papa. Rather than a set of cultural practices untainted by modernity, intangible heritage emerges as fluid and open to change. This chapter examines these issues in the context of the Vanuatu Cultural Centre (VCC) in Port Vila, the capital of the Melanesian island state of Vanuatu. Over the last decades the VCC has been an institution of an important standing in Pacific museological literature (Stanley 1998; Jolly 2001; Bolton 2003, 2006, 2007; Geismar 2003; Geismar and Tilley 2003; Kasarherou 2007). Drawing on the VCC's complex colonial history, the involvement of international researchers in its development as an institution, and its more recent grassroots projects, the chapter explores how intangible heritage is adopted in the VCC to serve its postcolonial Indigenous museology (see Stanley 2007).

Heritage negotiations in Vanuatu unfold largely against the backdrop of the local discourse on kastom[1] (see Keesing and Tonkinson 1982; Philibert 1986; Jolly and Thomas 1992a; Linnekin 1992; Jolly 1994; Bolton 2003). *Kastom*, the Bislama[2] word for precolonial customary ways of life, spans the cultural heritage spectrum of tangible and intangible heritage and establishes a different dichotomy based on the distinction between colonial and precolonial practices. In Vanuatu the preservation of kastom has been one of the main narratives of nation

Intangible Heritage and the Museum: New Perspectives on Cultural Preservation by Marilena Alivizatou, 77–103. ©2012 Left Coast Press, Inc. All rights reserved.

building in the postcolonial period, expressed in efforts to document and revive local and customary traditions and ways of life. Recent debates around kastom and development (for example Stanley 1998; Regenvanu 1999, 2005; Bolton 2007) hint at further critical negotiations of cultural heritage and tradition. After the country's independence in 1980 and with the input of foreign researchers, including anthropologists, linguists, and ethnomusicologists, the VCC has worked closely with local communities across the archipelago on issues of kastom preservation. The establishment of the Oral Traditions Project in the 1970s has been one of the main activities of the VCC and reveals an un-museum-like interest in the preservation of practices and traditional ways of life rather than the conservation of material culture (Kaeppler 1994; Huffman 1996; Tryon 1999; Bolton 2003).

Rather than a collections-based museum, the VCC has been conceptualised more as a "peaceful *nakamal*,"[3] a meeting house dedicated to cultural preservation and identity work with an increasing focus on local, economic, and social development. Unlike Te Papa, which foregrounds the idea of ethnic and cultural diversity, here the national mobilisation on intangible heritage reveals how distinct cultural traditions are engulfed in a broader post-independence ni-Vanuatu narrative.

VCC: THE PEACEFUL NAKAMAL AND THE GLOBAL HERITAGE ARENA

Previously known as New Hebrides[4] and administered since 1906 as a joint British and French condominium, the island nation of Vanuatu proclaimed its independence in July 1980 after a decade of sociopolitical mobilisation (Bolton 2003:12–22). Eight years after independence, with the Vanuatu National Cultural Council Act the Parliament predicted "the establishment of the Vanuatu National Cultural Council, for the preservation, protection, and development of various aspects of the rich cultural heritage of Vanuatu." By the end of the 1980s the VCC was the principal national executing body that would implement programmes to achieve the Council's objectives. In what follows I examine key moments in the VCC's pre- and post-independence history, tracing how the organisation evolved from a small colonial museum into a paradigmatic Indigenous cultural centre, and how it has since emerged as a key player in the global heritage arena.

Bolton (2003) and Tryon (1999) situate the foundation of the Port Vila Museum, the ancestor of the VCC, in 1956, as part of the celebrations for the fiftieth anniversary of the condominium. Mainly sustained by diplomatic employees in their spare time, the museum was initially located on the main road of Port Vila and soon developed a collection of both ethnographic objects and natural history specimens. Quoting

Woodward, the political secretary at the British embassy in charge of the museum, Bolton argues that the museum was primarily used as a storage place for objects that were either donated to or collected by colonial officials and was rarely visited by ni-Vanuatu (Bolton 2003:33–34).

Today the VCC is an umbrella organisation that includes the National Museum, the National Library, the Film and Sound Unit, the Historical and Cultural Sites Survey, and the Oral Traditions Project. The remit of the VCC is not limited to the collection, conservation, and presentation of material culture; rather, it extends to wider issues in the areas of education, social inclusion, and cultural preservation, engaging local communities and individuals through different grassroots programmes (Regenvanu 1999). In addition, it monitors research in the archipelago, acting as the fundamental link between local communities and international researchers. Departing from the traditional understanding of the museum as a repository of material culture, the VCC is also an active agent in civil society. For example, the Women's Culture Project that was established in 1994 (Bolton 2003, 2006, 2007) contributed significantly to the empowerment of ni-Vanuatu women, while the Young Peoples Project established in 1997 (Mitchell 2002) sensitised national policy towards the effects of recent changes in demographics[5] and the social, professional, and financial difficulties encountered by younger generations. Both programmes, which are currently sustained by the VCC, were initially administered by international researchers in partnership with local communities, with the aim of benefiting the latter.

This begs the question of what led to the transformation of a rather marginal colonial museum described as a storage place into the country's (if not the region's) most popular and dynamic cultural centre/nakamal. The engagement of local communities has featured in VCC's work well before the country's independence and can be traced to the activities and initiatives of non-Native researchers conducting fieldwork in Vanuatu in the 1960s and 1970s, as well as the involvement of international and foreign agencies and institutions, including for example UNESCO and the Australian National University (Huffman 1996; Bolton 2003). The recruitment of Kirk Huffman, an anthropology student conducting research on the island of Malekula, as curator of the VCC in the 1970s significantly altered the historical course of the institution. As Bolton remarked, "Huffman's emphasis was always more on the ideas and practices of the ni-Vanuatu in their own communities than on anything that was kept in the museum" (2003:38). Huffman's concerns were instrumental in informing the VCC's continuous focus on living and intangible rather than material culture, ultimately defining its community-oriented perspective.

With funds from the South Pacific Commission and UNESCO and the intellectual input of Huffman as well as of ethnomusicologist Peter Crowe and linguist Michel Charpentier, the Oral Traditions Project was put into practice in 1976 (Huffman 1996:290). The project started as a wish "to get Melanesians interested in the documentation and revival of their traditional cultures" (Bolton 2003:36). Based on the rationale that Western influences endangered traditional customary practices, it aimed at training selected ni-Vanuatu from throughout the archipelago, subsequently called fieldworkers, in documentation techniques and at encouraging dialogue on ways for sustaining and reviving traditional culture. Local fieldworkers were trained in ethnographic methods like dictionary making, the recording of genealogies, and the documentation of specific customary practices in their islands (Regenvanu 2003:2). Under the guidance of Kirk Huffman, the programme gained wide momentum on a national level: by the time of my research the number of fieldworkers had grown from the initial two men to one hundred individuals, forty of whom were women. The Oral Traditions Project, with its strong preservationist connotations, is one of the nodal moments in the history of VCC, defining the organisation's turn to grassroots research and informing local conceptualisations of intangible heritage.

As acknowledged by VCC staff, being a fieldworker is an honour and as such fieldworkers do not receive wages. They convene every year in a series of workshops taking place in the VCC in which they discuss their research. The recordings and information that they collect are kept in the VCC's Tabu Room, access to which is restricted to VCC staff and community representatives. For Huffman,

> the project is purely ni-Vanuatu oriented, and is seen as one of the many ways to assist in the local preservation, promotion and development of Vanuatu's rich linguistic and cultural heritage . . . The aim is to build a bank of kastom to be used by future generations of ni-Vanuatu wishing to reach their roots, and to retain and develop their own identity. [1996:291]

Anthropological researchers and other social scientists have influenced the scope of the Oral Traditions Project in terms of both subject matter and methods. Reflecting on her own impact on the VCC kastom discourse, Bolton wrote:

> Darrel Tryon, a linguist, leads the men fieldworkers' workshop every year,[6] and when the women fieldworker's group was established I brought my own anthropological understanding and training to the task of teaching that group. All of us have contributed our own understandings of culture and of kastom to the fieldworkers' discourse and have introduced them to fieldwork methodologies from our disciplines. [1999:5]

The conceptualisation of kastom in the fieldworkers' project has been significantly informed by Western methods and research questions, and as such themes of salvage, loss, and cultural preservation are particularly strong. This requires a more focused examination of the history and meanings of kastom.

Kastom

Retracing the history of discussions on kastom in the pre-independence period, Regenvanu has remarked the intensity of "the ideological struggle between custom . . . and the representations of the colonial regime" (2005:40). He argues that the demonisation of traditional practices by Western missionaries and colonial agents led to extensive loss of knowledge and practice and to the devaluation of precolonial culture, which came to be referred to in Bislama as "time of darkness." This, Regenvanu claims, has led to a "psychology of dependency" on "what is not or from ourselves" (2005:38–39). As such, Walter Lini's[7] commitment to "establishing a state based on 'Melanesian values', practicing a 'Melanesian socialism'" (2005:40) demonstrated a will to self-determination based not on colonially imposed values, but on local kastom. The 1980 Constitution's acknowledgement of traditional ownership of the land by local communities substantiated the value of kastom in the formation of the new state.

Two years after Vanuatu's independence, the publication of a special volume of the journal *Mankind* entitled "Reinventing Traditional Culture: The Politics of Kastom in Island Melanesia" (Keesing and Tonkinson 1982) sparked discussions among anthropologists about the manipulation of kastom in the post-independence period. Keesing remarked that "the leaders of Melanesia often idealize the pre-colonial past . . . appeal to a nationalist sentiment and seek to fashion a positive sense of identity with rhetoric about the Melanesian Way" (Keesing 1982:297). In the same tone, Tonkinson commented on the unproblematised use of kastom on local and national levels: while locally it seems to be "defining differences and marking boundaries among competing groups," nationally it "forms the basis for a pan-regional 'Melanesian Way', vaguely defined but clearly different from, and in some respects opposed to, modern Western culture" (Tonkinson 1982a:302). Similarly, drawing on discussions about invented traditions in the "fetishization of the past," Philibert observed that "nation-building in Melanesia has required an indigenization of the state," conceptualised and implemented by "Western-trained Vanuatu bureaucrats, ex-churchmen, and civil servants who have promised to build a modern country molded onto traditional ways and values," adding that although this "Westernised elite . . . knows least about kastom [it] is busy inventing it" (1986:7–9).

Similar comments about the invention of tradition were also expressed in the 1980s regarding the revival of Maori art and culture, and, as Jolly and Thomas have remarked, are often translated as "saying that a tradition is false or fabrication" (1992b:243). Keesing's statement that "the ancestral ways of life being evoked rhetorically (by Melanesian leaders) may bear little relation to those documented historically, recorded ethnographically and reconstructed archaeologically" (1989:19) seem to devalue ni-Vanuatu claims to cultural continuity as inauthentic fabrications compared to the Western scientific record. In the following years and with the imposition of the moratorium on anthropological research in 1985, discussions on the invention and spuriousness of kastom toned down and researchers became more reflexive on the ethnocentrism of their judgements.

However, discussions on kastom cannot be situated only in the post-colonial search for roots and identity of the 1970s, but need to be contextualised within the early days of colonisation. The arrival of Western settlers and missionaries in the nineteenth century and the introduction of new languages and religions increasingly made people "self-conscious of their way of life" (Lindstrom and White 1994:1). Although the impact of colonisation was felt differently in different islands, many were the islanders throughout the archipelago who changed their "religious, economic and political life to conform to European models" (Jolly 1993:341). While ni-Vanuatu were faced with major changes brought about by their contact with the West, including conversion to Christianity and massive dislocations, which led to the diversification of their ways of life, their "traditional culture" became progressively the focus of study by anthropologists travelling in Melanesia and the rest of the world in order to "salvage" the customs, traditions, and material culture of "disappearing races."

Starting in the late 1800s and throughout the twentieth century a series of anthropologists and other social scientists have conducted research on different aspects of social and cultural practice (for details see Bolton 2003:xxviii). These fieldtrips not only resulted in the collection of artefacts and audio and photographic records from the archipelago, held today by many museums and research institutions around the world,[8] but also established a certain way of looking, talking, and thinking about local customs and ways of life. The political use of kastom in the late 1970s then has been significantly influenced by the research of the previous decades, including anthropological research conducted on different aspects of kastom.

For example, in 1996 the English publication of Felix Speiser's *Ethnology of Vanuatu* (originally published in 1923), one of the first detailed ethnographic accounts of the archipelago, was forwarded by

Iolu Abil, who was the ni-Vanuatu minister of home affairs at the time. Speiser's observations, such as "the culture was already in a sorry state of decay almost everywhere, and I probably arrived only just in time to salvage what was left" (1996:2) are dismissed as "ethnocentric comments . . . of those early times." Instead, he remarks that "the amount of ethnographic and photographic material he collected is of great value to our new nation," adding that Speiser's work has "often assisted our people in the revival of certain traditional art forms thought to have been lost forever" (1996:vii). By foregrounding local ways of knowledge and practice, anthropological research becomes a means of counteracting the "psychology of dependency" (Regenvanu 2005), instilling pride in and raising the profile of traditional culture. As such, the preservationist work of the VCC as a guardian of the "rich cultural heritage of Vanuatu" is strongly informed by anthropological approaches towards what constitutes kastom. In the last decade, however, kastom is negotiated in Vanuatu within the parameters of another and often competing discourse: the one about development.

Development

Visiting the VCC in the late 1990s, Joy Hendry mentions that "foreign anthropologists, including those who helped establish it, had been expelled for a period after independence and it was running according to local ideas" (2005:86). Taking on the directorship of the VCC in 1995, Ralph Regenvanu's objective was to "mainstream the issue of culture and cultural heritage in national development" (2005:42). As Bolton observes, while Huffman was more concerned with the revival of traditional customary practices and as such practiced a more conservationist approach towards kastom, Regenvanu's approach aimed at raising "the profile of kastom and drawing it into the unfolding process of Vanuatu's national development" (2007:24). Kastom was thus conceptualised not only as vulnerable aspects of traditional life in need of preservation, but also as knowledge and practice stemming from the past that could be mobilised to serve the present and future. Ideas of cultural authenticity that surrounded early approaches to the Oral Traditions Project were gradually replaced by an approach that acknowledged the fluidity and adaptability of kastom to present conditions.

The adoption in 1992 of the Cultural Research Policy, which resulted in the lifting of the moratorium on foreign research, reformulated the terms on which researchers were welcome in Vanuatu. As Regenvanu remarked, the objective of the policy was not to "rejuvenate academic discourse about Vanuatu's culture," but to ensure that "at other levels more relevant to their own lives, ni-Vanuatu can perceive research as an exercise over which they can have some control, in which they can meaningfully participate and from which they can benefit" (1999:99). The policy states that "there must be maximum involvement of Indigenous scholars, students and members of the community in research, full recognition of their collaboration, and training to enable their further contribution to country and community" (Vanuatu Cultural Council 1992 §7); that "where research is undertaken with a local community, the research will include a product of immediate benefit and use to that community" (§8.1); and that "the National Cultural Council may request any researcher to provide certain products or perform certain services additional to their research work" (§8.3).

Through this process the VCC has not only been active in reframing the scope of foreign research in the archipelago, but has also become a key administrator of that same research on both national and international levels. I mentioned earlier how the Oral Traditions Project was established with funds from UNESCO and the Australian National University, channelled in Vanuatu primarily through foreign researchers. Today, the VCC and its staff have established programmes and partnerships with major institutions such as the British Museum, the Cambridge Museum of Archaeology and Anthropology, the Field Museum in Chicago and the National Museum of Australia to promote research for the benefit of ni-Vanuatu. Moreover, the VCC has become active in the global heritage scene administered by UNESCO and its various networks, with heritage projects relating both to intangible heritage and to the World Heritage Centre.[9]

One such example is the proclamation of the practice of *sandroing* (sand-drawing) as a Masterpiece of Intangible Heritage in 2003 (Zagala 2004). Mostly practiced in the northern and central islands of Vanuatu, sandroing is a complex communication practice of writing or drawing geometric and abstract pictures on the ground, sand, volcanic ash, or clay. The master drawers' skills are assessed not only in terms of their ability to make aesthetically impressive or complex designs, but also with regard to the narration of relevant stories. The proclamation of the sandroing is celebrated in the museum with a large panel and a permanent interactive display. What is interesting to note is how the VCC buys into the formal UNESCO approach towards the preservation of intangible heritage and marriages this with calls for development; how, for example, the practice is described as an intrinsic part of ni-Vanuatu identity threatened with abandonment; and how an action plan, including sandroing festivals and competitions, formal and informal education and a database of designs, has been predicted for its safeguarding (www.vanuatuculture.org). In this sense, intangible heritage emerges not only as kastom that needs to be safeguarded, but also as a tool for soliciting international attention and aid towards the benefit of local communities. As Regenvanu observed in an interview, "it is true that we collaborate with many overseas museums and organisations and we take on a lot of their knowledge and categorisations. If it works we use it, if it does not, sometimes we change the meaning of it." In this context, the VCC has adopted the idea of intangible heritage to conflate kastom and development, and in so doing suit the ni-Vanuatu heritage lexicon. The VCC is both a museum and a nakamal run by local people and for the benefit of local people by combining local and external methods, techniques, and understandings of heritage. The actual museum space of the VCC provides an interesting setting for examining these issues further.

THE MUSEOLOGY OF THE VCC

The VCC is situated off the centre of Port Vila, on a small hill facing the National Parliament. Its different sections are housed in the National Museum, which is part of a wider construction complex including the National Council of Women and the Malvatumauri or Council of Chiefs (Figures 4.1, 4.2). Initial plans included the construction of several more buildings, but funding limitations at the time of my research had put

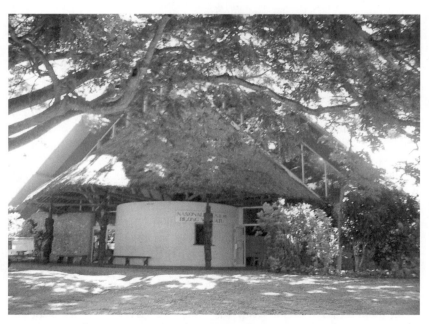

Figure 4.1: The Vanuatu Cultural Centre. (All images in this chapter published with permission of VCC.)

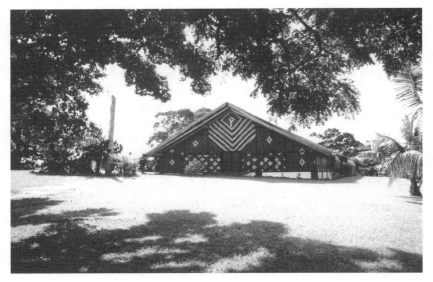

Figure 4.2:   The Malvatumauri, or Council of Chiefs, Vanuatu Cultural Centre.

a stop to their erection. The complex also includes a ceremonial open space (*nasara*) for the performance of different events, celebrations, activities, and meetings.

The VCC moved to its current location in 1995. Prior to that, it was based in the centre of Port Vila and, according to different sources, in a not so inviting building (Bolton 2003:32–34). Visiting the old museum in 1984, Kaeppler remarked, "I was surprised by the cavalier treatment of the quite extraordinary objects on display. Most objects were not in cases, including such fragile items as sculptures made of tree fern and earth colors. Objects can be touched and labels were at a minimum, if they existed at all" (1994:40).

While in the 1980s the conservation and interpretation of objects were apparently not among the top priorities of the VCC, the subsequent training of staff in museum practices in the 1990s had resulted by the time of my research in a more mainstream museological approach, with glass cases and labels accompanying the artefacts. As pointed by Jimmy Takaronga Kuautonga, VCC curator, the museum made an effort to mainstream exhibitions and object conservation areas and align them with Western museum work by training staff in basic collections management skills in Australia.

Reaching the museum from the southeast, passing in front of the Malvatumauri, the architectural similarities between the two buildings with their wide roofs almost touching the ground are obvious. Although both were constructed in the 1990s, the tradition-inspired architecture links them to ni-Vanuatu culture, underlining their contemporary roles as "guardians of kastom." My first impressions of the VCC were much informed by my meeting with Eddie Hinge Virare, VCC guide and master sand-drawer, who introduced me not only to the museum displays, but also to different expressions of local kastom, such as songs and sandroings. In our discussions, he extensively talked about aspects of local kastom, often making jokes about past practices no longer part of ni-Vanuatu life.

At the entrance to the museum, a big panel introduces sandroing in French, English, and Bislama (Figure 4.3). The panel bears the stamps of UNESCO and of the Vanuatu National Cultural Council; after describing the tradition and its meaning, it concludes by stating:

> On Friday 7, October 2003, UNESCO proclaimed Vanuatu sandroing a Masterpiece of the Oral and Intangible Heritage of Humanity. This international distinction honours the most remarkable examples of oral traditions and forms of cultural expressions in all regions of the world. The UNESCO jury awarded Vanuatu an additional prize as recognition of sandroing's outstanding cultural value and to encourage the people of Vanuatu to sustain and protect this unique practice.

Next to the panel is a permanent interactive display in the form of a board containing sand. Eddie Hinge Virare made several sandroings representing the storm, the yam, the turtle, and love (Figure 4.4), and narrated local myths about the meaning of each. He also played a flute and sang two songs: the first one about an old man in search of a wife

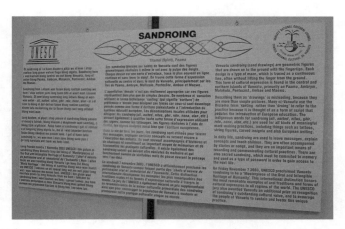

Figure 4.3: At the museum's entrance a large panel written in English, French, and Bislama introduces the practice of sandroing and its proclamation as a UNESCO masterpiece.

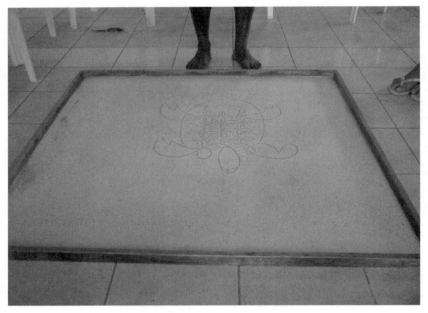

Figure 4.4: The permanent interactive display for making sandroings at the National Museum.

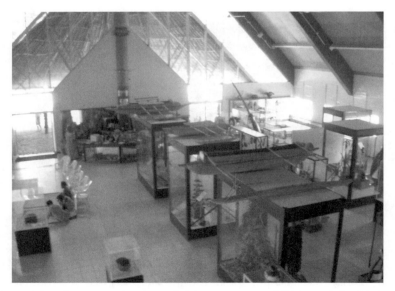

Figure 4.5: A panoramic view of the permanent exhibition of the National Museum with local people making sandroings in the lower left corner.

and the second about a boy mourning the loss of his parents. He then took me around the museum displays, explaining the origins and meanings of many objects and talking about the different islands of Vanuatu. A key theme of his talk was the idea that by preserving kastom the VCC preserves people's sense of identity (Figure 4.5).

Further into the exhibition, the artefacts that grab attention next to the sandroing panel are a carriage and a flag of New Hebrides containing the English and French flags. Eddie Hinge Virare explained that these items represent the colonial period in the history of Vanuatu. The carriage stands for the introduction of wheeled vehicles, and the flag stands for the emergence of nationalism in an island archipelago that only in the last century emerged as a unified entity. Behind these, several display cases contain findings from archaeological excavations proving that the islands were inhabited for several centuries prior to the arrival of Europeans. Great emphasis is given to the Lapita, early inhabitants of the islands, and to the presentation of ceramic findings from archaeological excavations. Central to the display are materials from a royal tomb, allegedly that of Chief Roi Mata, discovered by French archaeologists. According to Eddie Hinge Virare, local legends and oral traditions about a powerful chief who was buried with his wives and servants about four hundred years ago led archaeologists to excavate the northwest regions of the island of Efate in the 1960s.[10]

After the presentation of the archaeological material, the narrative moves to artefacts that were primarily collected in the twentieth century and that make up the museum's ethnographic collections. As Geismar and Tilley have observed, islands that are particularly famous for the production of certain types of objects take precedence over the rest (2003:176). For example, large slit drums, also known as *tam-tams*, from Ambrym feature prominently on the northern wall of the exhibition, together with graded figures from Malekula. A label near them, entitled "Graded societies and societies based on title: Forms and rites of traditional power in Vanuatu," explains the two types of political power, "chiefdoms based on hereditary titles and chiefdoms based on achievements," adding that the latter is "going through something of a renaissance, especially in islands like Ambae, Pentecost and Maewo."

Next to them is the reconstruction of a men's house from Malekula containing an effigy. Eddie Hinge Virare explained that when important persons died, they were not buried but kept in their houses. He noted that the presence of the dead ancestor was a form of spiritual guidance, adding, however, that such practices were no longer performed for hygienic reasons. Facing the men's house is a display case showing the "statue of a dead chief" from Malekula. Contrary to New Zealand and the USA, the display of human remains is still practiced in Vanuatu. A label nearby explained that "in South Malekula skull masks were made from skulls of important men or of a dead person that was particularly loved," adding that "there was generally no great fear of death and a belief in the temporary survival of the soul, the duration of which depended on the grade of the dead man."

Not far from the dead chief's statue, a separate display case containing different weapons, like clubs and spears, presents a different story. Here it is not the museum curator who is speaking but rather Chief Willie Bongmatur, who narrates the "History of the fighting club" (Figure 4.6).

This club belonged to my ancestor Malsagaveul. It was made somewhat around 1913 or earlier, the time there was fighting at Deep Point, West Ambrym. When Malsageveul died, the club was given to another of my ancestors, Melewun Tare. Melewun Tare smoked the club over a custom fire to make it strong for use at the time of war. The same club was used for a long time by a chief when he stood up to talk on the nasara or at a ceremony, he held onto the club, as security for himself and for his people. There is also a song connected with the club used at the time of war. The song says "When you hit me you miss me, I will hit you." This song gives more power to the club to enable it to kill plenty of people. This club was cut from a strong old piece of oak, not using whiteman's tools, but using a stone axe and shells to cut it. In order to cut down the oak tree, they burnt it with fire. Today very few people know how to make a club like this. After Independence, my uncle Paul Temakon, sold the club to a Frenchman called Peko, from Olul. I was not pleased when I heard this news, so I bought back the club from him. At this time I performed a

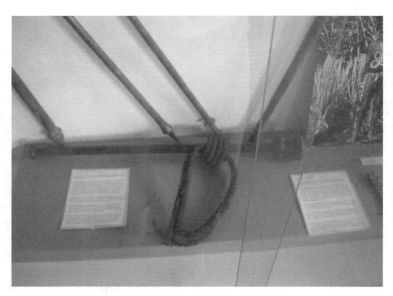

Figure 4.6: The story of the fighting club.

custom ceremony to take back the club and then I took it to Vila. I will go back to Ambrym and talk with my uncle, Paul, in case he has some more stories or historical information about this club. What I have told you is what my father told me. Now I am the new owner of the club. After the customary ceremony I performed I thought it would be good to put the club into the National Museum in remembrance of my ancestors.

Chief Bongmatur's account of the club's story as it passed from one owner to the next recounts the life of the artefact and reveals its multilayered trajectory. The fact that it was deposited in the VCC in remembrance of the ancestors highlights that the VCC is regarded not as a storage place for objects collected by anthropologists or excavated by archaeologists, but instead as a community space, a public meeting house, and a place for safekeeping cherished artefacts and commemorating local history. The narrative underlines the chief's will to make visible the club's history as a political process of representation and cultural reification. As such, the club stands as a symbol of history and a link with the ancestral figures that owned and used it.

The museum makes several efforts to allude not only to aspects of contemporary life, but also to changes in customary practices incurred through contact with Western culture. For example, the section "Ornaments and Beauty" describes in detail the practices of head elongation and female tooth extraction, but as Eddie Hinge Virare stressed in our discussions, as something of the past that is no longer performed following concerns over the violation of fundamental human rights. The display of *goulong* masks from Malap in South Malekula further illustrates the idea of cultural revival and renewal of tradition. In the late 1990s Marcelin Abong, who became director of the VCC in November 2006 after Ralph Regenvanu's resignation,[11] took photographs of earlier goulong masks displayed at the Parisian Musée des Arts d'Afrique et d'Océanie. As Eddie Hinge Virare pointed out, local clan members made the goulong masks currently on display in the VCC after seeing the photos that Marcelin Abong brought back from Paris. According to the label, the new masks were used as part of the Luan Veuv dance "performed on the occasion of the Catholic Church celebrations of St. Pierre Chanel in Lamap." The revival of traditional dances within a Christian context reveals contemporary dimensions of tradition, providing thus a more fluid framework for negotiating kastom (see also Bolton 2003).

Similarly, the label that accompanies a display case about the ceremony of Nalawan Nevenban and the associated ritual object reads:

Nalawan Nevenban was brought here after a ceremony which was performed by Chief Mathias Batik. After the ceremony Chief Batik gave a custom chief title to the former director of the VCC Mr. Ralph Regenvanu on the 17th of November 2006, after he resigned from his position as director. The custom title given to Mr. Regenvanu by Chief Batik is "LIBELHAMEL TAHA TAMATA," which means "he who looks after the Nakamal (meeting house) that always has peace in it" . . . This title has been given to Mr. Regenvanu after all the excellent work he has done within the VCC up to the standard it is in today.

Here, the VCC celebrates and commemorates an important event of the community. The fact that a customary title is given to a person that has been primarily concerned with "streaming development into the discourse on kastom" hints at new ways for thinking about kastom beyond the idea of preservation per se and in terms of community benefit.

Another important issue emerging from this display is the conceptualisation of the VCC as a nakamal, or meeting house. Just like the label with the chief's account of the war club's history, here as well the VCC emerges not simply as an artefact storehouse, but as a collective space for cultural transmission and nation building. The fundamental role of the VCC in bringing communities and people from the different islands together was stressed in most of my interviews with the museum's staff. The title given to Ralph Regenvanu, the caretaker of the peaceful nakamal, underlines his role as a guardian of the VCC, and the VCC's pivotal role in the building of a united nation with a rich kastom, but also in dialogue with the rest of the world. Past, present, and future, kastom and development are brought together in the discourse of the peaceful nakamal.

Moving further into the exhibition, another significant point alluding to the recent history of Vanuatu is the collection of photographs and documentary material from the early 1980s and the struggle for independence. Decorated with yellow, green, and red ribbons, which are the colours of Vanuatu's flag, a large panel contains photographs portraying the marches for independence, the transfer of power from colonial authorities, and Father Walter Lini, who was the president of the Vanua'ku Pati and the country's first prime minister. While the carriage and the colonial flag were presented in the beginning of the exhibition, this section seems to mark the end of museum displays. Key moments in the islands' history, like the beginning of the colonial period and the country's independence, frame the display of ethnographic material, bringing together history and kastom.

The final section of the display, in the museum's southwest corner, is the natural history collection, which was donated to the museum in the 1960s by German naturalist Heinrich Bregulla (Bolton 2003:33) and makes a subtle reference to the colonial origins of the VCC. This is mostly comprised of taxidermy specimens and seashells. Much like the natural history displays of Te Papa, this corner of the VCC underlines the bonds between nature and culture.

Despite the limited financial resources of the VCC, its exhibition narrative is regularly updated. As Jimmy Takaronga Kuautonga, VCC curator, explained, a new exhibition on canoes and the subject of "kastom transportation" would soon be mounted in the museum's mezzanine, accompanied by canoe-carving workshops and demonstrations. Moreover, in early 2008 objects and documentary material from World War II and the Condominium administration were added to the permanent exhibition, casting light on the more recent history of the archipelago. These recent additions demonstrate the responsiveness of the VCC to community concerns and its willingness to engage with historical rather purely kastom-related themes.

Apart from objects, the main museum space also contains photographs and posters revealing the range of activities undertaken by or in collaboration with the VCC. Two large photos, one of the female and the other of the male fieldworkers, hang from the wall, pointing to the less visible aspects of VCC work. Also, posters from the festivals held throughout Vanuatu after independence decorate the walls, reminding the cultural revivalist efforts of the 1970s and 1980s (Figure 4.7). The audiovisual equipment at the entrance of the hall is used to present recorded material, including ceremonies and local practices to international tourists, but primarily to local visitors interested in finding out more about traditional practices (Figure 4.8).

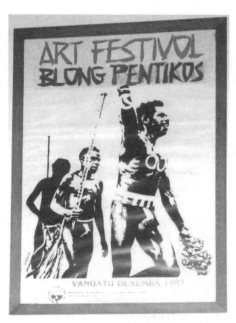

Figure 4.7: A poster of the Arts Festival of Pentecost that took place in 1985.

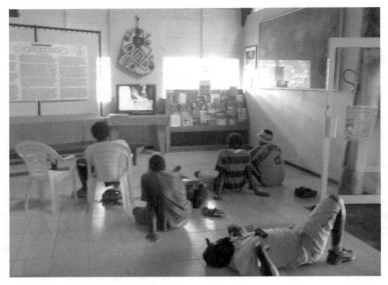

Figure 4.8: Recordings and films made in the context of the Oral Traditions Project are presented on special screens to local communities and young people living in Port Vila.

Overall the permanent museum space provides interesting perspectives for thinking about intangible heritage locally. Dominating the entrance to the museum, the sandroing panel foregrounds the UNESCO terminology in the VCC space: "outstanding cultural value," "sustain," and "protect" are key terms that define the practice and people's relationship with it. On the one hand, therefore, intangible heritage emerges as the UNESCO-based conceptualisation of kastom that needs to be safeguarded and passed on to future generations; on the other hand, Eddie Hinge Virare's approach towards the permanent displays offers alternative perspectives, whereby traditional practices such as head hunting, tooth extraction, and head elongation appear as defining aspects of ni-Vanuatu kastom that, although respected, are no longer practiced and are even the subject of jokes. Kastom seems to be a cultural asset that can serve current processes of local and national development. In this context, it emerges as something that is not fixed and static, but rather impermanent and ever changing.

NI-VANUATU APPROACHES TO MUSEUM WORK AND INTANGIBLE HERITAGE

My talks with the VCC staff highlighted the institution's role in sustaining traditional culture while at the same time balancing national development with cultural preservation. My informants are ni-Vanuatu that have worked at the VCC for several years and have extensively collaborated with expatriate researchers. In conversations with VCC staff it became evident that Western-derived notions of research and epistemological categorisations are filtered through the ni-Vanuatu context so as to serve local needs. What emerges is a holistic approach to heritage preservation, enacted by local engagements with museological concepts and techniques. In the context of the VCC, intangible heritage emerges both in subtle and in more direct ways as a particularly Melanesian framework for responding to ideas of preservation, identity, and development, empowering local people, as in the case of the sandroing, to act globally.

Jean Tarisesei, head of the Women's Culture Project, became involved with the VCC in the early 1990s and was trained in ethnographic methods by anthropologist Lissant Bolton, who at that time was working at the VCC to establish the project and also conduct her doctoral research. In the 1980s and early 1990s, kastom involved primarily practices and traditions performed by men.[12] Since 1991 and the establishment of the programme, Bolton and Tarisesei have been declaring that "women have kastom, too" (Bolton 2003), providing thus a more gendered approach to kastom and heritage. This has not only revealed a new dimension regarding the scope of kastom, but has also raised the profile of women on issues involving the safeguarding of local knowledge and traditional culture (Bolton 2007). The Women's Culture Project takes place every year since 1994 in the form of workshops, in which women fieldworkers meet to discuss their findings and identify future areas of research. Past themes have included food preservation, mat production, and marriage customs. Both men and women fieldworkers work independently in their islands and communities, collecting data for a year and then discussing them during the annual workshop. As Tarisesei remarked in an interview, "there is not always enough money to give them cameras and recording equipment. Some have video cameras, others use audio recordings or photographs and others write their data. We write a report for each workshop and keep all that in our stores."

Data collected from the research of men and women fieldworkers are kept in a special area of the VCC, the Tabu Room or oral traditions archive, situated in the backside of the building. Sam Kapere, who heads the VCC Film and Sound Unit, is responsible for administering the Tabu Room. As director of this unit, he is in charge of working with the fieldworkers, filming customary practices around the archipelago and keeping records of them. Access to the Tabu Room is controlled and restricted to VCC curators and community representatives, while copies of all recordings are sent back to the communities. For Sam Kapere, the "Tabu Room is like a traditional bank, where we archive the traditional knowledge of this country." The contents of the archive include post- and pre-independence recordings made in the context of the Fieldworkers' Project, but as Kapere underlined, the VCC, mainly with the help of Huffman, "managed to get the copies, masters and originals from the first films that were shot in Vanuatu in 1911 and 1925 . . . Our collection is very big and probably one of the biggest in the Pacific." Some of the recordings are disseminated over the radio and television, and others are used for publications and educational programmes. For Sam Kapere, notions of heritage preservation largely define the scope of the Tabu Room as a collective memory bank ensuring that kastom is never again lost or misappropriated.

For Jimmy Takaronga Kuautonga, the video, sound, and written records kept in the VCC archive are valuable not only for present communities and future generations, but also for a very important audience—the young people living in Port Vila. As he underlined, "the VCC is not only about the educated, but also about the jobless youth in Vila . . . The recordings and information gathered from the different islands are for ni-Vanuatu that do not know their culture, roots, and kastom." For him, traditional knowledge is a valuable asset that needs to be safeguarded, but that can also serve the public benefit.

For example, the Young People's Project[13] was initiated through the collaboration of the VCC with anthropologist Jean Mitchell. As Jean Tarisesei remarked talking about many young people throughout Vanuatu,

> when they finish school, they come into town to find work. But when they come most of them they don't find anything. Some of them, after school, they don't succeed in going further. So, they don't have work and their families and relatives are back in the islands. So, many of them have problems like stealing and having problems with other families living in Vila. The project tries to deal with these young people. We want to find what their intentions for coming into town are. We want to find out the expectations of these young people and how we can help them.

In the late 1990s, the VCC established the Juvenile Justice Project to set a special legal framework for dealing with young offenders. Today, the project aims to equip young people with the skill to advocate their interests and sensitise communities and government towards their concerns. While at the VCC, I met several younger ni-Vanuatu spending time in the museum, chatting with staff and watching videos of traditional ceremonies in the main museum space. For many, the VCC is a place where they come to learn more about island traditions and customary practices. The engagement of the VCC not only with tribal chiefs and elected fieldworkers, but also young unprivileged people demonstrates its commitment to serve all ni-Vanuatu. This transforms it from a museum and research institution to a dynamic cultural centre in tune with local and regional concerns. In parallel, reconnecting young people with kastom emerges as a central mission of the museum.

Ideas of social and cultural advocacy permeate also the work of Martha Kaltal. She is head of the Historical and Cultural Sites Survey, which in her words endeavours to "protect the historical and cultural sites for the people and the nation." The project, which was initially established by expatriate archaeologists, involves the documentation and excavation of sites and monuments. For Martha Kaltal this means that "we are collecting sites, but also the stories that are associated with them." As she explained, the survey includes historical sites, comprising mostly sites of the early European era—the 1600s of the traders and planters and the colonial era—and cultural sites, which are "sites of cultural values" and include "rock art caves, table stones, and special trees that are part of special ceremonies." Recent calls to modernise the islands by building roads, a new airport, and bungalows for ecotourism have threatened important sites in different islands. Working with community representatives from the islands of Malekula, the VCC managed to divert the new road that would pass from the nasara, the traditional meeting grounds and ceremonial spaces. For Kaltal, "development is okay, but we need to work together to make things work for everyone." Evident in her commentary are the conflicting values between kastom and development and the VCC's efforts to reconcile them.

Kastom and Development

A multidimensional personality—artist, anthropologist, barrister, and more recently member of parliament—Ralph Regenvanu served for more than a decade as the VCC's first ni-Vanuatu director. During his work at the VCC, a key priority for him was to support local development with a focus on sustainability and community benefit. In answering my questions, he repeatedly stressed the need to retain traditional culture against the growing pressures for social and economic growth. As he remarked, "we need to take development and empower culture, rather than destroy it." For Regenvanu, the "pressure to develop" is "a lot about destroying culture," as if saying that "what you have is not good enough and you need something better." It also prioritises aspects of living, such as "certain types of knowledge, having money, and consumerism," which "go very much against traditional culture." The VCC staff shared the concern that traditional ways of life were being abandoned in favour of Western ways of life. As Martha Kaltal observed, "the times are changing for the people in the islands. Modern life is coming in and many people don't see the importance of keeping their culture." As these comments reveal, economic development was increasingly problematised by the museum's staff. In an effort to promote national development with a focus on traditional culture, the year 2007 was declared the Year of Traditional Economy, and its key theme was how to achieve development by mobilising local knowledge, tradition, and expertise (see Huffman 1996).

Education and economy have become key arenas where the dynamics between traditional culture and development are played out. Jean Tarisesei noted that "our system and belief is that whatever knowledge you have, you pass it on to your children and grandchildren. But now children go to school and they don't spend that much time at home. This is why people are afraid that our kastom is disappearing." Since 2003 the VCC has been making efforts to inform school curricula with the knowledge about traditional culture gathered over the fieldworker's research of the last two decades. "We want the education system to teach our kids that you have Western knowledge, but you also have local knowledge, and that the two are equivalent. It is not that the one is better than the other," explained Ralph Regenvanu. In this context, in February 2008 the VCC launched the Urban Youth Kastom School to encourage young people to learn more about traditional culture, use vernacular languages, and develop skills that make use of available local resources in order to generate income.

Efforts to bring traditional culture into the lives of young people are also made on other levels. As Sam Kapere explained, the VCC produces once a week a radio programme and twice a month a television series on "Kastom and Culture." For Martha Kaltal, "people are changing and having a more modern life influenced by Western culture. But we have many activities in the museum to inform children about kastom. There is a music festival that lasts three days. Also every Saturday we have a children's programme with kastom dances, weaving, and sandroings. We also have a treasure hunt and traditional food preparations." For her, the VCC supports kastom education by coming up with new ways to transmit knowledge to younger generations through performance and practice. This hints at new engagements with kastom outside the traditional sphere of the family and tribe and at the formalisation of the VCC as a kastom school.

Along the same lines, the VCC is actively promoting the idea of a kastom economy (see also Huffman 1996). For Jean Tarisesei, "kastom economy is about retaining the ways our ancestors lived in the past . . . When we learn agriculture in the Western style, we need to buy spades, fertilisers and other equipment. But with the traditional way of gardening, we don't need anything. We make enough to feed our families." Sam Kapere expresses a similar opinion:

When the British and French came here, they told us to stop using canoes and they introduced cars. But we do not want to be dependent on oil prices. This could be devastating for our people . . . The introduction of Western lifestyles can eventually be very harmful to ni-Vanuatu. For example, if the international economy falls and prices rise, we won't be able to import rice. This is why we encourage people to live according to our kastom economy, cultivate the land, and use canoe to travel.

Kastom is thus put in the service of local sustainable development, which is eventually the objective of kastom economy and education. In this sense, reconnecting with kastom is a tool for reviving traditional ways of life and empowering local knowledge.

The Peaceful Nakamal

As we have seen, the VCC is actively involved in different aspects of social and cultural life. "We are out in the community. Assist them. Facilitate. Record. Document. Dialogue about what communities want to do," noted Ralph Regenvanu. "The government does not always reach people in the rural areas," noted Sam Kapere, "but we want to make sure that everyone is the same. Even though they are different and speak different languages, we want to make sure that they get the same service and equal benefits."

While the Vanuatu government has been criticised for catering to the needs of only a minority of citizens living mainly in Port Vila, through the fieldworker's network the VCC is reaching out to the different island communities, expressing pan-island concerns and preoccupations. It is thus negotiated as a peaceful nakamal, a space where ni-Vanuatu meet and discuss issues of identity and history. Its focus is more on the engagement of local communities and the revival of traditional ways of life through projects aimed at the social and economic benefit of local groups, rather than on the preservation and display of material culture. As a nakamal, the VCC is the guardian and the repository of collective memory about kastom, and its responsibility to ni-Vanuatu is to ensure that kastom is preserved in the future for the benefit and sustainable development of the community. Its interregional network of fieldworkers and international network of research partners have transformed the VCC into a quasi-political space serving local concerns and acting as a diplomat to the international community. The case of the sandroing and the Roi Mata site reveal not only concentrated efforts to mainstream kastom and development, but also the significant role of the VCC as a cultural agent in the international heritage scene of UNESCO and foreign institutions.

Fieldworkers

Rather than through international aid workers and NGOs, the preservation and revival of kastom are actively performed through the mobilisation of local participants. The fieldworkers' network emerges as a fundamental component of the VCC work, enabling the institution to reach all ni-Vanuatu, even the ones that live in the more isolated islands, facilitating communication between foreign researchers and local people, and ensuring that research projects run according to plans.

For Ralph Regenvanu, the Oral Traditions Project, which is administered by the fieldworkers, is a key example of how the VCC safeguards intangible heritage (2003:1). As he noted in an interview, "the fieldworkers are our cultural activists in the communities . . . They are the way through which we talk with communities about what they want for their heritage, they facilitate work to do with recording traditional knowledge, sites, oral tradition, and they also get resources from international museums to the communities." Similarly, Sam Kapere referred to the broader scope of the fieldworkers' role by underlining that "fieldworkers are not just documenting rituals and ceremonies; they also document their own language, traditional laws, and governance." This hints at a more inclusive understanding of traditional culture as the wider context of peoples' ways of life; in parallel, it also reveals that the title "fieldworker" adds a modern twist to traditional social grading systems, as fieldworkers constitute powerful players in local preservation initiatives to the benefit of local communities.

It is important to stress here that the scope of the fieldworkers' research area is largely defined by accepted gender roles and restrictions. As Martha Kaltal acknowledged, "we have men and women fieldworkers, because we have kastom that belongs only to men and kastom that belongs only to women . . . A man fieldworker would not do research about weaving, and a woman fieldworker would not do research about fishing; we respect the gender roles." Discussing the same topic, Jean Tarisesei argued that "there are some things that women do and don't talk to men about them, and also there are things men do and don't talk to women about them." The issue of gender roles in Vanuatu (Jolly 1993; Bolton 2003) is highly contested, especially with regard to ways of displaying and handling ritual objects that contrast significantly with Western approaches (see chapter 7 and Latour 2007).

Cultural Loss and Digital Repatriation

Another central theme in the narratives of VCC staff was the issue of cultural loss. As Jean Tarisesei remarked:

> Some of our things were lost a long time ago. They are now kept in museums around the world. Some of the researchers that come here to work

with us bring photos of these objects from the museums that they are now. We know where these objects come from and we give these photos back to the people. If they have lost the ways of doing things, then we can give them photos and they try to revive their ways and skills.

Similarly, Sam Kapere noted that "older recordings are taken back to communities and they take it to old people to identify the meaning of the songs. They listen to it, they practice it and then they dance to it."

Digital repatriation, as is nowadays called the practice of taking back to source communities photographs of objects and audio and visual recordings held in Western museums,[14] is increasingly encountered among the activities of museums and research institutions in Europe, USA, and Australia (for example Herle 2003; Murphy 2007). Often related to a postcolonial politics of recognition (Rowlands 2002), according to Ralph Regenvanu this practice benefits both parties. Talking about a recent collaboration with the Australian Museum, he stated:

> We are embarking on a new project with them. We try to bring the intangible elements of the artefacts to them. We make high-resolution images of the artefacts available to the communities that they can have as a resource back. These are images of their own pieces. In exchange of that, they tell us more of what they know about the pieces. Then this information goes back to the catalogue of the Australian Museum. So, we try to reconnect those collections with the people. In this way, both the museum and the communities benefit.

The idea of taking pictures of objects or people back to communities counteracts the feeling of cultural loss experienced with colonisation. Just like the case of the goulong masks on display at the museum, old photographs and recordings are used by communities to revive traditions, knowledge, and skills. Ralph Regenvanu even observed that "images are much more important to local communities than the artefacts," suggesting that reclaiming original objects is not as important as the establishment of mutually beneficial partnerships between foreign institutions and communities. Such partnerships eventually lead to the revival of ceremonies in which new cultural artefacts are created that empower local people to act globally.

Debating Materiality

In my discussions with the VCC staff, the artefacts on display in the museum were always connected to the ceremonies and practices in which they were used. In this sense, their physicality is less important than their ability to allude to the people that created them and to the broader context of their use. Sam Kapere, for example, observed that "these objects are alive. They are made and used in ceremonies. They are accompanied by special songs and languages. They are alive, they are not just dead objects." Similarly, Martha Kaltal noted:

> Some of the artefacts on display are alive, because they have been through a traditional ceremony, so they are taboo. We have a living culture in the people, in our traditional knowledge that cannot be destroyed. For example, some of the headdresses in the museum they have been to a traditional ceremony. When this is finished they have to destroy the headdresses. You destroy it because it is a living culture. You don't keep it. If you destroy it, the spirits go back to the place in the people for the next ceremony. It is taboo. You have to destroy it. Every headdress has to be destroyed. Even the most beautiful have to be destroyed.

The value of artefacts in the VCC is assessed in terms that are different from those suggested by mainstream approaches to museum objects. Headdresses or masks are not valued so much for their physical dimensions, but rather for their deeper meanings and associations, the role they play in ceremonial moments, and the knowledge or images that they convey. Preserving them physically for the future is often superfluous, because in the following year other masks will be made as part of the same ceremonies. Unlike mainstream curatorial practices that treat such objects as the material culture of a distant people, living in distinct ways, VCC curators often approach ritual objects as living entities with specific life cycles and belonging to certain ceremonies, recalling the processes of erasure, renewal, and impermanence examined in chapter 2. Objects are seen as part of wider processes of cultural transmission with limited life spans, in contrast with the Eurocentric notions of artefact authenticity and preservation.

PRESERVATION AND RENEWAL AT THE VCC

The group of ni-Vanuatu contemporary artists that was established in 1989 adopted the name Nawita (octopus), a word that could also describe the VCC: a central organisation operating a variety of projects in different areas bringing together the local and the global. Like an octopus, the VCC has tentacles that work independently or in collaboration with each other and feed back into the central body. As Bolton has observed, "few museums have the opportunity to make as much impact on the nation they represent" (2007:35). This chapter has demonstrated that the VCC is not only a museum, but an active cultural centre, a nakamal inviting local participation and at the same time a national institution that consolidates a unified national identity and monitors research on an international level.

In this context intangible heritage seems to be negotiated in both explicit and implicit ways, through an official preservationist approach and a more subtle and nuanced understanding that hints at a heritage of impermanence, fluidity, and change. The Oral Traditions Project and the work of the Film and Sound Unit, for instance, are characterised by fears of cultural loss and subsequent loss of identity, leading to the creation of a "bank" of intangible heritage expressions, which is the Tabu Room. Here, intangible heritage is the local kastom that is threatened by modern civilisation and needs to be revived through a kastom education and a kastom economy. Yet cultural revival also emerges, more subtly, as a space for subversive renegotiations. In my discussions with Eddie Hinge Virare, for example, it became clear that kastom is not fixed, but is often reworked so as to stay relevant in peoples' lives. With humour he explained that as headhunting is no longer practiced by ni-Vanuatu, population trends are growing and Vanuatu is the "happiest place in the world."[15]

Moreover, intangible heritage emerged as a framework for cultural preservation with a view on community development. In this sense, the celebration of the sandroing as a masterpiece of UNESCO protects, legitimises, and reworks the traditional practice locally, nationally, and internationally. The new regimes of visibility of the practice in the context, for example, of the sandboards of the National Museum, and the national or international festivals and commercial products enable local communities to create new utterances of tradition and invest kastom with contemporary meanings. This underlines preservation and transformation as a framework for rethinking intangible heritage, at the same time revealing its politicisation and entanglement in local and national objectives. The next chapter explores these last issues at the National Museum of the American Indian.

Chapter 5

Intangible Heritage at the
Living Memorial of Native Americans

> We could have chosen to look through our eight hundred plus thousand objects to find the most superlative, the most wonderfully beautiful, the most representative of each culture and just display that—which in some cases might have been a better idea. Instead, we took a chance to try and do something new.
>
> —José Barreiro, NMAI assistant director for research

"NMAI is not just about the past and certainly not about the dead or dying. It is about the living," announces a plaque outside the Alexander S. Hamilton Custom House in New York's lower Manhattan. Part of this early twentieth-century building, with the monumental statues of four female figures representing Africa, Europe, America, and Asia on the front, is occupied as of 1994 by the George Gustav Heye Center, the NMAI's New York site (Figure 5.1). During my fieldwork in the United States, I conducted research at the three sites of the NMAI: the New York museum, the museum on the Washington Mall, inaugurated in September 2004, and the Cultural Resources Center in Suitland, Maryland, which opened in 1999. Ideas of survival, renewal, cultural continuity, and pride in identity are prevailing throughout the NMAI and constitute the foundation for the development of a "new Indian museology" (Lonetree 2006b:636).

Based on its founding Act—the National Museum of the American Indian Act, proclaimed by U.S. Congress in 1989—the NMAI is required to be a living memorial of Native American cultures. Taking forward the discussions on the politics of representation presented in the previous chapters, I examine intangible heritage in the context of the dynamic between the living and the dead that is inherent in the idea of a living memorial. With its most famous site on the Washington Mall, the collective memory space and the heart of U.S. public life, the NMAI is fundamentally a political project bound up in painful memories of genocide and injustice. In this sense the idea of a living memorial stresses the dual

---

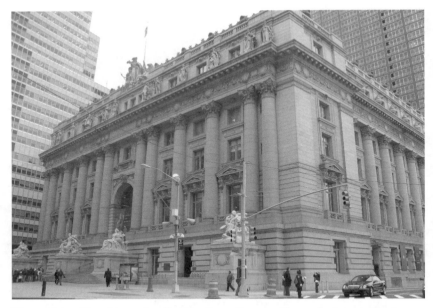

Figure 5.1: The Alexander S. Hamilton Custom House in lower Manhattan houses the National Museum of the American Indian in New York. In front of it the statues of four seated women represent America, Europe, Africa, and Asia.

purpose of the NMAI: coping with the past and celebrating the present and future. It is largely in terms of the latter that intangible heritage is negotiated as a bottom-up intervention much informed by processes of recognition and identity work in the context of a wish to represent, as was explained by NMAI staff, "the totality of the Native experience."

This presupposes on the one hand the active participation of Native communities, and on the other the development of new museum competencies, such as community engagement and cultural advocacy (Rosoff 2003; Sullivan and Edwards 2004). Given the painful history of museums as agents of plunder of sacred objects and desecration of Native graves, several questions have been raised about their contemporary role as mediators of memorialisation and community advocates (West 2000). Following the adoption of NAGPRA[1] in 1990, which resulted in the substantial return of sacred objects and human remains to Native communities (Simpson 1996; Nash and Colwell-Chanthaphonh 2010), the NMAI invites Native tribes of the Americas to become involved in museum work by curating exhibits, interpreting historical objects, and celebrating contemporary identity. For a growing number of museum critics (Fisher 2004; Rothstein 2004a, 2004b; Lujan 2005; Jacobson 2006; Zimmerman 2010), however, partnerships with communities often lead to a politicisation of the museum narrative that lacks scientific authority and turns exhibitions into a tool for political engagement.

In what follows I explore the representational strategies and discursive context of the NMAI and trace how the idea of a living memorial informs understandings of intangible heritage. Drawing on my findings from New Zealand, this chapter further examines self-representation and participatory work as avenues for the implementation of Indigenous museology, and problematises the role of the museum as a performative space of contemporary Native identities at the seat of the U.S. government. Unlike the bicultural, inclusive, and reconciliatory narrative of Te Papa, the NMAI is a monument to the survival of Native American cultures, the scars of colonialism, and contemporary Native identity. As such, far from being a "palace of collections" (West 2007), the museum emerges as a battleground for the negotiation of cultural rights and the advancement of a politics of recognition.

NMAI: Origins

Although the NMAI is celebrated today as a living museum in tune with the late twentieth-century postcolonial context (Simpson 1996; Kreps 2003:79–113), its roots can be traced to the first decades of the twentieth century and to the controversial personality of George Gustav Heye (1874–1957). A wealthy New York financier, in 1916 Heye founded the Museum of the American Indian Heye Foundation on upper Manhattan's Broadway and 155th Street. In the course of his life, he collected Indian artefacts throughout the Americas and Europe and financed a multitude of archaeological excavations and anthropological expeditions (Volkert et al. 2004:14–15) in the hope of salvaging the traces of the continent's disappearing races (see Jacknis 2006). In retrospect it has been acknowledged that "he collected wholesale; rather than carefully choosing one or two of the finest items in an assemblage, he would scoop up the entire lot" (Lenz 2004:95). As such, today the NMAI holds among its vast collections of eight hundred thousand objects about five thousand moccasins, most of which were collected by Heye in the early twentieth century.

Heye discouraged the collection of "tourist material" and was interested in "old" artefacts, such as hunting and fishing outfits, costumes, masks and ceremonial objects, household utensils, stone and pottery dishes, talismans, hunting charms, and ivory carvings, all of which ought to be carefully documented (Lenz 2004:105). Much in the context of salvage ethnography, he was concerned with the assemblage of "authentic" artefacts and the documentation of Indian traditions that had not been "spoiled" by modern civilisation. Heye confessed that he became interested in collecting Native artefacts when at twenty-three he came in contact with Navajo Indians that were working on a bridge-building project:

One night I noticed the wife of one of my Indian foremen biting on what seemed to be a piece of skin. Upon inquiry I found that she was chewing the seams of her husband's deerskin shirt in order to kill the lice. I bought the shirt, became interested in aboriginal customs and acquired other objects as opportunity offered ... In fact, I spent more time collecting Navajo costume pieces and trinkets that I did superintending roadbeds. [Lenz 2004:89]

Although Heye at least once in his life responded positively to claims for the repatriation of sacred objects,[2] it was not until after his death in 1957 and the sociopolitical mobilisation of the times that the museum's profile and approach to Native communities changed (Simpson 1996:218). In the decades that followed, it was increasingly felt that the state of the collection in the upper-Manhattan museum was deteriorating (Molotsky 1989) and that the presentation was "inadequate" and "overcrowded" (Simpson 1996:168). After long negotiations, the Museum of the American Indian was dissolved in 1988 (Howarth 2004:137), and the first National Museum of the American Indian was established as the Smithsonian's sixteenth museum with the 101-185 Public Law approved by the U.S. Congress. In this context, the NMAI emerges as a political project that cannot be separated from the civil and Indigenous rights movements of the 1970s and 1980s (Simpson 1996; West 2000).

The NMAI Act was innovative in several respects. First of all, by establishing the new museum as "a living memorial to Native Americans and their traditions" (Section 3), it acknowledged the importance of Heye's collections, but also more significantly that of the people from which these collections originated. Moreover, sections 12 and 13 dictated the establishment of two special committees to inventory, identify, and return the Indian and Hawaiian human remains and funerary objects held in the museum, and sections 14 and 15 declared that special grants would be provided to members of Native American tribes, museums, cultural centres, and organisations to travel to the NMAI for consultations about human remains and the museum's facilities.

The foundation of the NMAI as part of the Smithsonian signified a new period not only for the presentation of the collections, but also for the relationship between the museum and Native communities (West 2000; Jacobson 2006; Lonetree 2006a). Apart from the three permanent edifices in New York, Washington, and Maryland, the establishment of partnerships with Native museums, cultural centres, tribes, and individuals across the Americas has been labelled as the NMAI's "fourth museum" (Simpson 1996:169). The planning of the NMAI involved hundreds of consultations with communities and tribal representatives that lasted for several years (Volkert et al. 2004:17). The outcome was the foundation of a new museum that in many respects was very different from previous museological practices. The museum's aim was to fight racial stereotypes by presenting self-told stories of Native American tribes through a variety of media, combining oral history, myths, and historical accounts, and by redisplaying in this context the old nineteenth-century collections (see Conn 2006; Isaac 2008).

The NMAI was an outcome of longer processes of political and diplomatic negotiations. As discussed in chapter 1, its birth is embedded in the foundation of community and tribal cultural centres and museums throughout the 1970s and 1980s (see Coody Cooper and Sandoval 2006), like the U'mista Cultural Center (Clifford 1991) or the Anacostia Museum (James 2005), but its creation has also been much inspired by the personality of its founding director, Richard W. West Jr.,[3] who led the organisation for seventeen years. His imprint on the museum narrative is manifested in the institution's activities, debates, publications, and even displays, with his portrait featuring among those of other Natives Americans in the permanent exhibition Our Lives.

NMAI IN WASHINGTON, MARYLAND, AND NEW YORK

In his editorial of the NMAI's Spring 2007 quarterly produced magazine, after announcing his retirement from the museum's management, West acknowledged that "for me the NMAI is not merely a place to work or visit—it is an idea about who we are as a people. An idea whose time has come" (2007:17). With that statement he summarised a key philosophical principle of the NMAI, the idea that it expresses the identity of the Native peoples of the Americas and turns a new page in museological history and cultural representation. The NMAI is not so much about late nineteenth- and early twentieth-century collections, but rather about the cultural dynamism of contemporary Native Americans coping with loss and colonisation. This framework of loss and continuity provides an interesting context for rethinking intangible heritage locally.

Arriving at the NMAI on the National Mall, the museum's distinctive appearance becomes evident. The curved sand-coloured stone building, which was described by an NMAI staff member as "the only woman on the Mall," stands in great contrast to the white, neoclassical U.S. Capitol in its proximity. Long consultations with tribal representatives had suggested that the new museum should not perpetuate practices of cultural objectification that had characterised Native American displays in U.S. museums for most of the twentieth century (Jacknis 2006); instead, it should be a Native place, a theme that was interpreted in both practical and conceptual ways by the Native American architects, designers, and planners.

The museum building, which contrary to the other museums on the Mall faces east, is surrounded by a Native environment featuring Indigenous wetlands, a hardwood forest, a crop area, and cascading waters[4] (Figure 5.2).

The idea of a Native place is also expressed in the museological discourse of exhibitions, programmes, and activities. In each of the three permanent exhibitions—Our Lives, Our People, and Our Universe—representatives of eight tribes have been invited as cocurators to give voice to the Indigenous perspective. A strong interpretative framework in the form of written information, audiovisual installations, and graphic design expresses this participation, often at the expense of the presentation of material culture. This has been a source of dispute between the museum and its critics. Edward Rothstein, art critic for the *New York Times*, for example, observed that "most museums invoke the past to give shape to the present; here the interests of the present will be used to shape the past" (2004b). Along similar lines, Marc Fisher from the *Washington Post* described the NMAI as "an exercise in intellectual timidity and a sorry abrogation of the Smithsonian's obligation to explore America's history and culture" (2004). The NMAI's preference for the Indigenous perspective of survival and continuity over the scholarly curatorial voice of anthropologists, historians, or archaeologists is deplored as a lack of objectivity and poor museum work (Fisher 2004; Rothstein 2004a, 2004b; Lujan 2005).

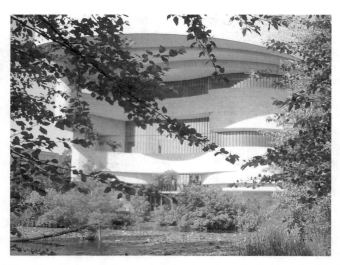

Figure 5.2: The National Museum of the American Indian on the Washington Mall is surrounded by a Native environment of wetlands, waterfalls, and croplands.

The museum has also been criticised by academics and members of the American Indian community. While for some its postcolonial, multivocal narrative fails to adequately portray the complexities of the colonial encounter (Atalay 2006; Lonetree 2006b), for others the unproblematised celebration of the survival of Native cultures ultimately "refuses to disrupt the mythologies of the noble and savage Indian" (Carpio 2006:627). These controversies reveal the competing voices at play in cultural representation and the complexities of participatory museum work in choosing what to remember and what to forget.

THE MALL MUSEUM

The museum on the Mall extends over five levels, overlooking the central space of the Potomac atrium on level one. On the same level are also the Rasmuson theatre, the Mitsitam café, and the Chesapeake museum shop. Level two features a small exhibition on the tribes that used to live in Chesapeake Bay, entitled "Return to a Native Place: Algonquian People of the Chesapeake Bay," and the second museum shop, named Roanoke. On level three, the first major permanent exhibition Our Lives is located next to the temporary exhibition space. On the same level is the research centre and library with computers, books, and other reference material. Level four presents two more permanent exhibitions, entitled Our Universe and Our People, and also the Lelawi theatre, which features an audiovisual programme introducing the museum and its philosophy and focuses on the resilience of Native Americans and their strong ties with nature. Different artefacts from the museum's collections are presented in special display cases, called Windows on Collections, on levels three and four. Level five, which is not open to the public, houses staff offices and meeting rooms.

Entering the NMAI from the main entrance, the Potomac atrium, a large, circular space, dominates the whole museum (Figure 5.3). As Rongomaraeroa is the heart of Te Papa, so the Potomac is the heart of the Mall museum, and the space is used for a variety of activities, including cultural performances, gatherings, workshops, or discussions. Moreover, it carries strong symbolic meanings and references to Indigenous beliefs. Like many Indigenous architectural forms, it is circular and faces east to greet the sun, while the "axes of the solstices and equinoxes are mapped on the floor with rings of red and black granite" (Martin 2004:35).

On my first day in the Mall museum, a children's chorus from Hawaii used the space and the entire building was filled with chants and music. As Howard Bass, cultural arts manager at the NMAI, later explained, the particular group had travelled to Jamestown to welcome Queen Elizabeth in her tour for the commemoration of the five hundredth

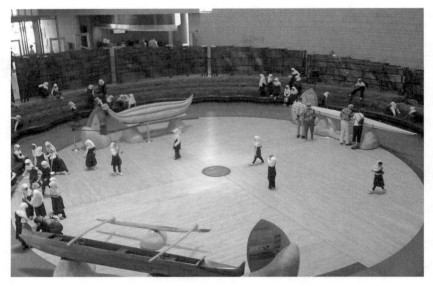

Figure 5.3: The Potomac atrium is at the heart of the Washington NMAI and hosts different activities and performances by Native American communities.

anniversary of the British colony. The group's performance at the NMAI had not been planned in advance: this further stresses the ties between the museum and Native communities and how the museum is seen as a space for performing a shared sense of identity.

The chants of the Hawaiian chorus accompanied my discussion with Gabrielle Tayac, curator at the NMAI. Being a member of the Piscataway tribe, which suffered major dislocations and loss of language and knowledge over the last five hundred years, she is particularly sensitive to the social aspects of museum work. Talking about the Potomac, she noted that occasionally, when there are no performances taking place, "it can feel a bit empty." This emphasis on community participation at the expense of NMAI's rich collections has been the object of several critiques (Fisher 2004; Rothstein 2004a; Berry 2006).

A further critique of the museum architecture is that levels one and two have very few displays and the spaces are taken over by the two museum shops selling among other things jewellery, pottery, books, toys, CDs, DVDs, t-shirts, beauty products, and chocolates. The large variety and amount of artefacts on sale is not atypical of U.S. museum shops; however, it hints at an increased commercialisation of Indigenous culture, ironically referred to as "from ritual to retail" (see Luke 2002:96).

Just like the museum shops constitute displays of contemporary Native arts and crafts, the Mitsitam Café[5] provides a glimpse into Indigenous culinary practices, revealing further negotiations of the museum as a living memorial of Native culture. Traditional recipes from South, North, and Central America include salmon dishes, tacos, and fajitas. Labels on the tables provide information on Native approaches to food. For example, one label reads: "Native Americans in the Northwest Coast region consider Spring the most important time of the year because that is when the salmon begin to migrate up the rivers to spawn. For many tribes, salmon are seen as supernatural beings that live in their own villages beneath the sea and have their own rites and ceremonies."

The Mitsitam Café is presented as an aspect of Native identity that is central to contemporary living culture. Tribes might have been robbed of their sacred objects, but traditional practices, like cooking, have been retained as a dynamic component of Native culture. The next section examines how the Native experience is presented in the museum's permanent and temporary exhibitions.

MALL MUSEUM EXHIBITIONS

The NMAI's inaugural exhibitions Our Universes: Traditional Knowledge Shapes Our World, Our Peoples: Giving Voice to Our Histories, and Our Lives: Contemporary Life and Identity have a similar structure. A main area introducing key issues and themes lies at the centre of each exhibition. This is surrounded by eight individual exhibition spaces, each one representing a tribe and cocurated by museum and community curators.

Our Universes

The introductory label of the Our Universes exhibition, signed and dated by NMAI curator Emil Her Many Horses, reads:

> In this gallery, you'll discover how Native people understand their place in the universe and order their daily lives. Our philosophies of life come from our ancestors. They taught us to live in harmony with the animals, plants, spirit world and the people around us. In Our Universes, you'll encounter Native people from the Western Hemisphere who continue to express this wisdom in ceremonies, celebrations, languages, arts, religions and daily lives. It is our duty to pass these teachings on to succeeding generations. For that is the way to keep our traditions alive.

Our Universes presents Native cosmologies, beliefs, and practices that while rooted in tradition remain a vital element of contemporary Native identities. The exhibition has a dark, almost mystic atmosphere. The main area presents ritual ceremonies like the Dia de los Muertos in Mexico, other annual practices like the North American Indigenous

Games and the Denver March Powwow, and audiovisual programmes about Native American creation stories, like "The raven and the sun" or "The star that fell in love." Objects representing the stars, the moon, and the sun, such as masks, beaded vests, and dance clubs are also presented in the main exhibition area, alluding to the Native spiritual world.

The main area is surrounded by eight tribal galleries where Native communities—the Pueblo of Santa Clara (New Mexico), Anishinaabe (Canada), Lakota (South Dakota), Quechua (Peru), Hupa (California), Q'eq'chi'Maya (Guatemala), Mapuche (Chile), and Yup'ik (Alaska)—present their tribal philosophies about the universe (Figure 5.4).

For example, Hupa curators have structured their gallery around the Jump Dance:

> When they leave this world, all the Ki'xanay [ancestors] go to a place where they dance forever. So when we pray, we ask them to come back and dance with us. During this time, the world is being remade and all the ancestors are with us. During our Jump Dance, the spirits of the ancestors watch from behind a cedar-plank house. When we conclude our portions of the dance, it's the ancestors' turn to dance.
>
> Mervin George Sr., Community Curator, 2000.

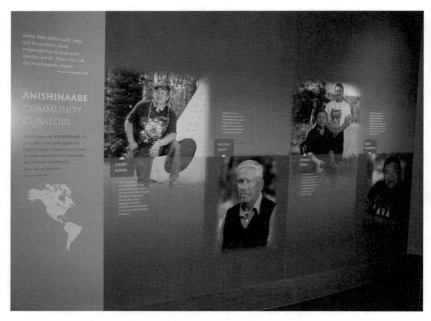

Figure 5.4: The Anishinaabe community curators were among the tribal representatives actively involved in the realisation of the twenty-four community exhibitions presented at the NMAI.

Further down the exhibition, Mervin George Sr. explains: "Our Jump Dance drives bad things away. We sing, stomp the ground and pray that everything bad will go up in the smoke from the fire. We hope that the bad things will get on a black cloud and go over to the east—over the mountain and away." The strong community narrative and the first-person interpretation highlight that traditions are part of tribal life in the twenty-first century.

In the Yup'ik gallery, six community curators give their own inter-pretations of the artefacts, masks, and ritual objects on display. Talking about the use of masks in dance festival in Alaska, Theresa Moses, com-munity curator, remarks in a label that "masks were used during dances to honor the fish and the animal and to ask for more in the coming season." Another community curator, Paul John, is quoted as saying "masks were used in healing a sick person. When masks were used in prayers for abundance, they also honored the winds and asked for good hunting weather." Community exhibition narratives are thus predomi-nantly based on traditions, popular myths, and beliefs that have been passed from one generation to the next and are today a vital part of tribal peoples' lives. These narratives, which are presented on text panels or audiovisual installations, express in an unmediated way the voices of different communities. Absent, however, are references to more compli-cated issues of intercultural exchange and colonisation.

Our Peoples

Facing Our Universes is the second inaugural exhibition, Our Peoples. The aim of this exhibition is to encourage "viewers to consider his-tory not as a single, definite, immutable work, but as a collection of subjective tellings by different authors with different points of view" (Volkert et al. 2004:50). The NMAI curatorial team led by Paul Chaat Smith and Ann McMullen introduces the key themes of "disease, guns, Bibles, and foreign governments" as forces that changed Native lives for-ever. Entering the exhibition, a large display case with golden artefacts, including plates, masks, swords, earrings, and other ornaments, grabs the visitor's attention. The accompanying text, entitled "Wealth, power, abundance," explains:

> The first 150 years of contact witnessed one of the greatest transfers of wealth in world history. Gold, silver and labor from the Americas cre-ated and transformed international economies and permanently linked the Western Hemisphere with Europe and Africa . . . Perhaps 20 million Indians died as a result of Contact. Tens of millions more perished of disease. Little of the gold made by Native people before Contact survives in its original form. Museums and collectors hold most of what remains.
> Paul Chaat Smith, NMAI, 2003.

The polemical and self-reflexive tone of this label is repeated throughout the exhibition, which narrates stories of loss, adaptation, and survival through the living memory of the tribes. Equally striking is the story of Inca ruler Atahualpa, also signed by Chaat Smith and presented on a label next to the gold and silver artefacts:

> In 1532, the Spanish Conquistador Francisco Pizarro seized the Inca ruler Atahualpa and held him hostage. From across Peru gold and silver arrived on the backs of people and lamas. They trudged along the empires four highways, carrying the largest ransom in world history. It took eight months. A room twenty-two feet long, seventeen feet wide and eight feet high was filled with gold. Two more rooms were filled with silver. When the rooms could hold no more, Pizarro became one of the world's richest men. He then ordered Atahualpa strangled.

In this context, the trauma of colonisation emerges as a key theme of the exhibition and the golden artefacts acquire new, contested meanings.

Further into the main area, another large display case contains guns, dollar notes, and different editions of the Bible. The label next to it introduces the concept of *survivance*: "These forces (guns, churches and governments) shaped the lives of Indians who survived the massive rupture of the first century of Contact. By adopting the very tools that were used to change, control and dispossess them, Native peoples reshaped their cultures and societies to keep them alive. This strategy has been called survivance."

This display stresses the agency of Native people in response to colonial forces of change, celebrating the survival and renewal of Native culture through adaptation. As critics have noted, however, treating objects of death and cultural annihilation as agents of survivance is part of a postcolonial discourse that politicises the museum narrative according to present-day concerns rather than reflecting the complexities and true proportions of colonisation (Atalay 2006).

George Catlin's nineteenth-century portraits of Native Americans are presented in a secluded area not far from the central display (Figure 5.5). Among them, a video screen the size of a painting presents Floyd Farel, a twenty-first-century American Indian, wearing a contemporary outfit. He introduces the exhibition by saying:

> This museum rests on a foundation of consultation, collaboration and cooperation with Natives. It has shared the power museums usually keep. The place you stand in is the end product of that sharing, a process of giving voice. What's found here is our way of looking at the Native American experience. What is said and what you see may fly in the face of much you've learned. We offer self-told histories of selected Native communities . . . Here we have done as others have done—turned events into history. So view what is offered with respect, but also scepticism. Explore this gallery. Encounter it. Reflect on it. Argue with it.

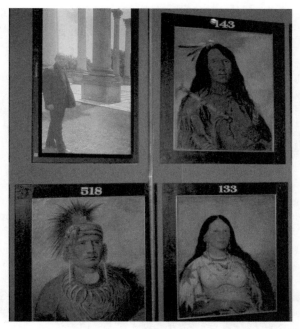

Figure 5.5: In the exhibition Our People, next to George Catlin's nineteenth-century portraits of American Indian chiefs a digital screen presents the story of a contemporary American Indian.

What follows is a presentation of the past events that shaped the present of each tribe. The eight tribes that narrate their histories are the Seminole (Florida), Tapiraré (Brazil), Kiowa (Oklahoma), Tohono O'odham (Arizona), Eastern Band of Cherokee (North Carolina), Nahua (Mexico), Ka'apor (Brazil), and Wixarika (Mexico). Each of these tribes rehearses nodal moments of its past drawing on oral history and knowledge passed on from the ancestors as well as written sources and historical accounts. Hardships, displacements, cruelties, and injustices are narrated and supported with evidence, while material culture is presented in ways that serve the community narrative. "We will never surrender—We will survive," reads the main panel of the Seminole gallery, where community curators narrate the struggles of their tribes against the American forces. For example, one panel with a Seminole woman on the background reads:

> When I was growing up I heard stories from my elders about atrocities that happened when troops removed our people to Oklahoma and Arkansas. These stories can't be found in books and one stands out, The Day the Ocean Turned White. During the wars they wounded up our people and

put them on ships. Once they put all the women on one ship. When they were far from land, the soldiers raped the women and tossed their bodies overboard. We didn't understand this story until we got older. Then it made us angry.

Ronnie Jimmie, 2001.

In the Ka'apor gallery (Figure 5.6), tribal curators explain their first contacts with colonial settlers and their move to the Amazon forest. This section features stories of violence and enmities that resulted in peace, including the presentation of the ongoing struggles between the Ka'apor and the Brazilian logging industry. As Ann McMullen remarked in an interview with me, Ka'apor curators were keen to take part in the exhibition development. For them, this was an opportunity not only to present their material culture, but also to publicise their disputes and sociopolitical struggles and to sensitise the broader American public towards their causes. The exhibition as a space for aesthetic contemplation is thus transformed into a present-day political tool for dealing with collective trauma, contesting rights, and raising awareness. As such, a political narrative often takes precedence over the artefacts on display.

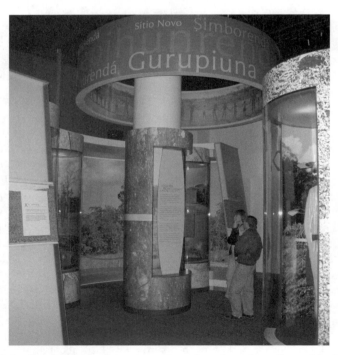

Figure 5.6: In addition to the presentation of artefacts the gallery of the Ka'apor community discusses the community's history and relationship with the Brazilian government.

Our Lives

On level three, the third inaugural exhibition, Our Lives, which was curated by Gabrielle Tayac, Jolene Rickard, and Cynthia Chavez, addresses the issue of Native American identity in the twenty-first century. The entrance to the exhibition is a short corridor with two large screens on each side. Each one projects footage of people walking by. The label next to it reads: "Anywhere in the Americas, you could be walking with a 21st century Native American." The introductory label explains that "the central areas of the gallery look at key elements that have affected Native identity, such as definition, social and political awareness, language, place and self-determination. These areas reveal that identity is not a thing, but a lived experience."

Unlike the two previous exhibitions, the central area of Our Lives does not present any objects. It is, however, rich in textual information and photographic material. The first part of the main area consists of the display of contemporary portraits of Native Americans (Figure 5.7) in green, purple, orange, and white tones—including, as mentioned above, that of the NMAI director Richard West.

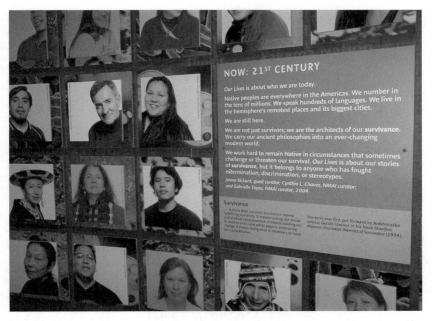

Figure 5.7: Portraits of present-day American Indians are presented on the introductory panel of Our Lives. Among them is that of the former Director of the NMAI, Richard W. West Jr.

The label on the wall reads:

> We are still here. We are not just survivors; we are the architects of our surviv-
> ance. We carry our Native philosophies into an ever-changing modern world.
> We work hard to remain Native in circumstances that challenge or threaten
> our survival. Our Lives is about our stories of survivance, but it belongs to
> anyone who has fought extermination, discrimination, or stereotypes.

Rather than just narrating historical events, the main area raises questions. A screen inserted in a portrait frame projects images of Native
Americans, either as late nineteenth-century portraits or as collages of different contemporary pictures. A panel with the title "Fully Native" asks:

> Who is an Indian? A Native American? An Indigenous person? American
> Indian, First Nation or Aboriginal? All these labels are used, but none is
> entirely correct. Who decided? Are you a full blood? Half blood? Quarter
> blood? The question of how much "Indian blood" you have . . . began with
> European contact. This colonial way of thinking continues when we keep
> defining ourselves by blood. What part of you is Native? Is it your head?
> Your heart? Maybe it is your thoughts. But it is not just your blood. We are
> all the sum of our parts. All human. One hundred percent. And fully Native.

Introduced by the question "Is my identity in how I look?" a copy
of Franz Boas' paper *The Half Blood Indian: An Anthropometric Study*
(1894) brings under scrutiny the role of scientists in the objectification of
Native Americans. This question is also raised by the large photograph
of the performance artist James Luna and his installation "The Artifact
Piece" (1987) in the Museum of Man in San Diego, in which he lay in a
nineteenth-century display case as if a dead specimen of his race. Next to it
the portrait by artist Luis Gonzalez Palma of a young Guatemalan with a
measuring tape around his head, entitled "Critical Gaze" (1998), criticises
the way Native people have been studied as anthropological specimens.

The final part of the main area introduces the theme of self-determination. This section presents images of the 1990 ride organised by the Lakota
people to commemorate the centenary of the Wounded Knee Massacre; of
the 1989 Paddle to Seattle, where Native people from the Northwest coast
revived traditional seafaring skills; of the 1991 anti-Columbus demonstration in Guatemala; and of the establishment of the 2002 UN Permanent
Forum on Indigenous Issues. The text display nearby reads:

> Self-determination means control of our lives and our land, knowing our
> traditions and understanding our relationships to each other, insisting on
> our rights to be who we are. We are ancient nations seeking recognition
> and respect from modern nations. We know that our future depends on
> integrating traditional knowledge with the modern world. One without
> the other is a world out of balance.

Here, survival is negotiated not only in terms of the celebration of tradition, but also with respect to ongoing claims and contested rights. As such, tribal galleries are transformed into spaces of civic and political engagement. These galleries feature the Campo Band of the Kumeyaay Indians (California), the Urban Indian Community of Chicago (Illinois), the Yamaka Nation (Washington State), the Igloolik (Canada), the Kahnawake (Canada), the Saint-Laurent Metis (Canada), the Kalinago (Carib Territory, Dominica), and the Pamunkey (Virginia). Key themes emerging from the community exhibitions are ideas of survival, agency, and traditional beliefs as constituent elements of contemporary identities, tribal lore, and ethnic self-determination. For example, the Kahnawake curators introduce themselves with the following words:

> We are Kahnawa'kehro:non—People who live by the Rapids. We also call ourselves Kanien'kehaka—People of the Flint, and the language we speak is Kanien'keha. Others know us as Mohawks. As part of the Iroquois Confederacy we are "Keepers of the Eastern Door," protectors of the territories in our regions. As "People of the Flint" we are hard and enduring like the stone and can provide spark to light the fire. When something happens, we react in a way that asserts our self-determination as a people and sovereignty as a nation.

The impact of European colonisation and the subsequent construction of urban centres on Native identities are emphasised in the gallery of the Urban Indian Community of Chicago. As the community curators highlight in their introduction, "Our community is different from the other Native communities you have encountered in Our Lives. For one thing, we represent many different tribes from all over North America. For another, we are urban Indians—residents of one of the biggest cities in the U.S."

By the early 1900s, the migration of Native people to Chicago led to the establishment of new communal bonds, relations, and institutions for the growing Native American communities in urban settings. The gallery presents a map with the different Native homelands along with recreations of contemporary urban Indian dwellings. The message expressed by the label is clear: "The foundation of our community rests on Native values. They keep us strong." The celebration of contemporary Native American identity at the interface of the traditional and the new is central to this display.

Temporary Exhibitions: Identity by Design

As we have seen, in the three inaugural exhibitions the display of artefacts was often sidelined by the narrative, stories, beliefs, and opinions of Native American communities as sustained or revived in the present.

Partly due to negative press reviews and partly due to institutional discussions, it was felt that an exhibition showcasing the rich collections of the NMAI would add a new dimension to its museological discourse. In response to this need, at the time of my research a temporary exhibition entitled Identity by Design: Tradition, Change and Celebration in Native Women's Dresses was opened in the temporary exhibition space facing Our Lives.

This exhibition was different from the ones discussed so far. Several costumes were presented, ranging from late nineteenth-century dresses from the Great Plains to contemporary dresses and the famous Ghost Dance Shirts. While the Native perspective still remains strong, with quotes, photographs, and videos of American Indian women making and wearing the dresses, visually the exhibition placed a greater emphasis on material culture. As observed by Richard West in an interview, in this particular exhibition an effort had been made to showcase Native dress by tracing at the same time the links to the makers and wearers. While the three previous exhibitions revolved around community myths and stories, here Native material culture took precedence over the community's perspective, hinting at a return to a more traditional and less political museum practice.

This shift reveals that in the last years the role and responsibilities of the NMAI as a living memorial of Native American cultures have been rethought. Initially conceptualised as a meeting space for all Native and non-Native people to fight stereotypes and celebrate identity, today the museum seems to be increasingly thought of as a space for the presentation of historic collections.

CULTURAL RESOURCES CENTER, SUITLAND, MARYLAND

The Cultural Resources Center (CRC) is located in Suitland, Maryland, about half-an-hour train ride from Central DC. For many staff, this is the heart of the entire organisation, because it is where the bulk of the collections reside. Alluding to the natural world, the building is shaped like a seashell and surrounded by trees, plants, running waters, and bronze sculptures of Native Americans (Figure 5.8). The collections occupy three stories. Unlike the general practice of storing collections in dark, crammed basements, at the CRC the collections area is spacious, with high ceilings and windows overlooking the gardens.

Patricia Nietfeld, NMAI collections manager, explained to me the large efforts made by the CRC staff to respect the wishes and concerns of Native communities regarding the care and documentation of collections. Artefacts are stored according to tribal affiliation and not according to material. They are kept in an upright position, or in the way they would

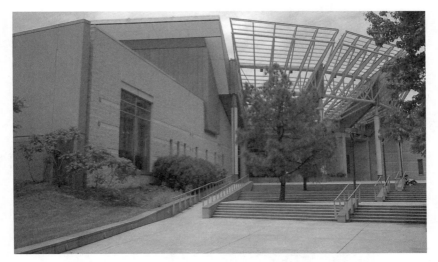

Figure 5.8: The Cultural Resources Center of the NMAI in Suitland, Maryland.

have been used, even if this means that they occupy more space. Sensitive and religious objects, such as medicine bundles, cloths, or ceremonial artefacts are usually kept in higher shelves as opposed to everyday arte-facts that are kept in lower ones. If requested by tribal representatives, such potent objects can be wrapped in muslin cloths. Muslin cloth is also used in cupboards instead of solid metal doors to allow artefacts to breathe. Moreover, the staff respect Indigenous protocols regarding who should handle objects (Figure 5.9).

The treatment of artefacts against pest infestations further reveals the concern and respect CRC staff hold for Native beliefs. The fact that many artefacts are made out of organic materials, such as skins, feathers, leafs, or wood makes them a source of attraction for insects. However, the use of pesticides on animate objects is regarded as disrespectful, and therefore alternative, non-toxic methods are used, such as freezing or placing artefacts in carbon dioxide tents. Respect of Native beliefs invites alternative practices in technical areas of museum work, such as collections conservation and management (see Clavir 2002).

The CRC has two spaces, indoor and outdoor (Figure 5.10), where tribal elders and representatives conduct welcoming or purification cer-emonies. Smudging is performed, whereby sage or sweetgrass is burnt in a shell to cleanse objects and people.

Such ceremonies have an important spiritual dimension for Native com-munities, who reconnect with and ascribe new meanings to the artefacts of their ancestors. They reveal the deeper significance of these objects, which

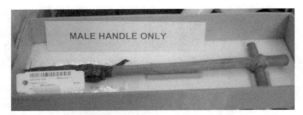

Figure 5.9: Label indicating gender restrictions regarding the handling of certain ceremonial or ritual objects, Cultural Resources Center, NMAI.

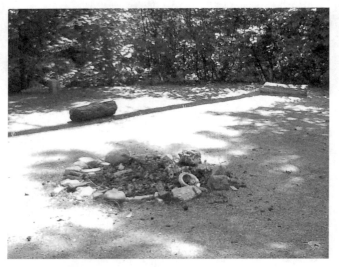

Figure 5.10: Outdoor ceremonial space for the conduct of purification ceremonies, Cultural Resources Center, NMAI.

are treated not as museum specimens, but as living artefacts. According to Hill (2004:128), "Native cultural leaders who visit the CRC sometimes leave water and traditional foods—for example, cornmeal or pollen from some of the Southwest tribes, salmon from the Makah people of the Northwest—as a sustenance for objects that are very much alive to them."

Community participation in NMAI activities from the care and conservation of collections to interpretation and programming is very strong. The NMAI's Community Services, which are also housed in the CRC, add a further dimension to the museum's engagement with Native American people. James Pepper Henry, associate director for Community and Constituent Services, and his colleagues Terry Snowball and John Beaver discussed with me the many ways in which the NMAI sustains collaborations with Native groups and individuals.

In terms of reaching out to communities, the "fourth museum" of the NMAI, special initiatives are taken on an annual basis. Among them is the Community Exhibitions programme, which supports tribal museums and cultural centres in the form of loans, travelling exhibitions, and collections research. Moreover, through the Native Arts and the Native Radio Programs the museum provides support to individuals and communities for art and radio projects and symposia. Similarly, the Film and Video Centre in New York supports Native American filmmakers and maintains a rich archive of Native films, documentaries, and radio programmes. Online resources like the Indigenous Geography website[6] and the Virtual Museum Workshops provide training in digital technologies and access to Native ways of life and philosophies.

Another dimension of the Community Services is the provision of internships for students in conservation, collections care, cultural arts, public affairs, and education, and of a training program for professionals working in tribal museums or cultural centres (see Zimmerman 2010 for a critical reflection on this). Also, through the Cultural Arts Program the NMAI invites musicians, dance and theatre groups, storytellers, writers, and artisans to present their work in the Mall and New York museums.

NMAI Community Services are particularly active in the area of repatriation of human remains and sacred objects to tribes. According to the NMAI Repatriation Policy:

> The NMAI is committed to the disposition, in accordance with the wishes of culturally based Native Americans, of (i) human remains of known Native American individuals; (ii) human remains of individuals who can be identified by tribal or cultural affiliation with contemporary Native American people; (iii) funerary objects; (iv) communally owned Native American property; (v) ceremonial and religious objects; and (vi) objects transferred to or acquired by the Museum illegally or under circumstances that render invalid the Museum's claim to them.

Since the NMAI's foundation more than two thousand human remains have been repatriated to about one hundred tribes. James Pepper Henry explained:

> We believe in the sanctity of humanity—meaning that we view the remains of Indigenous peoples as human beings rather than as specimens. We actually have a moratorium on any outside research; anybody from outside the museum wanting to conduct research like destructive analysis or invasive procedures. We even have a moratorium against research within our own institution, unless it is for the purposes of determining cultural affiliation to repatriate those remains back to their communities. We do not allow invasive or destructive analysis of the remains in our possession, unless the communities or the people that are directly affiliated with those remains

request it. Our goal is not to study the remains and draw statistics from them. Our goal is to return the remains for a respectful burial.

NMAI, GEORGE GUSTAV HEYE CENTER, NEW YORK

The third site of the NMAI is the George Gustav Heye Center, which opened in 1994 at the Alexander S. Hamilton Custom House in Manhattan's financial district. Located on Bowling Green, the city's oldest public square and not far from Ground Zero, the late nineteenth-century building housing the NMAI clashes architecturally with the corporate skyscrapers in its surroundings. With the exception of the marble Indian figure leaning over the shoulder of the statue of America in front of the Custom House, little else would suggest that this is a Native place. While the Mall museum seemed to be welcoming and filled with life, the overall atmosphere of the New York branch appears more sombre and less inviting.

During the first phase of my research at the museum, different exhibitions were taking place. Compared to the inaugural exhibitions of the Mall museum, the exhibitions at the NMAI were more focused on the presentation of tribal artefacts and art objects and on the aesthetic dimension of what was on display. For example, the temporary exhibition Off the Map presented paintings on canvases by contemporary Native American artists engaging with the idea of landscape. Similarly, Indigenous Motivations: Recent Acquisitions from the NMAI presented pieces that were created by Native artists after the 1950s and explored issues of cultural traditions and contemporary creation.

In a later period, the exhibition Listening to Our Ancestors: The Art of Native Life along the North Pacific Coast featured NMAI collections from the Northwest Coast and presented the eleven tribes from which these artefacts originated. These were the Coast Salish, Makah, Nuu-chah-nulth, Kwakwaka'wakw, Heiltsuk, Nuxalk, Tsimshian, Haida, Nisga'a, Gitxan, and Tlingit. When this exhibition closed, the eleven community galleries were displayed in their tribal homelands. Although the voices of the community curators were strong and clear, the focus of the exhibition was not so much contemporary life in the Northwest Coast, as the rich collection of late nineteenth- and early twentieth-century artefacts.

The three sites of the NMAI, in Washington, DC, Suitland, and New York, emerge as quite distinct localities for the realisation of the living memorial metaphor. The dynamics and tensions at play reveal that the NMAI on the Washington Mall, due to its symbolically charged location at the heart of the U.S. government, is dominated by a strong political narrative of self-representation. Here, it is the celebration of survival and contemporary identity that informs the display of objects, hinting that American Indian tribes are active agents in remembering the past and celebrating the future. The construction of a Native place facing the U.S. Capitol is a reminder that far from being extinct, Native Americans are dynamically present in public life.

This politically charged discourse is less strong in both the Suitland and New York sites. Not being open to the public, the Suitland branch is more focused on collections and community work. As such, the idea of the living memorial operates with respect to how objects are conserved and stored: not as dead museum pieces, but rather as living and sacred artefacts. Also, this site is more active in relation to the "fourth museum," in other words, in reaching out to Native communities across the Americas. These are hugely diverse groups often coping with much of the painful and detrimental consequences of colonisation. Museum work in this sense emerges as a new form of cultural advocacy, with museum professionalism driven as much by collections care and exhibitions development as by respect for the beliefs and wishes of excluded and marginalised communities.

The New York branch, on the other hand, emerges primarily as a space for the presentation of Native American art. Rather than narrating tribal stories, the exhibitions present the work of contemporary American Indian artists or artefacts from the NMAI collections. This means that tribal first-voice interpretation is relatively absent from the narrative, which is neutral and less charged. What is showcased, on the contrary, is a strong aesthetic discourse about traditional and modern tribal art.

INTANGIBLE HERITAGE AT THE LIVING MEMORIAL

In the course of my research in Washington I interviewed not only staff at the NMAI, but also people working at the Smithsonian's Center for Folklife and Cultural Heritage (CFCH), which, as discussed in chapter 2, has played a central role in the development of the intangible heritage preservation movement. Interviews at the CFCH reveal the close collaboration between the two institutions. In September 2004, the CFCH organised the opening festival for the NMAI, in which thousands of Native people from across the Americas came to the Mall to celebrate the inauguration of the new museum. The close collaboration between the two organisations underscores the adoption of intangible heritage by NMAI as part of its museological lexicon.

José Barreiro, assistant director for research, is an American Studies scholar, but also a journalist, novelist, documentarist, and political activist. In our discussion he described himself as "a reluctant scholar" searching knowledge in the library, but firstly in the community. For him, the NMAI emerged "within the Smithsonian at a time of fairly strong contest and activism from the Native communities" and "out of a more respectful idea about living cultures." A member of the Taino people from Cuba, he remarked that according to the Euro-American tradition his people were extinct. For him, as well as other represent-atives of Native communities, one of the main issues setting the new institution apart from earlier museums of Native cultures was the fight against racial and ethnic stereotypes.

Along similar veins, James Pepper Henry, assistant director for Community Services and Constituencies and member of the Kaw and Muskogee Creek Nations, noted that "many people still think that we live in *tipi* and ride ponies bareback causing trouble for the pioneers out there. No. We have not done that in some time." For John Beaver, cultural protocols specialist, member of the Muskogee Creek Nation from Oklahoma and doctoral candidate at the University of Chicago, one of the principles informing his work is "for people to learn that Native Americans are much more than the arrival of Columbus and Pocahontas."

The will to break away from stereotypes and celebrate the vitality of contemporary Native American cultures has influenced to a great extent the practice of the NMAI. "This museum is first and foremost a Native place that bespeaks the Native voice," underlined Richard West. The challenge for him is not only to present historic collections, but to capture and present "the totality of the Native experience." Similarly, Richard Kurin, director of the CFCH, talking about the opening festival of the NMAI, remarked that "the whole idea of opening the museum was not for it to be a monument or a memorial for the people that are dead, wiped out or killed, but rather a gathering ground for ensuring the continuity of Indian culture today." In this sense the NMAI emerges primarily as a contemporary space for the expression of Native identity rather than a monument to past violence, cultural annihilation, and loss.[7]

Recalling the opening of the NMAI and the six-day festival that the CFCH organised for the occasion, Richard Kurin noted:

> We started off with a massive procession . . . over six hundred tribes from all across the hemisphere participating in this Native Nations' Procession coming from the Washington Monument through the Capitol. The human-ity of it was great . . . you had people who were American Indian veterans, the beauty queens, people in their regalia, etc. It was massive. It was the largest gathering of Indigenous people ever in the Americas. On open-ing day there were about twenty-five thousand people processing; another fifty thousand observing and watching; over the course of a week there were close to six hundred thousand people. It was truly amazing. Just the diversity of all these peoples . . . Eskimos, Hawaiians. To me it was like,

hello, this is what living cultural heritage is all about. The message was very clear. We are still here. We are not here only as human beings, but as cultured human beings. You can see it in what we wear, in how we look, in our languages, in the songs we are singing.

According to Richard West:

The NMAI is profoundly about significant and beautiful collections of eight hundred thousand objects stretching from one end of the hemisphere to the other. But in its essence, the NMAI is not simply about the presentation of collections. This is not just a palace of collections. It is more like a cultural centre, because it is about the people, the communities. This is what we are doing and as such this museum is about tangible and intangible heritage.

Intangible heritage is thus connected to the vitality of Native cultures as they exist today, their empowerment and participation in museum work, reaching beyond the preservation of objects to the actual histories, traditions, and beliefs of communities.

Performing Identity

Howard Bass, cultural arts manager at NMAI further described the museum as a performative space. As he explained:

The main entrance is the Potomac, a large open area with a dance floor . . . for live activities, demonstrations and performances. Outside there is a small amphitheatre and inside there is a three-hundred-seat theatre that is used for performances, films, and discussions. Also, there is the outdoor plaza, where we present our outdoor music series in the summer. On the upper levels there are classrooms and other spaces that are wonderful for smaller scale performances and storytelling.

Howard Bass also highlighted the breadth of the activities and cultural performances taking place in the museum:

In line with the mission of the museum, we show everything that is relevant to Native people, whether it is ancient rituals, customs or traditions that go back hundreds of years to the most contemporary kinds of what may or may not on their surface seem anything like Native. You might hear rock, hip-hop, reggae or jazz . . . In some cases, you can see the ongoing traditions that stretch back to pre-contact times . . . Certainly some Latin American communities like the Quechua, or the people of the Ecuadorian Amazon are literally unchanged, or have clear or strong connections to pre-contact culture. They still speak their language, which is a strong component of cultural identity. But in the East Coast, there are communities that have lost their language and heritage . . . They find new ways to connect to their past through contemporary creation and to reclaim their Indian heritage that was suppressed for so long.

In this sense, cultural events, workshops, programmes, and performances presented at NMAI reveal the breadth of contemporary Native creation. Among the performances that were presented in the 2006–2007 season was the traditional masked performance of El Gueguense from the highlands of Nicaragua, a cultural performance that is recognised by UNESCO as a Masterpiece of Intangible Heritage, but also Shakespeare's *Macbeth*, partly performed in Tlingit by Tlingit performers. Tradition and its contemporary appropriations thus emerge as central dimensions for reclaiming and enacting Native identity at the NMAI.

As Atesh Sonneborn, associate director of CFCH's Folkway Recordings explained, the CFCH and the Cultural Arts Unit of the NMAI have worked together for the production of records and CDs of Indigenous music. For Howard Bass, the production of the CD *Beautiful Beyond* containing hymns and Christian songs sung in Native languages "speaks to language preservation through the singing of hymns . . . the NMAI is here to help communities perpetuate and preserve both their tangible and intangible heritage . . . even when we are dealing with potters and jewellery makers that produce tangible manifestations of culture, this still has to do with oral knowledge that is transmitted from previous generations."

Materiality and Spirituality

The cultural and spiritual connections of objects, cultural practices, and peoples constitute central themes of the NMAI. As Richard West noted: "As Native peoples we really don't distinguish between tangible and intangible heritage. In our cultures, it is all in one place, all in a whole . . . With Native Americans they all bundle up in one thing. Objects, for example, are nothing much without the intangible heritage that surrounds them: songs, stories, performances, traditions, and all kinds of non-material heritage."

Similarly, Gabrielle Tayac observed that

> the objects manifest the intangible, the intellect, and the mentalities of Indigenous people. So, it is not looking the object as the primary. It is looking at the thought. This is how the objects were selected; based on the thoughts that they represent, rather than because they are beautiful or pretty . . . In many ways, this museum has really a priority on the intangible.

The issue of the spiritual and cultural connections of NMAI collections also emerged in my discussions with the NMAI staff around the repatriation of objects to communities. Terry Snowball, cultural protocols coordinator and member of the Wisconsin Winnebago tribe, who is in charge of liaising with communities and conducting ceremonies and reburials, remarked that "it is essential for us to acknowledge the life-force of these artefacts." Concepts such as the life-force of artefacts or animate collections pose a new set of questions regarding the curatorial responsibilities of the museum in terms of collections care, but also exhibitions.[8]

Karen Fort, deputy assistant director for exhibitions and public spaces, has encountered these issues over the last seventeen years of her working for the NMAI. Talking about the wish of the museum to present exhibitions through Native perspectives, she acknowledged that

> when you are talking about the importance and value of an object in a museum, you are positioning yourself firmly in the Western way of looking at other cultures. What is in the museum has traditionally been the most beautiful, the rarest or the most unusual. One of the things that we are doing is trying to fight against looking just at the object isolated from its culture and its context. We are really trying to help the public understand the object from the Indigenous perspective; not from what we are so comfortably doing: "Oh, look . . . It is so beautiful." We try to see it as an Indian person would: a more cultural worldview, a more traditional way of behaving . . . The way we tried to bring intangible heritage forward is partly through the voice of community curators . . . The other thing that we did is that we relied a lot on multimedia . . . Part of the reason we did that was to make the Native voice stronger, more apparent and also to have more living Native Americans present in the museum.

Story-Driven Museology and Community Participation

Like at Te Papa, the empowerment of communities to become curators and interpreters of collections has resulted in a story- rather than object-driven approach. Gabrielle Tayac explained:

> The community was contacted through the proper protocols, whether this was through the chief or the council. They were asked for representatives to be the intermediaries between the community and the NMAI. The people that were selected could go back to the larger community and ask for advice as to how the exhibition could be curated. This was a back and forth process between community representatives and us at the NMAI. They selected the objects, they talked about what they wanted, they gave us the concepts, such as "these are the seven virtues of life" and "this is how we can illustrate that." The Lakota, for example, have wisdom and fortitude. They have these different virtues and that to them was very important. They would select the object based on the virtue. These would be different for each tribe. The Quechua have a completely different way for looking at things. So they selected differently.

Discussing the process of working with Indigenous communities, Ann McMullen identified two main areas of concern: communication and autonomy. As she remarked:

> When we would ask people to come to Washington and work for an exhibit in the museum, one of their first reactions would be "What's a museum?" . . . So, for some of the people, members of groups from Brazil or rural Mexico, one of the first thing that we did, because this building was not built, there was no place for us to show them what a cultural exhibit might be like. They were taken over to the Natural History Museum and shown what those exhibits were sort of like, but at the same time saying "the NMAI won't make you look anything like this, but this is what museums are."

Referring to the amount of autonomy and almost repeating the same arguments expressed by Stephanie Gibson at Te Papa, she added that "one of the things that the NMAI sometimes did not succeed really well to explain was how much each side, museums and community curators, contributed to decisions about the ultimate product. Also, whether their work was advisory, whether they were in charge or whether the museum was in charge."

The unclear relations between museum and community curators, as described by Ann McMullen, hint at some of the problematic areas of exhibitions. According to José Barreiro,

> we have been criticised that our exhibits are too conceptual. But the problem is not that they are anti-object so much, but that the concepts are not particularly well grounded. This is my critique of that and I think that the conceptual framework is always necessary, but sometimes it does not have enough depth. It also does not really appreciate how this message is transferred to the general public that has never before contemplated these concepts . . . We went soft on history. It is not about one side being completely evil and one side being completely good.

In a similar self-critical vein, Ann McMullen observed, "If there is a prevailing American mindset and the museum proposes to correct that mindset by presenting a Native perspective, the question is whether it actually works by simply presenting the Native perspective as if it is true." The uncritical adoption of the Native voice as a tool for "indigenising" the museum proves to be a controversial aspect of participatory museum work. What emerges, therefore, is the realisation on the part of NMAI staff that the presentation of the Native voice needs to be incorporated into wider conceptual and more academic frameworks. This invites the realignment of the tribal perspective with a more mainstream museology, placing a stronger emphasis on the aesthetic aspects of material culture, as was the case with Identity by Design and the New York displays, and combining tribal and scholarly knowledge.

Native Voice and Scholarship

The exhibition Identity by Design emerged out of such concerns. For Richard West,

> this is a result of the accumulation of knowledge about how we remain as a matter of philosophy and mission absolutely consistent: a first person articulation voice in the exhibit, the Native women who stand behind those dresses, but also, at the same time we have tried to lure in, if you will, those who think they may be coming for an art exhibit. The presentation is beautiful. It is a stunning exhibition to look from an aesthetic standpoint . . . Regarding the criticism that comes from the art critics, we have done and can do certain things to alleviate their concerns . . . We can be more explicable without changing our philosophy, or departing from our mission.

With respect to the issue of scholarly research, as Gabrielle Tayac observed, "now that the NMAI is open and the inaugural exhibitions are in place, there is the long term plan of how the museum is positioned as a site of scholarship for Indigenous Studies." As she observed, this is not only about scientific research, but also much aimed to "indigenise the museum." As such, the research that is conducted is "not only books and publications, nor is it purely anthropological. It can be, for example, listening to peoples' points of view on global warming."

The foundation of the Research Unit headed by José Barreiro in 2006 shows this tendency to "intellectualise" the museum. This has required refocusing attention on material culture with a critical interpretative input from scholars and researchers alongside the narrative of tribal curators. As such, the Native place as a space for the celebration of survival and identity is reframed according to the idea of the museum as a research institution; something that potentially could be regarded as a depoliticisation of the museum narrative via a return to more typical museological practices.

REVISITING THE PAST IN THE PRESENT

As we have seen, the participation of Native groups in the planning of the new museum led to a critical examination of older museum practices. This new "Indian museology" involved the adoption of more appropriate approaches to representation, interpretation, and collections care, through processes of Indigenous curation, community multivocal exhibitions, and first-voice interpretation. Intangible heritage was thus negotiated in relation to a holistic and inclusive framework for capturing and representing the Native experience through an active engagement with source communities.

But how is intangible heritage negotiated in the context of museums that are not as close (both physically and in terms of their broader approach) to Indigenous groups? The next chapters pursue this question in two museums in the European contexts of London and Paris. By looking at how these two museums take on intangible heritage, their role as museums of world art and culture is reviewed. In an increasingly globalised world, where tribal communities no longer live in undisturbed societies but actively seek recognition and participation in the international heritage arena, older institutions embedded in European colonialism are increasingly asked to reinvent themselves. In this process the discourses of world art and collections-based museum work provide a critical framework for revisiting themes of participation and representation and the relations between living and material culture.

Chapter 6

Reinventing the Gift at the Horniman Museum

Frederick J. Horniman wanted to create a window on the world here in Forest Hill, something that people could enjoy without having a great understanding of. Now, many of our visitors come from these distant cultures . . . About 25 percent of our visitors are black minority and ethnic. Our visitors are related to our collections in a way that previously our London visitors would not be. This is increasingly reflected in our work.

—Janet Vitmayer, director of the Horniman Museum

The last chapters examined three museums that have emerged out of major political and civil rights movements and in this process actively engaged with issues of recognition, reconciliation, and development. In this context, intangible heritage constitutes an aspect of postcolonial museology related to the empowerment of previously marginalised groups and the revival of traditional knowledge, in contrast with Eurocentric heritage conceptualisations and museum canons (Byrne 1991, 2009; Kurin 2007). Building on these issues, the last two chapters look at how ideas around the definition, display, and preservation of intangible heritage are played out in European museology. Mostly viewed as a non-European heritage discourse (Smith and Akagawa 2009), intangible heritage seems to be at the margins of a more mainstream and object-based practice.

The Horniman Museum, for example, was founded in London at the end of the nineteenth century, a period characterised by the expansion of the British Empire and the birth of modern scientific disciplines (see Coombes 1994; Bennett 1995). Collections of objects and artefacts are the museum's first port of call and play a crucial role in defining exhibitions, research, and programming. In addition, the planning of exhibitions is based on curatorial and scientific research, often with a strong didactic perspective. More recently, however, changing London demographics have provided a new operational context for the museum. Since its reno-

Intangible Heritage and the Museum: New Perspectives on Cultural Preservation by Marilena Alivizatou, 135–158. ©2012 Left Coast Press, Inc. All rights reserved.

vation in 2002, and in some cases well prior to that, the Horniman has established partnerships with different ethnic, religious, and diasporic communities. As such, one aspect that sets apart the Horniman from its earlier practice is its annual community events programme. For instance, in July 2008 the Utsavam Fest, a festival of music, art, dance, foods, and crafts took place in the museum's gardens as part of the temporary exhibition Utsavam: Music from India. With different stages for performing traditional and contemporary music, dance, storytelling, and culinary demonstrations, the festival was a celebration of the vitality of Indian culture in the UK. This was expressed in the large participation of members of the UK Indian community, with people of all ages dressed in traditional costumes and modern outfits and performing traditional instruments like the sitar, but also dancing to the modern beats of R&B.

The aim of this chapter then is to examine how intangible heritage fits in a museology that has for the last hundred years been mostly concerned with the interpretation of material culture. The Horniman still remains much attached to the academic disciplines that informed its practice throughout the twentieth century, with exhibitions covering the areas of natural sciences, anthropology, and ethnomusicology. Yet, as a diverse range of communities becomes involved in museum work, the relations between material and immaterial, objects and living people are increasingly refashioned. In this process the museum is faced with calls to combine academic scholarship with community perspectives, much in the spirit of the participatory work taking place in Te Papa, the VCC, and the NMAI.

A HUNDRED-YEAR-OLD MICROCOSM IN FOREST HILL

Similar to the NMAI, which resulted from the early twentieth-century collecting of George Gustav Heye, the Horniman Museum grew out of the nineteenth-century collecting of London tea merchant Frederick J. Horniman (1835–1906). Today, after various changes and renovations, the latest of which was in 2002, the Horniman stands on the same location in Forest Hill as it did when it first opened its doors in 1901 as a gift to the people of London. Unlike the other museums examined in this book, in which the collections were moved from older establishments to new museums in an effort to break away from different colonial legacies, the Horniman has kept to the same name and building for more than a hundred years.

Retracing the early days of the Horniman collection in the Surrey House Museum (Horniman's private museum that opened in 1891), Nicky Levell (2000) provides a detailed account of Horniman's travelling and collecting in Egypt, China, Japan, Burma, and India in the broader context of late Victorian orientalism. London-based international exhibitions of goods, products, and curiosities from different parts of the world, like the 1851 Great Exhibition and the 1886 Colonial and Indian Exhibition, sparked an interest in international travel, incentivising affluent Londoners to embark on the discovery of the world. Between 1894 and 1896 Frederick J. Horniman made two extended trips in South and East Asia, during which he collected various objects. With the aim of increasing his collections, throughout the 1890s he also purchased African artefacts—for example several of the brass plaques removed from Benin City palace after the British Punitive Expedition of 1897—from dealers and auctioneers as well as missionaries and colonial administrators (Coombes 1994:150). A private collection of rare and highly praised artefacts gave prestige and social recognition to its owner (Shelton 2000:166).

In 1901 Horniman's private museum was renovated with a new building, designed by Charles Harrison Townsend (1851–1928) and donated to the London County Council for the "recreation, instruction, and enjoyment" of the people of London (as stated in a plaque on the museum's façade). The appointment of Cambridge anthropologist Alfred Cort Haddon (1855–1940) as advisory curator in that same year led to major changes in the overall profile of the new Horniman Free Museum. While previously Horniman's eclectic collections were displayed rather spuriously and haphazardly in a maze of twenty-four rooms (Levell 2000:230), organised around the main divisions of art and natural history (Coombes 1994:151), Haddon aimed at turning the new museum into a space of scientific knowledge and education. For him, "The day has passed when we can consider a collection of 'curios' as a museum. If properly arranged a museum is an educational institution of the greatest value, as information is conveyed visually with accuracy and great rapidity" (Levell 2000:316).[1]

In this spirit, efforts were made to bring the ethnographic collections up to speed with the latest theories and discussions in the emerging science of anthropology (Coombes 1994; Shelton 2000). For most of the twentieth century, the museum's ethnographic displays would be a stage on which academic and museum anthropologists would use material culture collected and donated to the museum from around the world, including rural areas of Europe, to support scientific arguments and methods. Early evolutionist and diffusionist typological displays of objects were subsequently followed by functionalist dioramas, often reducing collections to "paradigmatic representations contained by the straightjackets of simply constituted knowledge fields" (Shelton 2000:186). Unlike other European museums with similar collections that have adopted a more aesthetic approach (see chapter 7), ethnographic artefacts are still presented and interpreted in the Horniman through the eyes of anthropologists.

Equally important in defining the museum's approach has been its educational focus. This can be linked not only to the wish of the museum founder to contribute to the education of the citizens of London, but also to the fact that as of 1901 the museum has been accountable to a public body, and therefore has had to prove in concrete ways its relevance and benefit to the wider community. Unlike other major ethnographic displays of the time, like the Pitt Rivers Museum and the British Museum, that were primarily addressed to an academic and erudite public, from its early days the Horniman strove to appeal to a broader social spectrum (Coombes 1994:154), something that is manifested in the programmes and lectures accompanying the exhibitions. These included lecture series held in a purposefully built lecture room, publications of handbooks and guidebooks on the collections, and educational aids for pupils in the form of questionnaires (Coombes 1994:154–157).

Although the themes and narratives of the exhibitions have changed significantly over the last hundred years, the museum's commitment to community and education still remains unchanged. At the time of my research, the museum operated as a non-departmental public body, funded directly by the UK Department of Culture, Media and Sport with the mission "to use our worldwide collections and the Gardens to encourage a wider appreciation of the world, its peoples, their cultures and its environments" (according to the funding agreement the museum and the Department of Culture, Media, and Sport signed in 2005). A variety of exhibitions, public and education programmes, concerts, performances, and storytelling sessions take place throughout the year, attracting a diverse range of communities and building an important framework around which the museum's engagement with intangible heritage was negotiated. Over the course of the last century, with a continuously growing collection of 80,000 ethnographic and 10,000 archaeological objects, 250,000 natural history specimens, and 7,000 musical instruments, the Horniman has created an eclectic and unique microcosm in Forest Hill, a *lieu de mémoire* of the nineteenth-century museum practice that created it (see Bennett 1995, 2004). In what follows I explore how a nineteenth-century institution creates space for an emerging museological dialogue on intangible heritage in twenty-first-century London.

THE MUSEOLOGICAL SYNTAX OF THE HORNIMAN

The Horniman stands on a sixteen-acre plot of land in Forest Hill, a ten-minute train ride from London Bridge. Reaching the museum from the busy London Road, the first thing one sees is the clock tower of the 1901 building. Next to it, a large carved writing on the old stone building, above a mosaic mural, explains that this is the Horniman Free Museum (Figure 6.1). The external spaces are as eclectic as the museum's interiors. The wall mosaic, which depicts the allegoric scene of "Humanity in the House of Circumstance", makes an interesting contrast to the Native American Northwest Coast totem pole standing nearby.[2] Heading towards the pole, three new buildings have been attached to the old museum. One of them is made of wood and its roof is covered with plants and grass. This is an ecological construction built in 1996 that houses the museum's library. The combination of the Victorian clock tower, the classical antiquity-inspired mosaics, the Tlingit totem pole, and the ecological building stresses the multilayered history of the museum, which fuses the new with the old, the exotic with the European.

The museum stands within the Horniman Gardens (Figure 6.2). Here at different times of the year one can see trees, flowers, and plants from the UK, but also from Africa and South Asia. The gardens are divided into different sub-gardens, fields, and picnic areas. There is also an animal enclosure with goats, rabbits, chickens, and geese. In addition, several sundials can be found in different parts of the garden, and a late nineteenth-century glass and iron conservatory, formerly at the Horniman family home at Coombe Cliff in Croydon and now used for public and private events, stands just behind the main museum building. Various sculptures have been lined along the main path. One of them

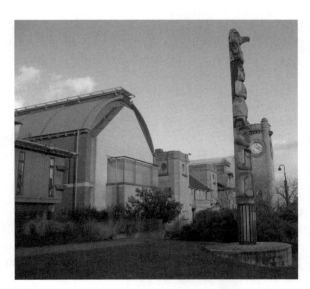

Figure 6.1: The Horniman Free Museum in Forest Hill, London. (All images in this chapter published with the permission of the Horniman Museum.)

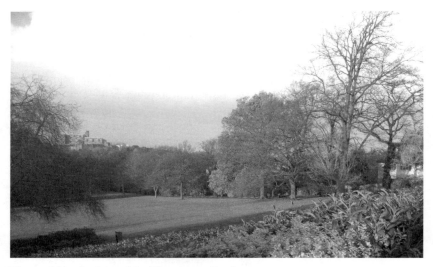

Figure 6.2:   A view of the Horniman Gardens.

depicts a bird hatching eggs and eating them, made by Zimbabwean artist Bernard Matemera. Unlike the unknown makers of nineteenth- and early twentieth-century objects in the permanent displays, makers of contemporary artworks are presented as named individuals. Over the last years significant efforts (like this type of garden gallery) have been made to reconnect the gardens with the museum. Much like at Te Papa, the NMAI, and the MQB, the museum makes direct links between nature and culture in its narrative. Unlike the British Museum, whose natural history and ethnographic collections were separated, the Horniman has retained its collections of *naturalia* and *artificialia*, which act as a reminder of the taxonomies and classifications defining early museology (Bennett 2004).

Entering the building from the main entrance on the West side, the first gallery after passing the museum shop and café is the Natural History Gallery. At its centre is one of the iconic objects of the Horniman, an over-stuffed walrus, surrounded by several evenly distributed Victorian glass cases that contain human and animal remains, fossils, and specimens (Figure 6.3). The Natural History Gallery with its arched roof is part of the old building and is surrounded by a balcony gallery. The appearance and displays of the Natural History Gallery have not changed much since the fifties, but the plans for its redevelopment will try to maintain its "historical quirkiness," as Victoria Brightman, head of learning, told me. The new gallery will also engage in discussions around biodiversity and sensitise the public on environmental issues, such as climate change.

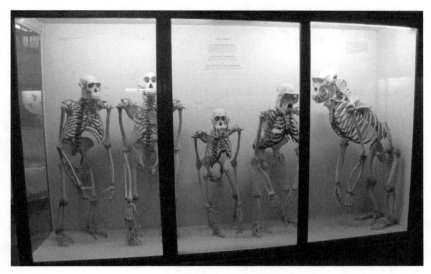

Figure 6.3: Victorian wood and glass cases are used for the display of human and animal remains in the Natural History Gallery.

"Bio" and "cultural" diversity emerge as key concepts that bring the Horniman in tune with broader social concerns and contemporary issues.

Biodiversity is also discussed in the adjacent Environment Room, where a fully operational beehive with living bees makes an interesting contrast to the skeletons and taxidermic specimens that can be found in the Natural History Gallery. Living bees are not the only live animals in the museum. In 2005 the aquarium reopened in the museum's basement, recreating habitats of swamps, Pacific reefs, and Amazonian rainforests and presenting different marine species, including sea horses, four-eyed fishes, and tropical monkey frogs. Treating these living animals like living objects stresses the eclectic taste of the museum and provides an interesting framework for thinking about living and dead museum pieces.

Lower Ground Floor Galleries

The separation between nature and culture is quite evident in the permanent exhibitions layout. With natural history displays on the ground floor, lower ground floor galleries are mostly about the presentation of the anthropology and musical instruments collections. Two out of the four galleries on that floor are part of the museum's 2002 extension. This also included the construction of the Gallery Square, a large open space used for public events and activities that provides access to the two new galleries and the existing Centenary Gallery. Each of these galleries lies behind heavy wooden doors; entering them, there is an instant change in the tone, lighting, and overall atmosphere. In the following pages, I examine in more detail the three permanent exhibitions, African Worlds, the Centenary Gallery, and the Musical Instruments Gallery, and two temporary exhibitions that took place during my research, Amazon to Caribbean (2006) and Utsavam: Music from India (2008).

African Worlds

The African Worlds exhibition is presented in a space not very different in size and shape from the Natural History Gallery: a large room with a high arched roof and balcony overlooking the lower floor. Entering the room, the statue of a lion in bright colours welcomes visitors. In front of it, a big blue panel introduces the exhibition. On the panel, a quote from African scholar Ali Mazrui celebrates the diversity of the African continent: "You are not a country, Africa. You are a concept . . . You are not a concept, Africa. You are a glimpse of the infinite." The panel further explains that African Worlds offers not one single, but different glimpses of Africa viewed "through the eyes of artists, diviners, anthropologists, drummers, elders and exiles."

In the spirit of postcolonial and participatory museology, African Worlds was created through the collaboration of an international group of curators, with input from members of London African communities (Shelton 2003). The introductory panel explains in a reflexive tone, "Some of the objects on display are only fragments of larger pieces; all have been removed from their original contexts. Although attempts have been made to, we can never give more than the most fleeting impression of the lives of these objects before they came to Europe." This last point hints at a curatorially perceived distance between African artefacts as museum objects and as used in their original contexts. In comparison with Te Papa, the VCC, and the NMAI, here material culture is far more removed from living communities.

The exhibition is strongly focused on the presentation of artefacts, with emphasis given to the display of masks from sub-Saharan Africa. It unfolds in three paths along which large display cases have been placed. The central path is elevated and separated from the rest by red and cream walls of different heights and shapes rising behind the glass cases. Objects in the cases are often hard to see, either due to low lighting or because they are placed in awkward positions, underlining the fact that in ritual settings access to them is restricted to certain individuals and museum visitors can only take a peek at them (Phillips 2002).

The exhibition creates an immersive environment that emphasises the vitality and spirituality of African cultures through video and sound installations. Occupying a prominent place in the main middle way are Bwa Plank, Bedu, and Dogon masks. Their imposing display, enhanced by the spotlights above, intensifies their formal elements, shapes, and colours. At their base, different interpretation media allude to their use and performance by their creators. For example, under the Dogon masks an early recording is projected that was made by French anthropologists Marcel Griaule (1898–1956) and Michel Leiris (1901–1990) in the 1930s. This shows the dance of the masks as people participate in local rituals, bending their heads and bodies to the rhythm of beating drums. As Hassan Arero, the museum's earlier keeper of the anthropological collection stressed, such recordings place the masks in their historical context and also allude to the performed tradition of which they are part. A similar screen accompanies the Bedu masks. Here, the recordings show how the particular masks were made by carving and painting the wood and were then used in local celebrations in Cote d'Ivoire.

A different interpretation strategy is used for the Bwa Plank masks. A large label contains three different readings of them. Firstly, a quote from Poboye Konate, an artist from Burkina Faso, explains that "the masks are carved with scars, like the scars on our faces. These are like the words on a sign that tell us how to live our lives. The signs are a language we learn in the bush that only those who have been initiated can understand." This local understanding of the masks is followed by a more extended reading by anthropologist Christopher Bay. Bay explains that Bwa Plank masks are "moving, living signposts" carrying the "religious laws" of the community. He also explains that the intricate carvings represent the "way of the ancestors," adding that their heavy weight means that only the "strongest young men who have strengthened their neck by months of practice can wear them." Finally, basic object information regarding the provenance, materials, and dating of the masks are included on the right side of the label.

This multiple reading of objects combining inventory information, academic interpretation, and local understanding is presented in several other displays. Agatha Okafor, a London-based solicitor of African origins, is pictured on a label under the Kuba Mingesh masks from the Democratic Republic of Congo next to a quote saying that "masquerades actually play games with women in that they run up and see if women are bold enough to stay. I have never seen a woman just stand there and wait for the masquerade, because some of them carry whips." Under her quote, the curatorial team explains that these masks are used in "male initiation ceremonies" and "represent nature spirits, *mingesh*, who dwell in forests next to springs, rivers and pools." A similar multilayered and multivocal interpretation accompanies most artefacts on display, including Yoruba, Gelede, Nkanu, Ekpo, Mende, and Gola masks and Mende and Temne society figures. Rather than presenting the African masks and sculptures as works of art, the exhibition interprets these artefacts within the context of an ethnographic analysis as parts of rituals, performances, and wider social practices. Although no longer performed and as such inanimate, ritual objects in the Horniman are displayed in ways that allude to their former lives. As such anthropological interpretative frameworks based on ethnographic fieldwork are particularly strong in African Worlds.

At the back end of the exhibition, the space is dominated by the gigantic *ijele*, the masquerade from Igboland in Nigeria. Anthropologists conducting fieldwork in Nigeria on behalf of the museum commissioned this enormous, multicoloured mask. A video on its side with photographs taken by the researchers that commissioned the masquerade and upbeat musical extracts explains how it was made and the contemporary context in which it is used, reviving the performative dimensions of the artefact.

Not far from this mask, on the exhibition's west wall, several cases with dramatic spotlights contain the Horniman's collection of another group of objects from Nigeria, the Benin plaques. A panel on their side signed by curator Antony Shelton explains their contested past as part of the 1897 Punitive Expedition booty and mentions contemporary claims "for a peaceful resolution of this shame of history." Moreover, the panel contains the photos of Nigerian curators Emanuel Arinze and Joseph Eboreimi and illustrates their collaboration with the museum for the interpretation of the pieces. Each plaque is placed in an individual high-security case of the kind used for the display of treasured objects. Under each plaque, a label provides information about the figures that are represented. The label contains quotes from different Benin aphorisms in local languages that are also translated in English. Local interpretations are thus mobilised to critically engage with the plaques' contested past, creating a dialogue of participatory museum work.

Next to the introductory panel, a video shows contemporary brass casting in Benin City. The video describes how the tradition has survived to this day, explaining the long work and different steps required in order to make a fine cast. Presenting brass casting in both its past and present dimensions suggests that this is not a tradition of a forgotten past, dispersed and abandoned after the 1897 British attack on the city's palace, but an important aspect of peoples' lives in present-day Nigeria, hinting that traditional practices are still alive.

Another important aspect of African Worlds is the treatment of religion. Islam is represented through the display of Koranic boards in a dark and sombre display case. African-rooted spiritual beliefs are also addressed on the east wall of the exhibition. Here, three altars have been recreated, showing the flourishing and transformation of three African beliefs in North and South America through the transatlantic slave trade: Candomblé in Brazil, Vodou in Haiti, and Vodoon in Benin. As explained by Antony Shelton on the introductory panel, "each altar has been recreated following the guidance of priests in Benin, Haiti and Brazil." Religious icons, posters, food, and drink are all put together to provide an image of the material culture of these complex spiritual practices. What is absent, however, are the actual practitioners, their voices, perspectives, and engagements with the practices as ongoing cultural phenomena.

Centenary Gallery

The same observation could be made regarding the Centenary Gallery. Entering the dark and silent room, the panel beneath the portrait of Frederick J. Horniman that faces the main entrance explains that "this exhibition puts on display some of the strange, colourful and exciting objects brought to the Museum during the late nineteenth and twentieth centuries . . . in the light of the theories and understandings of the people who brought them back to display in the Museum." This exhibition in a reflexive and critical tone rehearses key moments in the construction of anthropological theories based on the analysis of primarily non-European material culture. As such, it is very much about the appropriation of non-European objects by European collectors and anthropologists, mirroring at the same time the history of the museum.

The first section, entitled "The Gift: The Horniman Family" presents the "curiosities" collected and displayed by Horniman in his private museum. These include the Japanese merman, which is made up of papier-mâché and fish parts, a large collection of beetles, butterflies, and moths, statues of a Buddha and of Indian deities Shiva and Kali in battle, as well as Indian masks and papier-mâché caste heads from Rajasthan. The second section, "The New Museum: Illustrating Evolution," presents the reorganisation of the collections following Haddon's evolutionist approach, by which "different races were at different stages of evolution." The display case of this section presents mostly artefacts from the Pacific, including carved boards from Papua New Guinea, slit drums from Vanuatu, Maori carved figures from New Zealand, paddles from the Solomon Islands, and spears from the Torres Straits.

The third section, entitled "Material Culture Archive," refers to the archival aspects of museum work by presenting different ways for classifying objects according to their function. For instance, a label near a case with fishhooks from around the world explains that "they show how similar are the solutions found to the universal problem of how to catch a fish." Finally, the last section, "Scholars, Travellers and Traders," presents the more recent acquisitions of the museum, including contemporary objects that transcend ethnic categorisations, collected through the fieldwork of curators-anthropologists or through donations. Photographs of Antony Shelton and Ken Teague, previously keepers of anthropology at the Horniman, engaged in fieldwork are attached on a large panel, stressing the input of anthropologists in the work of the museum.

The Centenary Gallery is an exhibition showing a growing collection of objects and a museum that is constantly interpreting it. Its overall tone is in line with late twentieth-century anthropological reflexivity (see Clifford and Marcus 1986; Marcus and Fischer 1986), whereby the collections tell the history of anthropology and of the museum and underline the subjectivity of museum displays. Nevertheless, the objects remain silent as far as their makers are concerned, and references to the humanity of the material culture on display are absent.

At the far end of the gallery, much like the altars in African Worlds, lies the reconstruction of a Tibetan shrine. Like the Benin, Haitian, and Brazilian altars, not much information is conveyed about the makers of the altars or the practitioners of the religion. The exhibition is filled with material culture and its Western interpretation, but empty in terms of people.

Musical Instruments Gallery

The last permanent exhibition on this floor is the Musical Instruments Gallery, a space often full of music and sound coming from video projections, multimedia installations, and children running around. The display of musical instruments raises interesting questions about their presentation as material objects and vehicles for making music, and therefore about the relationship between the tangible and the intangible.

The exhibition is about musical instruments and music making as a social practice (Figure 6.4). A wide range of music traditions are presented, including Yoruba celebrations for the birth of children in Nigeria, music boxes and small music-making objects used as toys for children in Japan, wedding ceremonies in Uzbekistan, and teenage rock music from the UK.

The western wall of the gallery presents several hundreds instruments, displayed according to modern classification systems. Facing the rather crowded display are three music tables. Each of these contains a multimedia programme featuring selected instruments from the cases in front. By pressing a button, information is provided regarding the maker and the performance context of selected instruments. In addition, a short music extract in which the same instrument is played can be heard from loud speakers and headsets. The music tables allow for certain small or

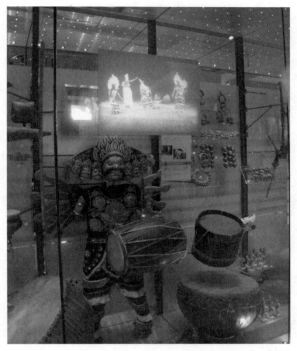

Figure 6.4: In the Musical Instruments Gallery, the Chau Dance Ceremony is presented through a combination of artefact and audiovisual display.

hard-to-find instruments to be singled out from the dark cases. Listening to the music made by the instruments addresses the exhibition themes in a more holistic manner. In this context, musical instruments are not presented as dead or beautiful museum pieces, but rather as objects used in social and symbolic practices.

Temporary Exhibitions

The third gallery on the lower ground floor is the gallery for the presentation of temporary exhibitions, which at the time of my research were Amazon to the Caribbean: Early People of the Rainforest (October 2005–January 2007) and Utsavam: Music from India (February–November 2008).

Amazon to the Caribbean

Amazon to the Caribbean, curated by Hassan Arero, aimed at tracing the links between Amerindian people of the Caribbean Antilles and mainland Northwest South America by presenting archaeological and ethnographic objects from the twentieth-century collections of the museum and also more contemporary artefacts collected by Hassan Arero during fieldwork in Guyana in 2004. The entrance to the exhibition featured sounds of the rainforest and a video with images of tropical birds and environments surrounding a rotating wooden carved figure by Guyanese artist Oswald Hussein. The replicas of an anaconda resting in a pond and a taxidermy specimen of a crouching leopard stood in the centre of the gallery, alluding to the fauna of the Amazonian tropics. Next to the entrance, a bright orange panel signed by Hassan Arero introduced the topic of the exhibition, emphasising the curator's fieldwork with the Wai Wai people in Guyana. The immersive environment of the exhibitions with dim lighting, sounds, and vivid colours as well as the combination of natural history and ethnographic objects recreated the broader context of the region.

Overall the exhibition had a strong educational focus and presented a wide range of objects, including archaeological finds like stone tools and pots, but also twentieth-century war and dance clubs, feathered headdresses, baskets, hammocks, and carved stools. A film projected on a wall next to a canoe addressed the theme of seafaring between Guyana and the Caribbean Antilles, and another film on the opposite wall showed aspects of daily life of the Wai Wai. A special "kid's zone" stood in a corner, with a canoe in the middle and tables for the children to draw, while another corner with sofas and a round table allowed adults to read the object catalogues.

In a rather prominent area of the space special reference was made to the community projects related to the exhibition. As Hassan Arero explained, different objects from the Horniman collection were used as inspiration for exploring the issue of Caribbean identity and were accompanied by comments and photographs of members of different London Caribbean groups. This reveals the museum's focus on working with ethnic groups and communities that historically have been excluded from the work of the museum and on making those partnerships visible in the context of the public exhibition.

Utsavam

Similar partnerships were also established with London Indian communities for the temporary exhibition Utsavam: Music from India. The UK-based Indian communities and cultural organisations consulted by curators were presented in two panels on a wall near the end of the exhibition and in extracts from recorded performances projected on a screen (Figure 6.5). Their contribution was also underlined in the introductory panel, placed against a red backdrop and next to a map of the

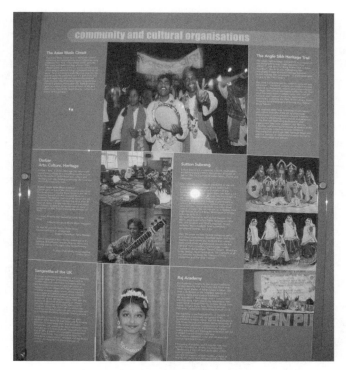

Figure 6.5: A panel introducing the community organisations that were consulted for the temporary exhibition Utsavam.

subcontinent highlighting the areas covered. In contrast to the Centenary Gallery and, to a lesser extent, African Worlds, the panel and map were surrounded by large images of people from different rural communities playing their instruments.

Next to this and lit by a spotlight was a *miravu*, a traditional drum from Kerala, placed on a pedestal and adorned with flowers. Above it, a video projected on the wall presented how the miravu is made and the blessing ceremony that takes place when the drum is first used. Interestingly, a small label on the wall next to the display highlights that the drum is "played solo or to accompany sacred dances, such as Kutiyattam, a form of Sanskrit theatre proclaimed as a masterpiece of intangible heritage by the international body UNESCO."

Much like the reference to the UNESCO proclamation of the *sandroing* as a masterpiece of intangible heritage in the VCC, the reference to the Kutiyattam alluded to the ritual performance of the object on display and placed it in a broader social and cultural context. Moreover, the UNESCO stamp seemed to validate the traditional practice, informing readers that oral culture and tradition are equally important expressions of cultural heritage as artworks and objects. Here, the miravu was singled out not in terms of its aesthetic value, its shape, or materials, but on account of the ceremonies that it represents and their spiritual meaning and significance.

Unlike the other galleries that were mostly object-focused, in this exhibit special attention had been given to the presentation of the people and communities from which the instruments originated, as well as the beliefs and traditions associated with them. As the introductory label explained:

> Most of the musical instruments in this gallery were made during the present century in rural areas of India. They were commissioned together with the audiovisual recordings during the course of collecting projects for the British Library Sound Archive and the Horniman Museum. The performance arts represented by the instruments and the films acquired during these projects are practised by communities in the states of Kerala, Orissa and Andhra Pradesh, Assam, Punjab and Arunachal Pradesh. Organisations within the UK that preserve and promote traditional music from India have been central to the development of the exhibition and their work is shown here.

The collaboration of the Horniman with the British Library Sound Archive has pointed to a more holistic approach as to what should be collected and displayed. New technologies enabled the recreation of the musical experience as performed by local musicians and recorded by curators in rural areas of India. In the absence of the actual performance, the instrument displayed in a glass case tells a fragmented story. Exhibition curators Margaret Birley and Rolf Killius placed significant emphasis on collecting both the tangible and the intangible related to traditional music from India. As one label explained, "Film is now exploited as a matter of course to illustrate technique, repertoire and cultural contexts for performance in most of the musical instruments collected for the museum." Moreover, an emphasis on the performative dimensions of certain pieces allows for them to be understood as social objects and vessels of deeper spiritual meaning.

UNIVERSAL MUSEUM AND MATERIAL CULTURE

Discussions with staff members highlighted that the history of the museum has been central to its current programmes. Janet Vitmayer, the museum's director, stressed that contemporary work at the Horniman is embedded in the museum's past:

> Frederick J. Horniman wanted to create a window on the world here in Forest Hill, something that people could enjoy without having a great understanding of . . . His big passion was to share the collections with

everybody. He was never an elitist. He wanted to share the idea of having an inquiring mind, being interested and very open to the world. This shaped a lot how the museum unfolded along the years.

She stressed that unlike many museums whose collections are dispersed in other institutions, central to the work of the Horniman is "the idea of a universal museum in which you can delve about all the aspects of the world, both cultural, natural historical and be able to have the wonders of the open space. It is a very holistic idea to create this all round institution."

The eclectic and multifaceted character of the museum and the aim to contribute to the benefit of the community are key facets of its practice. A related factor that has affected the articulation of the museological narrative of the Horniman has been the emphasis on the importance of the collections. Andrew Willshire, marketing and communications manager, talking about the public events taking place at the museum observed: "Everything that we do has a direct relationship with the collections. The collections are very much at the heart of what we do. They inspire us to do our programming and how we promote ourselves." Likewise, Janet Vitmayer noted: "A key for us is that always the collection is playing a central role. This is our linchpin . . . Even when redeveloping old galleries, like the Natural History, the objects remain the first port of call."

Anthropological Fieldwork

Equally important in influencing the museum's work has been the active fieldwork conducted by museum curators. "The Horniman is an intrinsically fieldwork organisation. It is the fieldwork nature of collecting that gives the character of the organisation and we have one hundred years of unbroken fieldwork," noted Janet Vitmayer, adding that "fieldwork links very well with intangible heritage." Hassan Arero described the importance of museum fieldwork as satisfying "the need to understand the context of objects and the stories surrounding them," remarking that "you can't do that by sitting in a comfortable armchair and musing about distant cultures. You have to go there."

Explaining how intangible heritage relates to fieldwork research, Hassan Arero used the example of African masks:

> Intangible heritage is what brings the object to life. It is what gives you deeper meaning; a deeper understanding of the object . . . Intangible heritage is a matter of the moment; you have to be there to capture that essence. The closest you get to that is getting a video or taping the sound of it. For example, you can see that in the African Worlds gallery. Next to

the Dogon masks, we have a video showing how they are used. We try to show their intangible elements. In a way, videos are a window into another world which the mask on its own would not be able to reveal.

Ethnographic fieldwork allows researchers to see the object in performance and find out more about the people that create and use it. As such, it uncovers the deeper meanings and symbolisms of material culture and is a way through which the intangible surfaces in the permanent museum.

Curating the Intangible

Intangible heritage is thus embodied in the knowledge, practice, and performance of artefacts, often viewed as something that can be collected and treated as an additional museum object. Discussing the planning for the Musical Instruments Gallery and Utsavam, Margaret Birley, keeper of musical instruments and curator of both exhibits, noted: "We thought it was very important to have video footage of people in source communities making music; to have this element of interpretation in the gallery. This gives a better idea of the complexity and sophistication of the musical traditions." A holistic interpretation of artefacts enables therefore a more profound understanding of displays.

Treating intangible heritage as a new category of museum collectibles, however, takes the discussion back to the debates about the preservation and the fossilisation of culture in static representations. Expressing his concerns about the tendency of museums to "fix things," Hassan Arero argued that museums "have to be able to understand these elements of dynamism and transformation of cultural symbols and forms . . . The same object that was used this morning as a cup can be used in a ritual and become a container of blood." Meanings of objects and practices are fluid, and fixing them in static representations fails to transmit the complexities of living cultures.

Living Heritage

Further discussions at the Horniman stressed the links between intangible heritage and contemporary cultural performances taking place in the museum. Combining elements of the traditional and the contemporary, these performances present by and large living cultural practices by actual practitioners and tradition bearers. Such performances are realised through partnerships between the museum and members of different communities with the aim of fostering participation rather than recreating authentic rituals or ceremonies. Referring to the importance given by the museum trustees to live performances, Janet Vitmayer observed that "what we always try to do is to have elements expressing the intangible heritage in our programming. It is intrinsic in it . . . Intangible heritage is in the gallery, but also in a live form that can only be transient."

During fieldwork I was able to observe the diversity of the events and performances taking place in the museum, usually within the context of temporary exhibitions such as Amazon to the Caribbean and Utsavam. Regarding the first, Hassan Arero talked at length about the significance of the residency of Oswald Hussein, a sculptor from Guyana, in the museum in October 2006. As he argued:

> Oswald told me once that he thought that people looked at him as if they were watching a football match. We had some of his pieces in the gallery already, but I did not see forty people standing around one of the finished pieces. But once the man is there, the whole process of transforming this material, the knowledge which he communicates with his hand and chisel, that knowledge, which is communicated by transforming this wooden piece, is so captivating, so intricate. Surely you can show a video, but actually living it is so different.

In the same context, in February and March 2008 several performances took place in the museum to accompany the opening of Utsavam. These, for example, included a *kathakali* performance by actress Kalamandalan Vijayakumar presenting a simplified version of the traditional performance. On the bright Sunday afternoon that I observed these events, the Gallery Square was packed with families and many people from London Indian communities and beyond (Figure 6.6). Discussing the operational framework of these performances, Andrew Willshire, who was in charge of their production, remarked that they gave "an opportunity to second or third generation Indian people in Britain to connect to their culture."

The wide range of performances that took place in the Horniman in relation to Utsavam also included concerts by the Raj Academy Ensemble and the London Sitar Ensemble, Punjabi sword dancing, traditional dances from Assam, and music performances by Indian and British musicians playing special instruments, like the *ghatam* (clay) pot and the Carnatic violin, as well as contemporary electronic music played by DJs. Presenting the diversity of the performing arts and traditions of India, these events aimed at showcasing the oral practices and performative customs that are still part of peoples lives. Against this backdrop, intangible heritage is largely seen as a way for transforming an object-focused museum into a performative and participatory space in which rather than Horniman's gift, it is communities that become the museum's port of call.

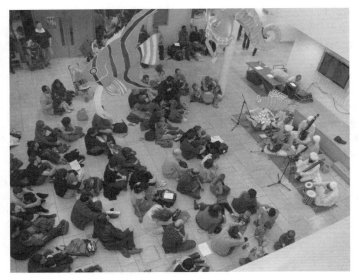

Figure 6.6: A music performance by the Raj Academy Ensemble at the Gallery Square in February 2008.

Intangible Heritage and Community Work

The presentation of local traditions and crafts of specific ethnic groups was much discussed during my research. Just like the Indian Festival, in the summers of 2006 and 2007 a Caribbean Festival took place in the Horniman Gardens. Andrew Willshire explained:

> A big event that we have been doing for the last years is an event in our gardens presenting Caribbean food, whereby we have had a big Caribbean cooking competition with other things like music, storytelling, and kids activities. The idea is that with events like these we draw people that do not usually visit museums. Whereas, if we had said, come and see this exhibition, it is about the historic connections between Amerindians and the African Caribbean communities, some people might be interested and some people might not be.

While Andrew Willshire is concerned mainly with one-off special events, Vicky Brightman oversees the work of the community learning team, which deals on a more long term basis "with families, community groups, adult learning, and community development, trying to bring in new audiences, non-traditional museum audiences, and focus on diversity." Among the activities that her team organises are storytelling sessions every Friday in the African Worlds Gallery, children and adult courses on African dancing and drumming, art and craft sessions, singing classes, and music appreciation sessions.

For her, "the Horniman is a community museum" working among others with ethnic minority groups, disability groups, and the elderly, and where "learning is at the heart of what we do." As she observed, however,

> community education is usually project-based because it is easier to fund . . . For the Horniman this is really dependent on our temporary exhibitions. For the Utsavam exhibition we are targeting lots of Indian communities. We also have an exhibition about Chinese textiles and we have a project worker for eight months to work with three different Chinese communities and develop an art installation that goes with the exhibition. So, you can see that it is collections and exhibitions driven, rather than saying we have got all these different people living around here.

Vicky Brightman and Andrew Willshire's comments reveal that Horniman community work is to a large extent driven by exhibitions and collections, something that raises questions about the depth, length, and sustainability of community involvement in museum work.

Curatorial and Community Knowledge

The community work of the museum is also strongly embedded in the exhibitions themselves. As the museum's director observed:

> We will take our collections into these communities or groups and they will use it in all sorts of ways. This will often lead to a creative output, textile, photographic, music, which we will then incorporate into our public displays. This brings a London contemporary output to our work. It is a win-win situation if you get it right . . . We have used this model with visual art extremely successfully in African Worlds, when we did a project with some groups. In general there is a pattern: objects, curatorial knowledge, and community involvement, but each project is very unique . . . What we have done more recently is trying to involve the curators. Previously the model would be that there would be education people, who have knowledge, but their knowledge is not as deep. The move is to put the curators more on the front line with these communities.

Both Hassan Arero and Margaret Birley have been involved in community work for the preparation of the exhibitions they curated. Explaining the importance of the Caribbean Identity Project that was planned together with the Amazon to Caribbean exhibition, Hassan Arero argued:

> We took some objects to communities and we asked them what they thought about them. People would bring back memories from their childhood, from living in the Caribbean. Such projects were particularly designed for working with communities, especially communities such as

the Caribbean that have been slightly isolated or put in the corner. Once we engaged with them, once they understood the idea, they took it up. It became their thing. And what we did is some of the objects they produced we put them in the main exhibition.

Community work seems to empower groups in terms of their participation in museum work, but it benefits the exhibitions, too. Discussing the partnership with a Somali community group in Croydon, to which the Horniman loaned some objects, Arero observed:

> The way they described and talked about the objects sounded very unscientific, but they knew what the objects were, what they were used for . . . The things that we look for as a museum are a bit different. It is mainly about presentation. For the community what was more important was getting the meanings out. So if we work together we can come up with a mythology that allows for both ideas to match.

Similarly, talking about the partnership with African curators for the interpretation of the Benin pieces in African Worlds, he noted:

> We took photographs of the Benin pieces to the communities and they rewrote history. The whole text was written by the originating community. It was their interpretation of history and who knows better than them? Most of the history of the Benin pieces was written by the conquerors, who wrote the story of masks and objects without involving the communities. But communities are the bearers of knowledge about these objects . . . Here we are assuming that we know everything, "a fetish, an African mask." But if you ask an African, he might say: "I don't want to look at it. It is a mask. It is a spirit." So you get into a very different interpretation of the same object. This is why working with communities enables a more profound understanding of objects.

As discussed earlier, however, community partnerships are fraught with power-related issues. In this regard, Janet Vitamayer observed:

> As a fieldwork museum, we have very particular types of knowledge. We have, for example, West Africa experts with fantastic fieldwork often commissioning collections. All that I think is very valid and absolutely necessary. I also think that the academic overview of someone like Hassan Arero who can look at a collection like the Wai Wai . . . and come up with a concept about Amerindian influences on the Caribbean is very important. Someone off the street could not come up with this concept. For me, those sorts of concepts are very important, because they revitalise and reinterpret your collections . . . What we have tended to do is always have a curatorial voice and be clear that we have one, but also use, if you like, individuals' experiences and voices . . . I think that the two can work very well together. I don't particularly like the one without the other . . . But focusing just on the perspective of communities would not stand well with the history of the museum and the way the collections have been built.

The combination of curatorial and academically grounded knowledge with personal interpretations by community members emerges as a key museological discourse of the Horniman, much in line with current trends of inclusion. There is little doubt, however, as to who is ultimately in charge of the exhibition content and narrative.

Community perspectives also inform the conservation and care of the collections. Louise Bacon extensively talked about how the museum is welcoming visitation groups, such as representatives of Native American, Australian Aboriginal, and Maori communities to inquire after collections. She also explained that the conservation team respects their opinions and traditions towards the collections. For example, she explained how certain objects cannot be X-rayed because of their spiritual dimensions, how using spit for cleaning objects is disliked by Maori groups and therefore not practiced on ritual objects, and how she had to ask people from the Indian temple if water and alcohol could be used for cleaning a sculpture of Nandi the Bull. She added:

> Conservators need to be really aware of ethical issues. It is a corporate responsibility. It is not only the director and the curator. There is no excuse for anyone working in museums for not knowing how to approach objects . . . I've been in conservation for many decades and there has always been much attention given to objects. Obviously in the last years what is different is the fact that we are actively consulting with groups and communities.

THE CENTRE AND THE PERIPHERY

For more than a hundred years the Horniman has been primarily concerned with the collection, display, and presentation of material culture to a predominantly white middle-class South London audience. Objects are the centrepiece of the museum, defining exhibitions, events, programmes, and even community work. Parallel to that, the curatorial and scientific voices have been central to its practice. Even in exhibitions that foreground community perspectives, like African Worlds, these have been largely filtered through the interpretative framework of the curator-anthropologist.

Against this backdrop, the multicultural and multiethnic makeup of London has invited the development of a more inclusive museology. Intangible heritage has thus been negotiated in terms of the narratives, opinions, memories, and interpretative frameworks of communities founded in traditional knowledge and inherited from specific cultural backgrounds. What emerges strongly, however, is that intangible heritage is mostly interpreted as something external to the museum's first port of call, which is the designated gift of Frederick J. Horniman and defines the museum's mission and fields of action. As such, community work, cultural performances, and events take place both in and out of the museum, but mostly in relation to the planned collections and exhibitions, revealing that the museum's work is still much defined by its founding bequest.

The final fieldwork chapter pursues the examination of intangible heritage in the musée du quai Branly in Paris. The MQB is a new museum that has tried to get rid of the label "ethnographic." As a consequence, and unlike the Horniman that is permeated by a strong anthropological discourse, it has been primarily concerned with the aesthetic presentation of "auratic" museum pieces, for which reason it has been significantly criticised. Tensions between anthropologists and aesthetes provide an interesting backdrop for reviewing the place of intangible heritage in French twenty-first century museology and in the local practice of a museum that aspires to refashion contemporary museum work.

Chapter 7

The Dialogue of Cultures, *Laïcité*, and Intangible Heritage at the quai Branly

> The musée du quai Branly is not in the business of representing cultures. This collection does not represent anything except itself.
>
> —Anne-Christine Taylor, MQB director for research (2005–present)

> It could be said that we tried to dissolve our colonial past in this aesthetic universalism.
>
> —Emmanuel Désveaux, professor of anthropology at the Ecole des Hautes Etudes en Sciences Sociales, MQB director for research (2001–2005)

Conceived and inaugurated by former French President Jacques Chirac and designed by Jean Nouvel, the musée du quai Branly is as much a scientific as a political project addressing not only issues of object display and conservation, but also matters of cultural representation and postcolonial relations (de l'Etoile 2007b; Dias 2007, 2008; Price 2007; Desvallées 2008). As demonstrated by the number of publications, reviews, papers, and books dedicated to its examination, the MQB is one of the controversial museums of our times (Clifford 2007; Price 2007, 2010; Vogel 2007; Shelton 2009). Against the diverse feelings its foundation has provoked, in this chapter I am interested in tracing how intangible heritage and the ensuing debates on representation, recognition, and people-oriented museum work that have been key themes of my research at Te Papa, the VCC, the NMAI, and the Horniman are interpreted in this new space.

In an effort to distance the MQB from the antiquated ethnographic displays of its institutional predecessor, the Musée de l'Homme,[1] it was decided by its founders that it would not just be a museum of anthropology, but an interdisciplinary institution concerned with the arts and cultures of Asia, Africa, Oceania, and the Americas.[2] While at first the anthropological and the aesthetic approaches seemed irreconcilable, recent research in the field of the anthropology of art (see Gell 1998) has largely bridged the gap between the two and is increasingly adopted as a key discourse of the MQB (see Derlon 2007).

A comment made by Oceania curator Philippe Peltier, noting that intangible heritage is "at the limits of the museum," hints at the scepticism with which French museology engages with the dichotomy between living and material culture. During fieldwork I discovered that intangible heritage is not as marginal as initially expected, but is often related to audiovisual programmes, multimedia installations, and live performances that take place year round in the museum. However, unlike Te Papa, the NMAI, and the VCC, where tangible and intangible were unified and interconnected, here strong dividing lines separate the material displayed in glass cases, usually under a spotlight and with very little information, and the intangible present in the theatre or digital screens. Moreover, largely missing are the voices of people connected to the collections, like collectors and source or diasporic communities.

The MQB is the newest of the five museums examined in this book. Its approach to world art and aesthetic universalism represents the political will to refashion the relationship of France with the non-European world through the celebration of world material culture. By mobilising state-of-the-art technology, cutting-edge architecture, and a versatile programme of exhibitions, programmes, events, and activities, the MQB is not just a museum of old things (Choay 2006; Martin 2007). As I will argue, however, it remains largely distant from calls for postcolonial, participatory museum work, with the museum priorities being primarily defined by the public discourse of *laïcité* and the work of world art experts, dealers, and curators.

FOUNDING IDEAS

The MQB exists today mainly on account of two reasons: a collection of about 300,000 artefacts from Asia, Africa, Oceania, and the Americas, and Jacques Chirac's interest in it. Developing at the interface of anthropology, art, and inter/national politics, it is an arena of sociopolitical contestation between politicians, art dealers, anthropologists, and international culture brokers, with the source communities only marginally involved. The foundation of the new museum has been traced to the friendship of Jacques Chirac and art dealer Jacques Kerchache (see Price 2007:1–3).[3] For many, it was this friendship that led not only to the foundation of the MQB and the Pavillon des Sessions,[4] but also to the reappraisal of non-European material culture in the Parisian museum and art gallery scenes (Amato 2006; Dupaigne 2006; de l'Etoile 2007a).

In 1990 Jacques Kerchache published in the French daily *Libération* an article entitled "Pour que les chefs-d'œuvre du monde entier naissent libres et égaux" (So that the masterpieces of the entire world are born free and equal). Arguing for the inclusion of non-Western artefacts in the Louvre, this article was signed by a number of French anthropologists, art historians, journalists, and other intellectuals. It stressed the need to acknowledge the aesthetic value of non-European objects, claiming that their presentation in the context of ethnographic displays greatly diminished their appreciation as works of art and cultivated a racist attitude towards non-Western cultures. On the contrary, he argued, their inclusion in the Louvre, the most celebrated art gallery and museum in the world, would place them on the same level of aesthetic importance as the masterpieces of European art. The aesthetic discourse obtains universal qualities by transcending differences in terms of the means, materials, tools, and techniques for creating art. It, nevertheless, remains largely Eurocentric, since judgements for the selection and display of artefacts are made based on Western criteria (see Morphy 1992), in the case of the MQB defined by French art dealers like Kerchache.

Reflecting on the place of non-European material culture in French museology, Nelia Dias has observed that almost every fifty years since the early 1800s, a new museum has been founded in Paris to replace an older one, often by putting forward a new understanding of the same collections in great contrast to the one supported by its predecessor (2007). In this context, the new museum clashes significantly with its ancestors, the Musée de l'Homme and the Musée des Arts d'Afrique et d'Océanie.[5] While arguably these two expressed mid-twentieth-century anthropological ideas of a hierarchical categorisation of cultures (Price 2007:33–41,101), the foundation of the MQB expresses a seemingly paradoxical relation between cultural diversity and "aesthetic universalism" (Désveaux 2002).

Introducing the rationale of the new museum, Jacques Chirac observed that "it repudiates the concept of artistic or racial hierarchy, and celebrates the universality of human genius in the dazzling range of cultural expression shown in its collections" (2006:6). The new museum's motto, *là où dialoguent les cultures* (where cultures dialogue), reveals respect for the ideals of cultural diversity and intercultural dialogue, in tune with France's postcolonial international relations agenda (see Somé 2003; de l'Etoile 2007a) and UNESCO's strategic aims. However, the expression of intercultural dialogue is not always clear in the practice of the MQB (see Price 2007:169–178). On the contrary, what often directs the permanent exhibition is the celebration of world art dictated by the exoticising Western gaze (see also Chrisafis 2006; Gibbons 2006; Kimmelman 2006; Shelton 2009).

Treating cultural objects as world art rather than sacred or spiritual artefacts can be related to the fact that the museum, as a French public institution, is a secular space. This is encapsulated in the idea of *laïcité*, the canon that French public institutions, including schools and museums, are non-religious (see also Dias 2008). As the principle of *laïcité* is race-blind, it is not possible for the museum to have special relationships with groups and communities that are ethnically defined. As a consequence the museum does not approach objects as invested with sacred meanings or spiritual dimensions but is rather more inclined to view them as "dead pieces" or decontextualised universal artworks.

Devoid of sacred or spiritual meanings the collections seem thus to have been related to a discourse of postcolonial recognition. For Jacques Chirac, the new museum

> stemmed from the political will to see justice rendered to non-European cultures . . . In bringing to an end a long history of neglect, arts and civilisations that have long been ignored or underrated are being given their rightful place, and dignity is being restored to peoples who were too often humiliated, oppressed or even destroyed by arrogance, ignorance, stupidity and blindness. [2006:6]

As opposed to the ethnographic specimens displayed in shabby cases in the Musée de l'Homme, the objects are showcased in the new museum and its Louvre outpost as works of art, and their mostly anonymous creators are admired as universal artists. Aesthetic universality, albeit highly Eurocentric, is remarkably in compliance with calls for North-South equality. What is not clear, however, in the intercultural politics of the MQB is the level of participation and involvement of these communities in museum work.

In 2004, while at UNESCO, I attended the preliminary intergovernmental committee meetings that discussed the adoption of a new Convention for the Protection of the Diversity of Cultural Expressions.[6] The latter and the 2001 Declaration on Protection of Cultural Diversity featured prominently among the priorities not only of UNESCO, but also of Jacques Chirac (de l'Etoile 2007a:309–314; Price 2007:40).[7] Largely influenced by Lévi-Strauss's *Race and History* (1952), both instruments acknowledge the delicate condition of ways of life and cultural and artistic expressions around the world, underlining "the value of otherness" (Chirac 2006:7), in tune with the preservationist scope of the global development of intangible heritage (see chapter 2).

Against the homogenising forces of globalisation, mainly expressed in the "Americanisation" of the world (Price 2007:40), the French-supported approach urges UNESCO states to become key defenders of cultural diversity and to encourage exchange and dialogue between cultures. Extending this to the new museum, Chirac notes:

> Bringing together different cultures and civilisations is therefore a national progression for a country that is fully aware of its responsibilities on global and historical levels to promote communication between peoples and cultures in order to counteract the unacceptable face of contempt, hostility and hatred that exists in the world . . . The MQB also sees its role, perhaps above all else, as championing this cause. [2006:7]

The MQB is thus conceptualised not only as a place for the presentation of universal artworks, but also as a space for expressing France's political views on the international cultural and diplomatic scenes. Through the rhetoric of world art, justice, and intercultural dialogue, the MQB emerges as a strong and ethically concerned player in the global museum scene.

A further interesting aspect of the MQB is the role of anthropologists in the articulation of its museological discourse. The efforts to distance the new museum from a purely anthropological approach regarding the appreciation and display of collections have been expressed in the adoption of a more aesthetic way for presenting and interpreting collections and in the separation of *art* and *knowledge*. The uneasiness that the anthropological community felt towards the new museum was expressed in the heated debates surrounding the closure of the ethnographic section of the Musée de l'Homme (see Amato 2006; Dupaigne 2006), and compounded by the fact that since the museum's inception the post of director for research and learning has been occupied already by three anthropologists: professors Maurice Godelier and Emmanuel Désveaux, followed by Anne-Christine Taylor. This has raised several questions around the collaboration of anthropologists and the administration of the museum (see Price 2007:48–53).

The rest of the chapter examines how the separation between art and knowledge provides a context for thinking about the relationship between the tangible and the intangible. Although not "at the limits of the museum," intangible heritage seems to be somewhere between the museum's colonial origins and its postcolonial rhetoric.

THE MUSEOLOGY OF THE QUAI BRANLY

I arrived for the first time at the museum in July 2006, a few weeks after its grand inauguration. Earlier in June, a series of meetings had taken place, where academics, intellectuals, and museum professionals from around the world—including Te Papa's late Chief Executive Seddon

Bennington, VCC Director Ralph Regenvanu, Pitt Rivers Museum Director Michael O'Hanlon, and Professors James Clifford and Maurice Godelier—discussed key issues defining the scope and practice of the new museum. The minutes of these meetings reveal the breadth and complexity of the interests of the museum, covering among others issues of ownership, citizenship, international cooperation, intangible heritage, and authenticity (Latour 2007).

As hinted by its name, which defines its geographical location rather than its subject matter, the new museum stands on the quai Branly on Seine's left bank in the seventh arrondissement of Paris. Reaching the building from the right bank of the Seine and the Debilly footbridge, the museum is hardly visible behind the tall trees. From a distance what dominates the view is the Eiffel Tower. Coming closer to the site, two architectural features appear: the Glass Wall and the Green Wall. The former acts as a transparent barrier between the busy quai Branly road and the museum's world garden. Magnified pictures of objects, exhibition posters, and programme announcements are attached to it. To its right the Green Wall, which has also been described as a "vertical garden" (Blanc 2006:106–107), adorns the façade of the administration building to the north (Figure 7.1). In subsequent visits to the MQB I discovered that entire walls in the building's interior are also covered in plants. Interestingly, the interaction of nature and culture hints that, unlike modern Europeans, people whose material culture is presented in the museum live in harmony with the environment (see Latour 2007:97–100).

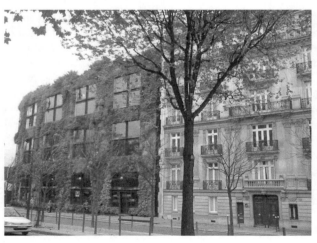

Figure 7.1: View of the Green Wall that covers the administration building of the musée du quai Branly. (All images in this chapter published with permission of the MQB.)

The nature and culture theme is strongly present throughout the museum, with several design and architectural references to the natural environment. Apart from the Green Wall, the MQB boasts a large garden above which the publicly accessible part of the museum, including the permanent exhibition, is suspended. The garden space features a variety of plants from the four non-European continents. According to its inceptor, its aim was to "break away from the European tradition dominated by order and symmetry" (Clément 2006:102). As such, the garden features meandering paths unfolding around trees, plants, and bushes, creating turtle-like shapes. In explaining the use of the turtle motif, Clément argues that it is a "mythical animal occupying a special place in the animist and polytheist cosmogonies, objects from which the museum welcomes" (2006:102). Elements from Native beliefs are borrowed to create a postmodern collage of the non-European in twenty-first century Paris.

Crossing the garden, visitors are invited to enter the main museum space, opposite of which is the entrance to the administration building and the museum store. These spaces have been decorated with ceiling and wall paintings made by eight Australian Aboriginal artists (Figure 7.2). As Philippe Peltier, Oceania curator and partly in charge of the project,

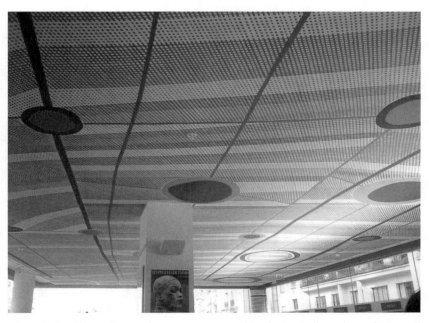

Figure 7.2: The ceilings of several spaces within the MQB have been decorated by eight Australian Aboriginal artists.

commented, "the MQB ceiling paintings should be considered like an embassy that demonstrates that Aboriginal society is alive and flourishing and showcases the great spiritual heritage of Aboriginal people," adding that the eight artists "have demonstrated their powers of survival and invention and their ability to express ancestral stories in a surprising and modern pictorial language" (2002).

Although the intervention of the eight artists has been heralded as a "bridge" in the diplomatic relations between the museum and Australian Aboriginal communities, little information is provided about their meanings. As a consequence, they are usually interpreted as decorative motifs rather than as interventions of strong sociopolitical commentary (Price 2007:132–139). Once more, non-Western traditions and beliefs, this time of Australian Aboriginals, have been inserted into a decorative narrative of intercultural dialogue with little effort to understand them.

Suspended on several pillars above the garden and partly surrounded by the administration and multimedia buildings lies the elongated main museum space. On the side facing the quai Branly protruding boxes of different sizes, dimensions, and colours hang from the building (Figure 7.3). These serve as private and secluded galleries in the interior

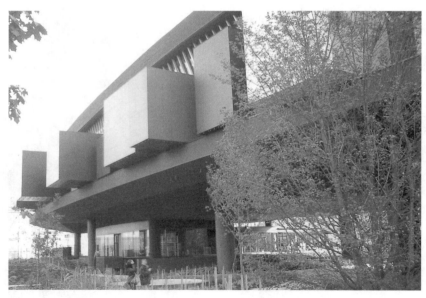

Figure 7.3: Twenty-seven boxes of different colours and sizes are attached to the north side of the MQB, creating secluded spaces for the display of important material.

of the building to display small artefacts, objects of important spiritual significance, and photographs. The south side of the building is covered with dark red moving panels that allow for the entrance of the sunrays into the permanent exhibition space. The architect has paid special attention to filtering the sunlight in the permanent exhibition. Apart from the panels on the south side, transparent images of tropical forests have been attached to the north side glass surfaces to create a naturally filtered "cave-like" environment (Nouvel 2006).[8] Under the dark red surfaces, a white curved construction with forward tilted white panels connects the north and south sides of the main museum building, delineating the exterior of the Garden Gallery. This design has been inspired by the movement of the "dress of a whirling dervish" (Lavalou and Robert 2006:77), another manifestation of the architectural intercultural inspiration.

In one of the folds of the dervish skirt lies the main museum entrance. Entering the building, the lobby is a white open area that provides access to the exhibition spaces, the auditorium, cinema, and education rooms in the lower ground floor, the *médiathèque* (multimedia library), and the library and reading room in the adjacent building. The lobby is minimalist in terms of design and features a few large artefacts, like a Haida totem pole from British Columbia, a *moai* statue from Rapa Nui (Easter Island), and the Music Tower, the MQB's visible storeroom containing the entire musical instruments collection.

This tower traverses vertically the different levels of the building, from the basement to the top of the permanent exhibitions. As Madeleine Leclair, musical instruments curator, explained, even before the announcement of the architectural competition, it was decided by the museum team that "visible stores" should be included in the museum so that visitors could get a glimpse of what museum stores look like and what is happening behind the scenes. However, the presentation of musical instruments in a visible store, with no explanation, sombre lighting, and poor visibility raises significant concerns about whether this is a successful way of displaying music. In order to bring these to life, stylised video projections of instruments are presented in small screens at the lower parts of the music tower. Moreover, a cutting-edge audio system acting as an "aural perfume" operates through vibrations of the glass tower, permitting the diffusion of musical extracts. New technologies are mobilised here to convey subtly the performative dimensions of the instruments.

On the same level as the lobby stands the circular Garden Gallery. This is a space dedicated to temporary displays showcasing artefacts from the MQB collections or travelling exhibitions. Also, from the lobby one can access the Jacques Kerchache Reading Room, named after the controversial friend of Jacques Chirac. This contains recent journals and books on the collections and is also used for temporary exhibitions and educational activities. Lifts connect this space with the multimedia library, the museum's photographic and video archive, and the library on the upper floors of the building. In contrast to the white lobby and bright study areas, the lower ground floor is particularly dark, with black and red walls and dim lighting. It is occupied by the Claude Lévi-Strauss Theatre, where several discussions, performances, and concerts take place, and by other smaller meeting and activity rooms as well as the museum's cinema. The exhibition and performance areas are clearly defined, demarcated, and separated.

A wide ascending and winding pathway unfolding along the Music Tower connects the lobby with the Plateau des Collections, the museum's permanent exhibition. This suspends above the Garden Gallery and is used to present video installations. During the first years of the museum's opening, images and short video clips of people from the four continents were projected on its white surfaces (Figure 7.4), along with images of their natural environments, such as snow covered mountain tops, tropical forests, and endless seascapes, stressing once more the bonds between nature and Native cultures. Moreover, words in different languages welcoming visitors are projected on the floor of the white ramp, hinting at

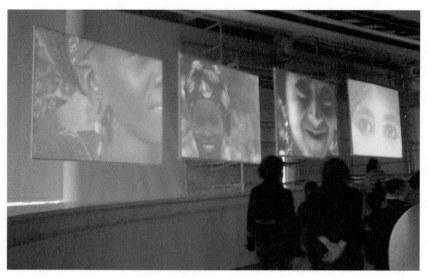

Figure 7.4: A series of audiovisual installations with images of people and landscapes from around the world decorated the ascending pathway leading to the Plateau des Collections.

the idea of intercultural dialogue. At the end of this cultural and natural diversity white path, a dark tunnel prepares visitors to enter into the main exhibition space, the Plateau des Collections.

The Plateau des Collections

The Plateau is the centrepiece of the MQB, the museum's permanent exhibition of mostly nineteenth- and early twentieth-century artefacts from Asia, Africa, Oceania, and the Americas. Built in the spirit of French museum *grandes galleries*, it is an elongated space with few partitions dedicated to the display of artefacts from the different continents. For Germain Viatte, in charge of the museology of the Plateau, "the first concern of the museum was to free the collections from our categories and labels and to place them in a situation where they could be considered as works on their own, not dependant on a discipline" (Viatte 2006b:29). Ethnographic contextualisation, like the one practiced at the Musée de l'Homme and most ethnographic museums, was regarded not only as outdated, but also as simplistic and no longer relevant to people living in highly interconnected and globalised worlds (Peltier 2000).

In explaining his vision for the Plateau, the museum's architect observed: "It was as important to me to give these works of art a real place of dwelling as it was to display them. It was thus with the hopes of dissociating the information about the objects from the objects themselves that I created the *grande gallerie*. I wanted each artefact to keep its power and its mystery" (Roulet 2006:62). Similarly, commenting on the appearance of the exhibition, Viatte referred to the architectural vision to create "an impressive landscape full of mystery and surprises" (2006b:28).

As opposed to the minimalist art gallery display of its Louvre outpost (Figure 7.5), with the bright open spaces and the well-calculated showcasing of selected pieces overseen by Jacques Kerchache, on the sunny summer morning of my first visit the Plateau seemed to me dark and chaotic (though in subsequent visits the lighting of the exhibition was much brighter). The dim lighting and the sunrays filtered through the transparent forest glass, along with the sounds of chants, music, and nature create an immersive scenography of "mystery and surprises," hinting at images from Joseph Conrad's *Heart of Darkness* and inadvertently reinforcing the colonial stereotypes that the museum purports to fight (Kimmelman 2006; Price 2007).

The exhibition has been conceptualised as a journey through the four continents starting with Oceania, moving on to Asia and Africa, and ending with the Americas. The four continents are traversed by an elongated space, the River, focusing on common intercontinental themes

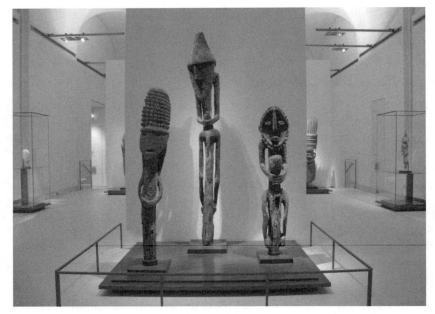

Figure 7.5: The Pavillon des Sessions, the outpost of the MQB in the Louvre, is characterised by the clinical display of objects against a white background and the lack of contextual information.

such as dwellings and the natural environment. Rather than linking the four continents, the River with its thick and high leather walls seems to cut through the permanent exhibition, a metaphor for the European force that brought most of the collections to Paris.

In the displays, contextual information is discreet and minimal. Artefacts are usually dramatically displayed in glass cases against a dark background and under spotlights, with the exception of larger objects, like the slit drums from Vanuatu, which stand on pedestals (Figure 7.6). Smaller labels discreetly placed at the far end of the cases or at the bottom of sculptures usually indicate place of origin, material, size, and previous owner or donor. Larger labels introduce geographical regions and provide basic information in French, English, and Spanish.

Oceania

In my discussions with the curators and museum professionals at the MQB, intangible heritage was often related to the performances and ceremonies projected in the multimedia stations and audiovisual programmes throughout the Plateau. Small screens with extracts from anthropological films and documentaries stand in proximity to the cases.

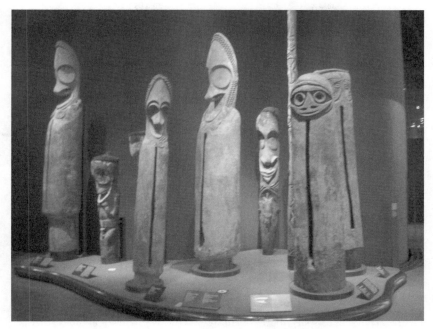

Figure 7.6: Slit drums from Vanuatu are dramatically displayed with little information about their use, significance, and history.

For example, not far from a case containing Melanesian war clubs, extracts from a documentary about warfare in Papua New Guinea are presented; near a case with moulded skulls from Melanesia, a short documentary shows how such skulls were made by moulding resin onto the skeletal remains and then painting or decorating them with seashells. The video extracts affirm human presence, hinting that most of the objects that are now dramatically displayed were part of broad and complex cultural traditions and ritual ceremonies. Interestingly, much like the idea of pure, authentic, and preindustrial objects, the films portrayed pure, authentic, and uncontaminated traditions unaffected by Western culture.

Nineteenth- and early twentieth-century artefacts from Polynesia follow the rich Melanesian collections. These include Maori woodcarvings, *hei tikis* (pendants in the form of human fetuses), Hawaiian feathered helmets and feathered gods, and distinctive fans and clubs from the Marquesas. The mode of presentation emphasises quite distinctively the formal elements of the artefacts through an almost theatrical display of dark background and spot-lit objects (Figure 7.7). As such, someone who had no experience of such objects would find hard to understand

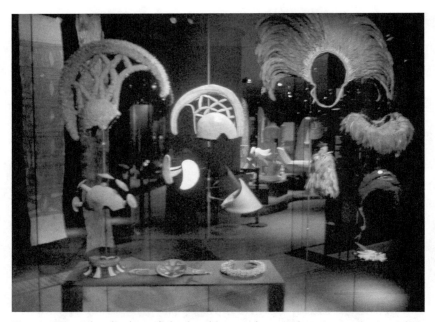

Figure 7.7: The display of the headdresses from Polynesia emphasises their aesthetic dimensions.

what they are, how they were used, and the processes through which they are now displayed in Paris. Unlike Te Papa, *iwi* voices are absent and no reference is made to ideas of traditional knowledge, such as *wairua* or *mana*. Maori *taonga* are thus largely divested from their spirituality and instead incorporated in the wider aesthetic narrative of the permanent exhibition. There are not many flows and connections in the Oceania cases, and objects are primarily organised geographically (Melanesia, Polynesia) and typologically (moulded skulls, weapons, masks).

The final section of the Oceania exhibit, behind the Music Tower, is Australia. Kupka's 1963 collection of Australian Aboriginal paintings on eucalyptus bark is displayed in a secluded, dark area, again with little information about their role and biography. Next to them are some of the few contemporary pieces displayed in the permanent exhibition. These are mid- and late-twentieth-century Aboriginal acrylic paintings on canvases, widely acknowledged nowadays as contemporary works of art (see Myers 2002).

Connecting Oceania and Asia is the gallery space covering the geographical areas of Indonesia, Eastern Malaysia, and the Philippines and presenting funerary sculptures, ceremonial objects, and golden jewellery. A treasure of golden ornaments gleaming against the black backdrop of the cases occupies a prominent place in this display. Also connecting the two areas is a *boite à musique* (music box), one of the twenty-seven boxes on the building's north side. This is a large dark room with film footage projections on the three walls and sound recordings of different chants, songs, and performances. The music boxes are one of the ways in which the MQB curates the intangible through the creation of immersive and multisensory environments.

Asia

While Viatte and Nouvel supervised the overall museological concept, a different team depending on the geographical specialisation of the curators was in charge of the display cases for each continent. Former Musée de l'Homme anthropologist Christine Hemmet curated the Asian section. Her approach to the presentation of the hugely diverse arts and cultures of Asia was quite different from the one adopted in the Oceania exhibit: as she noted in our discussion, "You won't see any pierced noses or naked bottoms in my section."

With the large collection of monumental sculptures from South-East and Central Asia and China at the Musée Guimet, the Asian artefacts presented in the MQB are largely objects of daily and rural life usually made of perishable organic materials, like Japanese prints on bark paper, one bamboo Vietnamese scarecrow, and animal skins or costumes made of silk and cotton. For Christine Hemmet, intangible heritage needs to be conceptualised in terms of perishable artefacts that are the outcome of living traditions, and not only in terms of performing arts. Therefore, she has tried to show the evolution of traditional practices by focusing on the people behind the objects. For example in the display of Vietnamese jackets, by presenting four different jackets made by women of four different generations in 1975, 1985, 1994, and 2004, she has tried to show the development of the practice and the incorporation of new patterns, colours, and materials, hinting thus that weaving traditions are not static but constantly reinterpreted by living communities.

Further down the exhibition, Asian spirituality (mainly, Buddhism) is addressed in one of the secluded boxes, with the stylised presentation of small statues of Buddha and ritual paintings. These boxes create confined spaces for the display of sacred objects. However, the MQB is a secular space, which often creates tensions between sacred and secular understandings of material culture. This museological secularism is often seen as a factor divesting objects of their more profound social and cultural meanings.

The Asia section is the smallest of the four, mainly because of the relatively recent and small number of collections. Again, the displays follow the conventional geographical and typological path with little textual interpretation. The final part is devoted to the presentation of objects from the Middle East, which acts as a bridge between Asia and Africa. These include headdresses and costumes from Turkey and Palestine as well as sacred objects like Judaic amulets and objects from the Islamic world, such as a bowl engraved with verses from the Koran.

Africa

Objects from the Islamic world feature prominently in the African section, reflecting the complex relationships between France and North Africa. Reference is made to Islam through the presentation of the art of writing. Pages from the Koran are displayed in a secluded space decorated in the Islamic tradition and immersed in a religious atmosphere. Not far from that, costumes and objects from the nomadic people of Sahara, like the Tuareg, allude to the mobility and exchange between cultural groups and traditions. The African section features mostly artefacts from Central and Western Africa like masks, ceremonial objects, and sculptures—Fang, Dogon, Yoruba, Bedu, Senufo, and Baoule masks, Benin brasses, Nok terracotta,[9] and Kota figures. Once again, these objects are displayed in cases that follow a conventional geographical classification with very little information about the ceremonies in which they were used, the practitioners, how they got to be in Paris, or any claims for their restitution.

As an exception to the above, the video about the Dogon masks in performance recorded in the 1930s during the mission Dakar-Djibouti, also presented at the Horniman, is an interesting intervention because it is one of the rare occasions in which artefacts are linked to people. Another such occasion is the multimedia installation about the Sandogi divination by the Senufo in Cote D'Ivoire. This occupies one of the smallest protruding boxes on the building's north side, next to a case containing several divination statues. It forms a small cave with video projections of divination ceremonies on the three sides and the floor. Subtitles in French explain the dialogues between the diviner and the persons who solicited his help.

African masks and statues are presented in a very long and narrow section of the museum, which in days of large attendance makes it hard to get a good look of the objects without being squashed or pushed around.[10] Moreover, cases are placed in proximity to one another and it is not uncommon to bump into them.[11] This, along with the dark surroundings and the filtered sunlight coming through the images of the tropical forests on the windows, creates an atmosphere that impedes the contemplation of both objects and information.

On the contrary, the secluded boxes containing religious objects are easier to access. For example, a gallery displays the canvases removed from the Coptic Christian Church of Abba Antonios in Ethiopia by the

Dakar-Djibouti Mission in 1931. The canvases, which represent stories from the Orthodox religion, have been mounted on the three walls of the box, creating the feeling of being in a church. Just like the display of the Buddhist statues and Islamic material, sacred objects are displayed as artworks in a quasi-religious atmosphere. This, however, serves design and architectural purposes rather than their sacred nature. Again, there is no narrative of how Orthodoxy was reinterpreted in Ethiopia; moreover, the ethical aspects of the Dakar-Djibouti collecting practices have not been adequately addressed (see Clifford 2007; Price 2007).

Next to the secluded area containing the Coptic paintings, the second music box of the permanent exhibition presents video extracts from ritual dances and performances from India and other South Asian regions. The proximity of the music box and the Coptic paintings gallery-box means that music from the one can be heard in the other, creating an atmosphere that transcends geographic and cultural borders.

Americas

Such borders are also transcended in the section dealing with the impact of African heritage on the Americas, especially the Caribbean, Brazil, and Southeast USA. Like the altars in African Worlds at the Horniman, ritual objects—such as magical bundles decorated with Christian crosses that are used in Vodou ceremonies in Haiti and statues of Candomblé effigies from Brazil—underline the impact of the transatlantic slave trade on the culture of the Americas and also the adaptability and development of cultural practices and religions. More information on the slave trade and the cultural flows it initiated would provide a deeper context for looking at and understanding these complex objects.

This section is rather abruptly followed by the display of North American collections, comprised among others of Inuit artefacts, including Yup'ik and Alutiiq wooden masks and walrus ivory utilitarian objects, which in turn are followed by a totem pole, masks, and ritual objects from the Northwest Coast tribes Haida, Tlingit, and Tsimshian. Other nineteenth-century ethnographic collections are coats, capes, and dresses made from dear or porcupine skins by Indians from the Great Plains and different elaborate feathered headdresses, pectorals, and body ornaments from the Amazon. Much like the Oceania and Africa sections, artefacts are once more presented in dramatically lit cases with little or no contextual information.

Unlike the tribal exhibits of the NMAI, it is not tribal people who interpret the objects on display, and most labels are signed by Emmanuel Désveaux, professor of anthropology and former MQB director for research. The exhibition narrative is informed by the idea of transformation. Drawing on Lévi-Strauss's understanding of the unity of Amerindian beliefs, as expressed for example in the different versions of the myth of the crow, Désveaux claims that "the principle of transformation can also be applied to objects" (2006:238). As a consequence, in one of the audiovisual stations a video is projected in which animal- or human-shaped containers from throughout the continent are transformed into different objects, like food storage jars, plates, or spoons.

Another interesting video is the recitation of Native American myths in Native language presented in a small screen not far from the displays of North American material culture. It is one of the few cases that present the actual people and traditions connected with the artefacts. Interestingly and much like the video with the New Guinean warriors, however, Native American traditions emerge as pure and uncontaminated from the influences of Western development. The communities that are represented are placed in an atemporal preindustrial space rather than in the same globalised and interconnected world as the viewers.

Following the geographical classification of nineteenth- and twentieth-century ethnographic collections from North and South America is the final part of the Americas section, which showcases pre-Columbian artefacts from the Andes and Central America. Pre-contact Andean objects from Peru, Bolivia, and Ecuador, like Inca deity statuettes, urns, and goblets are among the objects on display. Finally, the exhibition ends with an array of Mesoamerican artefacts, including terracotta sculptures from Costa Rica, polychrome ceramics from Panama, Maya stone statues, artefacts from Teotihuacan, and Aztec deities. The displays employ the black background and spotlight effect emphasising the formal and aesthetic dimensions of the objects; again, little reference is made to the post-contact cultural transformations of Native American cultures.

The River

The River is a long and narrow path traversing the four continental areas and demarcated by thick walls covered in light brown leather. On one side, it presents key French explorers and anthropologists, like Louis-Antoine de Bougainville (1729–1811), Michel Leiris (1901–1990), Marcel Griaule (1898–1956), and their collecting missions. One of the most interesting parts of the River is a deformed map of the world showing the size of countries (usually colonial territories) in proportion to the objects in the MQB collections. This map is a rare reflexive instance of the permanent collection as a colonial product.

On the other side, it offers comparative glimpses of how world cultures respond to living habitats and interact with nature. Being planned for people with disabilities, the light brown leather walls of the river present information in Braille. On the backsides of the wall, bordering the permanent displays, benches and multimedia stations allow visitors to sit and learn more about the collections. This is part of the broader idea of separating art and knowledge that permeates the museology of the MQB.

From the above it becomes apparent that the permanent exhibition is primarily about the aesthetic display of the 3,500 artefacts with selected contextual information in the dispersed multimedia stations, labels, and panels. The aim has been to create a "visual hook", to "shock" and "excite" (Viatte 2006c) viewers through the dramatic display of artefacts, compelling them to seek more information in the multimedia stations. Interestingly, and in contrast with the general tone of the exhibition, one of the labels in the America section about Arctic people reads: "The Yup'ik and Alutiiq who inhabit the milder Bering Sea regions also belong to the Aleut Eskimo linguistic group, with highly inventive and spectacular rituals. Today, these people lay claim to a common identity and culture. In 1999 mobilisation on their part led specifically to the establishment of the autonomous region of Nunavut." Such comments about the historical and social struggles of the people related to collections are scarce in the permanent exhibition. Had they been more, they would have invited new readings of the collections beyond a purely aesthetic contemplation.

Multimedia Gallery

A key aspect of the permanent exhibitions is the separation of the *visual pleasure* of viewing the objects from the *knowledge* surrounding them. For this reason, it was predicted by the architect and planning committee that special areas would suspend above the Plateau and provide temporary exhibition spaces and a Multimedia Gallery for the presentation of additional information about the collections and the societies from which they originated.

The Multimedia Gallery is above the Africa section and comprises several small and larger screen stations with different types of recordings, like short musical extracts or performances, ethnographic film documentaries, and historic photographs. Unlike the small video screens next to the display cases showing programmes that last for only a few minutes, or the slightly larger screens attached to the River that visitors can consult for longer time sitting on benches, the Multimedia Gallery allows for a more concentrated understanding of the rich photographic and audiovisual material on offer. Among the issues that can be consulted through a combination of text, image, video, and sound are exchange and funerary rituals in Oceania, ritual cannibalism and headhunting in the Americas, knowledge and use of textiles in Asia, and masks in Africa.

The MQB possesses vast resources on traditional practices and ceremonies from the four continental areas. These present important information about the communities that created the artefacts on display and provide a space for the presentation of different expressions of intangible heritage. Interestingly, however, there are no connections to the material culture displayed underneath. Moreover, Asian, African, Oceanic, and Native American cultures are usually presented as the object of ethnographic research, rather than an expression of empowered agents in making self-representations. As such, the Plateau reinforces a Western way of researching other cultures, which emerge primarily as rural, underdeveloped, and outside the context of Western modernity.

Temporary Exhibitions

Surrounding the Multimedia Gallery from the west and the east are two additional suspending galleries for temporary exhibitions that overall engage more critically with the key themes of the museum. The Suspending West Gallery presents anthropological exhibitions lasting eighteen months and broadly offering comparative approaches to universal human themes. The first such exhibition was entitled Qu'est-ce qu'un corps? (What is a body?), and was presented from June 2006 until September 2007. The exhibition brought together artefacts from Central Africa, Papua New Guinea, Amazonia, and Western Europe in order to present multiple understandings and approaches to the representation of the body. This was followed by the exhibition Planète Métisse (Hybrid Planet) that dealt with issues of colonisation, globalisation, and hybridity. By presenting traditional ethnographic artefacts along with contemporary artworks, like films by Korean director Wong Kar Wai, Planète Métisse addressed more complex issues and clashed with the permanent exhibition below that favoured the "purity" of the artefacts.

The East Suspending Gallery presents a wide range of short-term exhibitions, each one lasting about three months. Several exhibitions have been presented in this gallery, mainly based on objects and documentary material from the MQB collections. For example, the work in Vietnam of French anthropologist Georges Condominas was presented, along with an exhibition about Ciwara, animal-like masks from West Africa. These were followed by an exhibition of the nineteenth-century photographic material taken by Désiré Charnay in Mexico, Madagascar, and Australia, and by an exhibition about the First Nations Royal Collections (mainly from the tribes Naskapi, Micmac, Huron, Mohawk, and Ojibway), brought in France from Canada by seventeenth- and eighteenth-century explorers. Among the other exhibitions presented here there were one about *ideqqui* (the Berber female practice of pottery making), another about traditional object conservation and healing methods in Africa, and even an exhibition with the provocative title the

Aristocrat and his Savages about the voyages of Count Festetics de Tolna (1865–1943) in the Pacific.

In addition to the above, a significant amount of temporary exhibitions takes place in the Garden Gallery on the MQB ground floor. These range from traditional museum exhibitions to contemporary art and new media installations. D'un Regard l'Autre: Histoires des regards européens sur l'Afrique, l'Amérique et l'Océanie (Visions of the Other: A history of European conceptions of Africa, America, and Oceania) offered a historical account of European appropriations of the non-West, starting with the cabinets of curiosities and the evolutionist museum and ending with the late twentieth-century inclusion of non-Western objects in European aesthetic canons.[12] This was a provocative exhibition examining European views on "the other." Another exhibition organised by the Ethnographic Museum of Vienna about brass and ivory artefacts from Benin was presented in conjunction with the exhibition Diaspora. There was an interesting dialogue developing between the two, as the latter dealt with the issue of African artists living away from their homelands and creating contemporary video, sound, and image installations, all presented in a dark area with individual tents and cubicles. The fact that there were no walls separating the two exhibitions but only a curtain facilitated the movement between the two spaces. The juxtaposition of the sixteenth-century artefacts from Benin with contemporary artworks alluded to an African continent with a rich past and creative future.

During the Rugby World Cup season in the autumn of 2007 a magnified portrait of the All Blacks[13] dominated a central part of the main hall. In addition, the museum's terrace had been converted into a mini rugby field that was named *la melée des cultures* (the scramble of cultures). Greg Semu, a contemporary artist of Samoan and Maori origins, had been invited within the context of the Rugby World Cup season events to work in the museum and create a new piece for its collections, displayed next to the All Blacks portrait. As MQB Director Stéphane Martin argued, such events brought into the museum people who do not typically visit museums of art and culture.

DEBATING INTANGIBLE HERITAGE IN PARIS

Through its permanent and temporary exhibitions the museum encourages a multiplicity of interpretative approaches to collections and addresses wider issues surrounding its thematic areas. The temporary exhibitions transcend and mix the boundaries of art, anthropology, social criticism, and history. This enables dynamic and multiple expressions of different perspectives—by academics, but also contemporary artists—and liberates the museological narrative from the often authoritative curatorial and scholarly voice. Less conventional approaches challenging traditional museum practice encourage alternative perspectives often in great opposition to the aesthetic discourse of the Plateau. What is still absent, however, from the MQB narrative is the active inclusion and participation of the originating communities, which would in effect be more relevant to the museum's motto of intercultural dialogue. My interviews with MQB former and current staff revealed why such partnerships have been resisted, but also critically rethought.

Art, Anthropology, and the Plurality of Discourses

Maurice Godelier is a prominent professor of anthropology teaching at the École des Hautes Etudes en Sciences Sociales in Paris. From 1999 until 2001 he served as director for research and learning at the MQB. During this period he was also partly involved in the planning of the permanent exhibition. Meeting him in his office at the EHESS, I was interested in finding out his opinion on the MQB project and further explore the objections that led to his resignation and the intensification of the art/science debate (Amato 2006; Dupaigne 2006). As he acknowledged, the MQB and the Pavillon des Sessions in the Louvre stemmed from the political will "to show, something which is right, that African or Oceanic artworks are as universal as the Venus of Milo," further underlining the museum's wish "to turn over to a certain extent the page of colonialism" as manifested in "Chirac's postcolonial inauguration speech." However, he also admitted that "the MQB was created in conflict. I gave an advice. Then, I was warded off because I demanded the union of the two dimensions, art and knowledge. But the people in charge preferred art and very little knowledge. The aesthetic tendency won."

Maurice Godelier's comments hint at a broader conflict faced by ethnographic museums today regarding the display of objects collected through colonial processes and interpreted and reinterpreted in different contexts and periods (de l'Etoile 2007a).[14] This conflict is something that the current administration of the museum tries to reconcile, as the museum's director, Stéphane Martin, explained. Unlike Maurice Godelier, Stéphane Martin is not an anthropologist, but rather a cultural manager who previously worked in the Ministry of Culture and headed the Centre Pompidou. Maybe for this reason, he quite openly acknowledged in an interview that "this museum accepts its holes and gaps and presents itself more as the museum of an ethnographic collection, rather than an ethnographic museum."

For him, this has meant that, unlike most ethnographic museums, the MQB has adopted "a non-dogmatic museology," being more of "a scene where dialogues and actors of different origins meet . . . We tried to reconcile the aesthetic approach that strangely scares anthropologists—a reaction that I find childish and naïve—with the scientific content, but with a humility towards this content and trying to avoid a dogmatic scientific discourse of the kind 'this is what you should know about these people.'" As a consequence, his aim is for the MQB not to be a "museum of anthropology," but a more inclusive cultural and intellectual scene addressing contemporary concerns, such as environmental issues and globalisation: "I see, for example, young people visiting the Amazon section with the problems of pollution and deforestation on their mind rather than Lévi-Strauss's work on parental systems."

The issue of the museological discourse of the MQB was raised in most discussions with museum staff. For Anne-Christine Taylor, "the MQB is not in the business of representing cultures. This collection does not represent anything except itself." In our discussion she acknowledged that traditional ethnographic museology, or "the idea that in a sense you could condense the essence of a culture and then represent it by exhibiting a certain number of artefacts," is parochial and against the wishes of the museum. Instead, she explained: "We choose visually spectacular objects and we use them as a sort of hook to capture people's attention and get them to engage with the idea of cultural diversity. We do not represent cultures, but we use these objects to introduce people to different ways for composing the world." For her, the MQB could be "a very good museum of the anthropology of art," with respect to addressing the issues of "artistic intention and symbolic meaning," adding that nowadays "this is a particularly vibrant domain of anthropology, so we kill two birds with one stone."

Both Stéphane Martin and Anne-Christine Taylor argued in favour of a "plurality of discourses" on the collections; indeed, most temporary exhibitions are planned by researchers on contracts and not by permanent museum staff, which explains the diversity of approaches and the frequency with which one temporary exhibition follows the other. Moreover, exhibitions are also accompanied by conferences, talks, discussions, and even the museum's open university, headed by philosopher Catherine Clément, which invites speakers to address topics such as the history of colonisation and universal human rights. A common theme often transcending these discourses and museological approaches is the acknowledgement of the aesthetic dimensions of material culture and their ability to overcome social and cultural barriers.

The power of artworks to convey universal meanings and the museum's role in facilitating this was also conveyed by Emmanuel Désveaux. He served as director for education and research from 2001 to 2005. For him the museum, via the display of spectacular objects, ultimately celebrates that "throughout space and time people have wanted to go beyond the banality of everyday life." As he acknowledged with reference to the colonial roots of French anthropology and ethnographic museums, however, "it could be said that we try to dissolve our colonial past in this aesthetic universalism . . . In a way by saying that this is art, we keep everyone satisfied."

The importance for the MQB of the universal artistic value of artefacts was effectively summarised by Philippe Peltier, curator of the Oceania section. For him, "a museum is about seeing; it is about memorising a number of objects, comparing, and finding out how they were made. It is an exploration of the eye; for me, it is a culture of the object."

Debating Materiality

Christine Hemmet, Asia curator at the MQB, has significantly tried to stretch the limits imposed on the museum's practice by this focus on the physical and aesthetic dimensions of material culture and to show "the people behind the objects." As she explained, "a priori, intangible is all that is perishable. So, it is not only performing arts . . . As far as perishable objects are concerned, the knowledge that comes with them is also perishable and this is something very relevant for museums today." Unlike the other sections of the permanent exhibition presenting monumental objects, Christine Hemmet worked with small and fragile artefacts, like costumes, rugs, wood, and bamboo, and included in the exhibitions images of people wearing and using these objects, referring to them not only as artworks, but also as parts of people's lives.

Hélène Joubert, MQB curator of Africa, seemed to be particularly attuned to the same concerns, although she was not directly in charge of the display of the artefacts in her section.[15] In our discussion, she expressed the wish to see the MQB becoming "a *lieu de mémoire* of this contemporary reality of multifaceted cultures that are neither monocultural nor monoethic. Especially in towns like Paris or London that are really multicultural we need to show this story that was not written, that was oral, but effectively left its traces in collections of objects, in poems, in myths, and in stories." This, she added, would "bring us, French, closer to Africa, a continent that we can barely draw and whose countries we can barely find on the map." For her, as for nearly all of the people that I interviewed, the permanent exhibition wants to excite peoples' curiosity about other cultures: "When people arrive at the museum, they get a shock. They are impressed and overtaken by the objects. The objects are beautiful and well placed . . . But then people start to ask, 'What exactly is this? What is its use? Where does it come from?' and then, they are directed to the multimedia." The use of multimedia applications on three different levels in the permanent exhibition has been translated as a way for conveying the intangible heritage surrounding the collections (see Bezombes 2006 for a full account of the MQB multimedia and intangible heritage). For Emmanuel Désveaux, "Intangible heritage embodied in myths and traditions has an important place in the MQB. For instance, near the section with artefacts from the Plains, we have put a multimedia programme about an American Indian elder reciting a myth. We think that this is heritage and it is not communicated through an object, but through video and oral transcripts."

As we have seen, the separation of art and knowledge is one of the fundamental museological principles of the MQB's permanent exhibition. Although against the aesthetic approach adopted by the museum, even Maurice Godelier observed that "it is important to separate the interpretation space from the space dedicated to the aesthetic and visual enjoyment of the objects . . . Understanding a culture means understanding a way of life and ways of thinking. So, artefacts need to be presented in a way that reveals these ways of thinking." Referring to the shark-shaped reliquary from the Solomon Islands containing a human skull that is on display in the Oceania section (Figure 7.8), he explained:

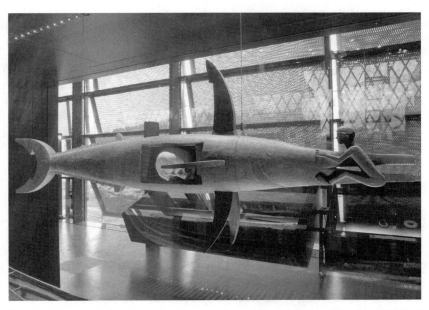

Figure 7.8: A shark-shaped reliquary from the Solomon Islands. (© 2012 musée du quai Branly, photo Antonin Borgeaud/Scala, Florence.)

In these islands in Oceania, people don't kill sharks because they think they are their ancestors. This is why the shark-shaped sculpture contains the skull of an ancestor. Unfortunately, this is not explained in the exhibition or in the multimedia. We see a beautiful object that surprises and excites and this is all. But many people would probably like to know a bit more. MQB is not really a museum of cultures. It is above all a museum of arts. This is a pity.

Comments such as this reveal once more that the museum's practice does not adequately address the complexities of the human and object relationships. Against this backdrop, intangible heritage is separated from the collections and is primarily related to the non-static and ephemeral, often embodied in the performances taking place in the museum theatre and the curation of music.

The Museology of the Intangible

Discussing the role of the intangible in the exhibitions at the MQB, Stéphane Martin remarked:

When we started planning the new museum, we wanted a theatre not only for conferences and discussions, but a centre for the visual arts, for the performing arts, and this is why we have a very dynamic programme in the field of music, song, recitation, dance, storytelling, and all that we can define as intangible heritage—everything that we can define as living... We are not so much interested in a historical heritage that is about to disappear, but rather in the transformation and re-appropriation of tradition... Intangible heritage is the richness of the living, not Bela Bartok collecting the last Hungarian folksongs.

The diverse programme of performances that take place in the MQB, including a contemporary version of the Indian epic Mahabharata, shamanic songs from Siberia, the performance of the Bwa Plank masks from Burkina Faso, and Korean hip-hop constitute an interesting approach on the part of the museum to engage with the idea of heritage as performance.

More in general, an important dimension in which intangible heritage is translated in the work of the MQB is through the curation of musical instruments and the presentation of music. Madeleine Leclair is an ethnomusicologist and curator of musical instruments. Her main responsibilities have included the display of the entire instruments collection in the Music Tower and the production of the music installations in the permanent exhibition. As she explained, presenting music in an exhibition is completely different from displaying objects, because "it requires special attention on the part of the audience not always used to such modes of representation." In making the music boxes, she wanted "to throw the visitor in the heart of a musical event with no beginning or end," where images are projected to accompany the music rather than vice versa: for her, "musical instruments are instruments that serve a musical repertory, but this repertory remains inaccessible if we only look at the object."

However, the presentation of such practices and live performances in a museum context raises several points for consideration: "How far can we go in showing on a theatre scene, things that don't take place on a scene? Should we change their form? Can we present rituals in a Western theatre setting?" are some of the questions that MQB staff face in their work, pointing at debates around the authenticity of cultural performances in the museum setting. Many of my interviewees expressed mixed feelings about the performances taking place at the museum. Philippe Peltier argued that "I am not really convinced by this. These performances are out of context and there is always a kitsch and folkloric side to them." For Emmanuel Désveaux, "there is always the suspicion that we are back in the 'human zoos' of the nineteenth century, when groups of people were brought to Europe and they were exhibited behind bars, just like animals," although he acknowledged that "today we are not at all like this, since people are very well informed about what they are doing."

At the same time, the museum staff defended the value of showing live performances notwithstanding their limits. For example, Anne-Christine Taylor observed that "we certainly don't pretend to show authentic rituals. Most of the spectacles that we show try to find a balance between the two." Similarly, regarding African performances Hélène Joubert remarked:

> It is an adaptation. It is an adaptation of a ritual in a space that is not at all the original space, for a public that is not at all the original public . . . But these performances are also a medium of recognition for [African] people . . . who have chosen themselves how they want to present their culture effectively through the representation of a moment, or a sequence of a ritual, or the dance of some masks . . . This is a collective identity card of cultural validation. I am absolutely fine with this, knowing that it is a spectacle, a way for mediating their culture, for making it known in its contemporary dimensions.

As mentioned earlier, the performance of cultural expressions in a Western museum context was debated at length in the meetings celebrating the inauguration of the MQB in June 2006. Several participants expressed the fear that the authenticity of cultural events would be undermined and that mainstream European audiences would find it hard to understand what they were being presented with. A serious concern was also raised on the part of the performers, who occasionally seemed to be "prisoners of their heritage" (Latour 2007:201–208). For example, having Siberian performers presenting their traditional music in France wearing fur costumes in the heat of August, just because European audiences had such expectations, raised important questions as to the notion of authenticity of cultural performances and the freedom of the performers to alter their traditions (Latour 2007:190–193).

A further issue raised in the meeting involved the dichotomy between tangible and intangible heritage. This was sparked by the contribution of Laurent Lévi-Strauss (see Latour 2007:219–221), deputy director of culture at UNESCO, who in addition to the notion of intangible heritage as performing arts referred to the intangible heritage of objects often neglected by museums. Drawing on that and criticising UNESCO and the wider Eurocentric heritage norm for advancing artificial categorisations of heritage, Eliane Karp de Toledo, the first lady of Peru, argued in favour of a Native understanding of heritage with no dividing lines between tangible and intangible, between the exhibition and the theatre (Latour 2007:227–229). This obviously constitutes one of the major differences between heritage conceptualisation in the MQB and in Te Papa, VCC, and NMAI, and points to the negotiation of intangible heritage as the empowerment of the Indigenous voice.

The Politics of Heritage and the Native Voice

The political aspects of intangible heritage were raised in several interviews. Maurice Godelier extensively talked about the difficult problems posed by the concept:

> People live their culture, they fish, they cook, et cetera. Culture as heritage or intangible heritage is a modern situation. Today people sell their culture like merchandise for tourists, or they defend it politically because they have lost their past sovereignty. Culture has become today a political argument for Indigenous people not only for the reclamation of land, but also for obtaining rights and power. People that live their culture without being dominated by other ways of life or by other societies don't consider their culture as something separate. Whereas now, in the modern world, culture as heritage exists in the sphere of politics.

The collaboration of museums with source and immigrant communities as a way for presenting alternative narratives and suggesting new interpretative frameworks for collections was also debated in my discussions with the MQB staff. Questioning the grounds on which such partnerships have taken place internationally, Anne-Christine Taylor observed that "this whole business started in countries that had a very severe internal problem, the USA and Australia, two countries in which local minorities were effectively highly oppressed and where it would be outrageous not to include them." Similarly, hinting at the political dimensions of a more participatory museology as occurring in the NMAI and Te Papa, Emmanuel Désveaux argued that "for reasons related to a politics of reconciliation and national identity, these museums have given

Native minorities control over their self-representation. This is absolutely legitimate and in the context of these countries and I understand it completely. But in France and in Europe in general, it is different."

Interviews also demonstrated a significant reluctance on the part of MQB staff to work in partnership with immigrant communities, on the assumptions that "they are not interested" or "do not have the competencies." Despite the fact that the museum is trying to develop a network of contacts with source communities, it was generally acknowledged that "there is very little admission of other voices for the time being." A key reason for this can be related to a discrepancy between Western scientific discourses and Native motivations in self-representation. For Emmanuel Désveaux, the first is bounded by "the ethics of academic scholarship in search of truth," while the latter "is motivated by political reasons at best to affirm the quality of Indigenous culture," further arguing that "it is quite possible that community representatives might become revisionists and say for example, that cannibalism never existed, or that this tribe is pacifist, while we know that they were warriors . . . Should the museum present truths verified by academic criteria, or should it present a remodelled vision of the past viewed from a favourable angle?" Similarly Stéphane Martin acknowledged that he felt uncomfortable with "claims that only representatives of a cultural group can speak for that group," and further explained:

> At some points in the NMAI in Washington it feels like historical reality is put aside and replaced by a discourse of reconciliation giving the speech first and foremost to the Natives . . . However, I am not entirely sure if Picasso would be the best curator of an exhibition about Picasso . . . The museum should construct its discourse starting with a dialogue with source communities and with other museums, because nowadays museums are less and less isolated and it is important to exchange opinions and to reply to the suggestions of others, but at the same time it needs to keep its own perspective and autonomy.

In a comparable tone, Emmanuel Désveaux noted that "we need to work towards the collaboration between the two perspectives (academic and Indigenous) without saying that the one is better than the other."

Laïcité

A further issue concerning the balance between autonomy and dialogue with communities revolved around the notion of *laïcité*, or whether the museum should be a secular or a sacred space. Stéphane Martin acknowledged for example that after consultations with Australian Aboriginal groups, it was decided that artefacts that were considered sacred by Aboriginal communities would not be put on display. However, he also acknowledged that gender restrictions held for example in Vanuatu as to who has the right to handle or view sacred objects could not be respected, noting that "it is obvious that this is something impossible for a museum that is in France and operates in a significantly different context." In this respect, Anne-Christine Taylor declared:

> We would never accept objects to be set up and worshipped, or be set up in ways that would suggest that they are in a sacred context. We specifically say, if these objects are here, they are not sacred, simply because the museum and particularly the French museum cannot be a sacred space . . . It would be complicated and embarrassing for the museum if someone for example bowed down and started praying or brought offerings for the statues. *Laïcité* is a principle that many people find hard to understand, but it is one of the basic tenants of French public space.

This line of thought explains why artefacts in the MQB are predominantly considered as desacralised or dead objects separated from their original environment and showcased as *objets d'art* or museum pieces. Unlike Te Papa, NMAI, and VCC, where objects are often regarded as "enchanted," living and animate vessels of cultural transmission, here material culture is largely divested of its spirituality—something that is also manifested in the museum's reluctance to engage more meaningfully with source or diasporic communities.

THE MUSEUM AS A CULTURE

The existing tensions between the secular identity of the museum and the sacred and spiritual meanings of some of its collections suggests that rather than a "dialogue of cultures," the MQB is more prone to establishing a French monologue. As Anne-Christine Taylor characteristically remarked, "We are entitled to our own culture. We are not a-cultural. Part of our cultural framework is the game we play. We play the game of anthropology, we play the game of museums, and we play the game of public, non-religious laic republican museums, which is a complete culture in itself. So be it."

Paraphrasing Taylor's comment, we can conclude that each of the five museums "plays the game" of intangible heritage locally, in accordance with the principles and rules set by national legislation, international influences, historical circumstances, and local complexities, and as such is "a culture in itself." In the last chapter I explore the broader implications of the issues that have emerged so far: the critical relations between the museum and intangible heritage, between material and living culture, and between preservation and erasure.

Chapter 8

Rethinking Cultural Preservation, Museum Curation, and Communities

This book has examined global and local perspectives on the safeguarding of intangible heritage and its museological articulations. A central underpinning was that top-down preservation measures risk decontextualising oral traditions and practices from their broader social and cultural environment. Recent research, for example, has revealed how processes of heritagisation project a global vision of cultural heritage that meets certain predetermined criteria set out by international expert committees (see Churchill 2006; Butler 2007; de Jong 2007; Bauer 2009; Joy 2011). Often fashioned in a formalised manner, these criteria do not always reflect the concerns of local practitioners, who then have to reconfigure their practices in order for these to make it to the relevant lists and international inventories.

Building on this critique, this study has argued for the need to rethink modern preservationism and the associated fears of cultural loss and homogenisation. The various conventions for the preservation of cultural objects, monuments, sites, oral traditions, and expressions that have largely defined cultural heritage throughout the twentieth and well into the twenty-first century express the international anxiety for the protection of the remains of the past and are often entangled in narratives of national identity and distinctiveness. Such approaches have prioritised a particularly Western European and North Atlantic valorisation of what needs to be safeguarded. Moreover, inherent in these preservation initiatives is a deeper notion of an endangered cultural authenticity: the idea that there is a pure essence and value of heritage embedded in objects, places, and practices that provides an unbroken connection with the past and needs to be preserved intact into the future.

Against this approach, this book has engaged with other paradigms of cultural transmission beyond ideas of loss, salvage, and authenticity. As David Lowenthal has observed, "what is deliberately withheld from the natural course of decay and evanescence . . . ceases to be part of a living entity and ends up a fragment surrendered from context" (1985:405). This raises the question of whether just like living entities, cultural heritage, objects, places, practices, and ceremonies can indeed follow a "natural course of decay and evanescence" and still allow for their meanings and values to be maintained, but also developed and changed into the future. Rather than the adoption of short-term preservation and documentation measures and action plans, this requires a consideration of heritage as a much longer-term process.

In my discussions with the curators in the five museums, but also in different events and activities, intangible heritage was often presented not as a set of preciously safeguarded and unchanged traditions, but as knowledge and practices inherited from the past and revived in the present. Practices that combined the traditional and the new, like a modern interpretation of a Maori marae and kapa haka, or the performance of sandroings for a broader tourist audience in Port Vila, reveal the persistence and adaptation of traditions in the face of modernity and change. This suggests that the transmission of cultural expressions should be led not by strict criteria and measures imposed by governmental institutions, but rather through the active and ongoing engagement of practitioners. In this sense, erasure does not suggest a *laissez-faire* approach leading to the total obliteration of traditional ways of life, but instead promotes their creative continuation based on local needs and responses.

Central to the exploration of how museums engage with intangible heritage has been the examination of their relations with diverse communities and more specifically with members of ethnic, diasporic, and Indigenous groups. This has raised questions about the implications of participatory museology. The five museums examined in this study have all engaged in different ways with various community groups. Such engagements have led to major reconsiderations of key museum activities, including collections care and curation, exhibitions and public engagement. The Indigenous curators responsible for the interpretation of Native American collections or the Maori elders acting as advisors and tribal hosts at Te Papa are examples of how museums strive to include tradition bearers in their work and in this process enable the expression of other voices, opinions, and narratives. The incorporation of customary knowledge systems, oral traditions, and tribal beliefs initiates a process of cross-cultural dialogue and empowers communities that have historically been marginalised and excluded. Participatory museology invites therefore a broader rethinking of the museum and its role in society. Envisioned like a cultural centre, a public space for sharing ideas and bringing people together, the new museum is based more on dialogue rather than on a one-dimensional dissemination of knowledge.

Here, participation, equality, and respect build the foundation of the museum as a democratic institution, often negotiated locally as a Native place or nakamal, and as a platform for social and civic engagement. As we have seen, while ideas of dialogue and participation direct the work of Te Papa, the VCC, and NMAI, a focus on historic collections and disciplinary fields does not permit the Horniman and the MQB to engage more dynamically with participatory practices.

A further implication of the participatory paradigm is the idea of performance as a defining feature of new museological work. All five museums provide an active space for the performance of living culture, in the form of community festivals, annual celebrations, world art spectacles, and national days. The Potomac atrium, Te Papa's marae, the nasara in front of the VCC, but also the Gallery Square at the Horniman and the Claude Lévi-Strauss Theatre at the MQB enable the presentation of living culture as a parallel avenue for engaging with contemporary cultural identities. In this sense the idea of the museum as a contact zone (Clifford 1997) or interactive theatre (Phillips 2005) acquires further meanings that go beyond notions of conflict and negotiation and address issues of survival and cultural change. Against this backdrop, intangible heritage emerges as an impermanent act of dynamically engaging with the past in the present and making traditional culture relevant to the contemporary global context. In the process, it is practitioners and community members who define authenticity, rather than experts based on top-down criteria.

Moreover, the participatory model provides a new context for thinking about museum collections and the relationship between the tangible and the intangible. Thinking about the tangible and the intangible holistically allows for deeper meanings and associations to come to the fore. In this context, historic museum pieces are re-enchanted and considered as taonga in Te Papa, while sacred Native American objects are returned to their originating communities or reinvested with spiritual meanings and ceremonially cleansed at the NMAI. Bridging the divide between material and living culture, then, fortifies the relationship between objects and peoples and foregrounds their entanglements, as was the case with the presentation of chief Bongmatur's fighting club through the recounting of his own ancestral stories at the VCC.

Exhibition work becomes a central area for exploring and negotiating these relationships. The idea of concept- or story-driven displays was a significant characteristic of the permanent exhibitions of the NMAI and Te Papa, where different media like interactive stations, film projections, text panels, and screens provided a different interpretative context for the collections. Against this multilayered interpretation, objects were often taken off centre stage or used as side illustrations in order to enable broader themes or personal and communal stories to be told. Yet this shift in attention from objects to ideas, community stories, and narratives has been met with resistance, especially from a body of critics who consider museology "a culture of the object." For many, exhibitions that have been curated by community groups lack scientific authority and become instruments of political advocacy and propaganda. This not only questions the scholarly content of exhibitions, but also the role of museums as scientific institutions. As my research has revealed, indigenising the museum through processes of cross-cultural curation, participation, and sharing is bound up in complex issues of rights and recognition that remain a central and controversial aspect in postcolonial societies. This raises further questions about the makeup of the different communities that participate in the work of museums and about who actually speaks for the community. Whilst the development of the collaborative paradigm is one of the most significant museological developments of the last years, its manifestations and articulations need careful consideration.

Taking forward ideas of erasure and the creative interplay of heritage destruction and transformation, this book has considered intangible heritage as cultural practices that are renewed and recreated by practitioners, providing a new approach to cultural dialogue and communication. Here, processes of globalisation and cross-cultural hybridisation often revive rather than endanger cultural heritage, allowing it to respond to contemporary multifaceted social and cultural environments. This enables heritage institutions, museums, and cultural centres to sustain the messages of the past by engaging with the realities of the present: something that reveals that these institutions are not fixed in perpetuity, but are living organisations shaped by their collections, social surroundings, and diverse communities.

Notes

Chapter 1

1. Taken into account that museums are highly complex and changing organisations, this is almost impossible even in single-sited research.
2. As I will argue in the next chapters, such artefacts have been interpreted by different groups in multiple ways as world art, curiosities, treasures, heirlooms, and living or sacred objects (see also Thomas 1991; McCarthy 2007).
3. During my fieldwork at the NMAI, the museum's Native communities outreach programmes throughout the Americas were described as the "fourth NMAI."
4. While the MQB collections include objects from Africa, Asia, Oceania, and the Americas, the Horniman is much more eclectic and has also a significant collection of artefacts from Europe as well as natural history specimens and living animals.
5. This collection of mostly African, Oceanic, Asian, and Native American artefacts from the nineteenth and early twentieth centuries has been designated of national significance.

Chapter 2

1. Major ethnographic expeditions took place in the late nineteenth and early twentieth centuries—among others, the Cambridge Ethnographic Expedition in the Torres Straits (Herle and Rouse 1998).
2. ICOMOS is the International Council of Monuments and Sites, a nongovernmental organisation advising UNESCO on the merit and conditions of the different nominations.
3. This was the theme of the 2003 ICOMOS General Conference in Zimbabwe. See http://www.international.icomos.org/victoriafalls2003/papers.htm (accessed January 23, 2011).
4. Despite its wide popularity among UNESCO member states, several countries—including Australia, Canada, Switzerland, United Kingdom, and the United States—still remain sceptical of the implications of the 2003 Convention. See Kurin 2007 for the United States, Smith and Waterton 2009 for the United Kingdom.
5. Derived from the English word "custom," the Melanesian term *kastom* refers to precolonial practices and ways of life. For Lissant Bolton, it is a local process of looking and talking about the past in the present (2003). For further discussions, see chapter 4 in this volume and also Jolly and Thomas 1992, Stanley 1998, Leach 2003, and Were 2005.

CHAPTER 3

1. The Treaty of Waitangi was signed in 1840 between Maori tribal chiefs and representatives of the British Crown. Although subsequently forgotten and repeatedly breached, today it is recognised as the founding document of the country, stressing the unity and equality between New Zealanders, both Maori (*tangata whenua*, or people of the land) and Pakeha, subsequent European settlers (*tangata tiriti*, or the people of the Treaty) (King 1985:151–167).

2. The nature and culture dynamic permeates the narrative of Te Papa as well as the other museums examined in the next chapters.

3. *Taonga* is the Maori word for communally valued treasures, comprising not only historic artefacts, but also people, traditional knowledge, and practices (see Tapsell 2011).

4. At the time of my research at Te Papa, on level three visitors could see the Egypt, Beyond the Tomb temporary exhibition. Interestingly, this exhibition was the subject of controversy at Te Papa because it presented a mummy and the display of human remains still remains a sensitive subject for Maori communities.

5. This is the Maori mythical place of origin (King 1985:74).

6. Moriori are the Indigenous group of the Chatham Islands in the south of New Zealand.

7. Te Papa has the policy of inviting every two years a different tribe to be the resident iwi. In this context, the iwi plans and organises a two-year exhibition; in addition, two kaumatua (elders) are invited to act as consultants to the museum. Among their responsibilities is the conduct of welcoming ceremonies.

8. It is interesting to note the ambiguous place of Pacific peoples in the Te Papa bicultural framework. Pacific islanders in New Zealand share a common ancestry and tradition with Maori, but they are placed in the tangata tiriti group.

9. After my fieldwork, Mana Pasifika and On the Sheep's Back were replaced by a new exhibition about people from the rest of the Pacific (Tangata o le Moana). The community exhibition at the time of my research was about the Italians in New Zealand, and was subsequently replaced by a new exhibition about the Scottish community.

10. This presents the founding story of Maori mythology, the physical separation of the sky father, Rangi, and the earth mother, Papatuanuku, by their children, which resulted in the making of daylight and the creation of New Zealand (see Tapsell 2011).

11. This points to a general critique of Te Papa with regards to the sacralisation of Maori and the trivialisation of Pakeha culture (Brown 2002; Goldsmith 2003).

12. In January 2008, representatives of Te Aitanga-a-Hauti gave a talk at UCL presenting "digital repatriation" as the core of project connecting tribal communities with their taonga in overseas institutions.

13. Topics included Waka: From Wood to Fiberglass; Body Adornment: Bone and Stone versus Gold and Silver; Weaving: From Harakeke to Plastic; Storytelling: From Oratory to Scriptwriting; and Dance: From Kapa Haka to Kinetic Choreography (see National Museum of New Zealand Te Papa Tongarewa 2006:5–6).

14. A variety of the performances that took place in Te Papa's 2007 *Matariki* can be found on YouTube (accessed July 28, 2008).

15. For an account of the dynamics and tensions between museum and communities in exhibition development, see Gibson 2003 and the response by Wood 2005.

CHAPTER 4

1. As argued in chapter 2, several researchers have discussed various controversial aspects surrounding the revival of kastom, including the invention of kastom in

Melanesia as a postcolonial tool for nation building bound up in the reinvention of the past (see Linnekin 1992; Were 2005).

2. Bislama is the pidgin *lingua franca* of Vanuatu and one of the country's three official languages—the two other being French and English.

3. "He who takes care of the peaceful nakamal" is the customary title given to Ralph Regenvanu after his resignation from the VCC's directorship in November 2006.

4. A name given by Captain James Cook (1728–1779) who visited the islands during his second voyage in 1774.

5. In 2005 more than half of Vanuatu's population was under eighteen years old, of which more than half was under the age of six (Regenvanu 2005).

6. The workshops have been conducted since 1981 (Huffman 1996:290).

7. Walter Lini was the first prime minister of Vanuatu. He was an Anglican pastor educated in the University of South Pacific. He is also called Father Walter Lini, having been "the father of Independence" (Regenvanu 2005:40).

8. These old collections of salvage ethnography are reinvested today with new meanings in the initiatives on cultural revival and digital repatriation by international cooperation organizations.

9. In the summer of 2008 the domain of Chief Roi Mata on the island of Efate was proclaimed a World Heritage Site.

10. This site was proclaimed a UNESCO World Heritage Site in the summer of 2008. Local communities have developed an ecotourism project around the legend and domain of Chief Roi Mata. See the Roi Mata Cultural Tourism Project at http://www.vanuatuculture.org/vchss/20060915_roimata-tour.shtml. (accessed September 20, 2008).

11. Ralph Regenvanu resigned in order to complete legal studies at the University of South Pacific. He remains actively involved in the work of the VCC.

12. See for example, the video documentary entitled *To Learn Who We Are* about the Arts Festival held in Malekula in 1985. This documentary, produced by Kirk Huffman, explains the revival and reconnection with different practices, such as dances, songs, body painting, magic, and sandroing, that are only performed by men.

13. For more information on the Young People's Project, see: http://www.vanuatuculture.org/ypp/index.shtml (accessed March 10, 2008). In 1998 the Project produced in collaboration with students from Griffith University in Australia the film *Kilim Taem*, portraying the problems faced by young ni-Vanuatu living in urban centres. See Bolton 2000.

14. See chapter 3 for the "digital repatriation" of taonga by Te Aitanga-a-Hauti on national and international levels.

15. This is one of the main characteristics of the tourism campaign of Vanuatu. See for example the BBC article "What's so great about living in Vanuatu?" http://news.bbc.co.uk/2/hi/uk_news/magazine/5172254.stm (accessed May 17, 2008).

CHAPTER 5

1. This is the Native American Grave Protection and Repatriation Act passed in 1990 by the U.S. Congress, which signified a fundamental change in the relationship between Native communities and museums and other academic institutions. See also chapter 2.

2. This was the case of the return of the Water Buster bundle to the Hidatsa people in North Dakota in 1938 (Lenz 2004:112).

3. Richard West Jr. is a member of the Cheyenne and Arapaho tribes of Oklahoma and has served as vice president of the International Council of Museums (ICOM), which makes him well aware of the intangible heritage debates on an international level.

4. An architectural idea that much like Te Papa's Bush City and the green walls of the MQB (see chapters 3 and 7) stresses the sustainable interaction between Native culture and nature.
5. *Mitsitam* in Delaware and Piscataway means "let's eat" (Martin 2004:39).
6. http://www.indigenousgeography.si.edu (accessed March 3, 2012).
7. On that, West has been quoted as saying "We do not want to make the NMAI into an Indian Holocaust Museum" (Lonetree 2006b:637).
8. The treatment of Native American sacred objects was the topic of a conference organised by the American Association of Museums and Harvard's Center for the Study of World Religions (Sullivan and Edwards 2004).

CHAPTER 6

1. Haddon's involvement in the Horniman was the first in the long and ongoing history of anthropological involvement in the work of the museum.
2. This totem pole was donated to the museum by Tlingit carver Nathan Jackson in 1985.

CHAPTER 7

1. This museum was founded in 1938 one year after the International Exhibition in Paris. It soon became a temple for anthropological research and came to represent the "scientific approach" in terms of presenting non-Western artefacts (Clifford 1988; de l'Etoile 2007a).
2. This was notably embodied in the contradictory term *arts premiers* (Degli and Mauzé 2000; Price 2007; Alivizatou 2008a).
3. Kerchache is a key figure in the art-versus-anthropology debate that led to the foundation of the MQB. He wrote against ethnographic museums and criticised their simplistic representations of complex cultures (see Kerchache et al. 1988).
4. This is the name of the gallery that opened at the Louvre in 2000, exhibiting about one hundred works of art from Asia, Africa, Oceania, and the Americas, and curated by Jacques Kerchache. This is a minimalist display aimed at showcasing the aesthetic dimensions of displayed objects; contextual information is absent from the gallery and presented in a small room on large video screens. Presently, it is the Louvre outpost of the MQB (see Figure 7.5).
5. This museum was founded in the late 1950s by André Malraux, but by the end of the 1990s it had become outdated (see for example Taffin 2000; Price 2007; Alivizatou 2008).
6. UNESCO eventually adopted this Convention in October 2005.
7. See details about his post-presidential foundation at http://www.fondationchirac.eu (accessed February 12, 2011).
8. Such allusions to a cave-like or jungle-like space for the non-European collections have met with significant criticism in the Anglophone press (see Chrisafis 2006; Gibbons 2006; Kimmelman 2006).
9. The Nok terracotta displayed at the MQB were the subject of legal debate and controversy due to their dubitable provenance (Dupaigne 2006; Price 2007).
10. This also applies to the Oceania section.
11. An exception to this is the white box containing the Dogon masks, which has been built in the traditional art gallery approach.
12. This exhibition, although much larger, had several themes in common with Horniman's Centenary Gallery.

13. This is the name of the New Zealand rugby team famous for their performance of the Maori *haka* before each game.
14. His position also hints at the scepticism with which a large number of anthropologists look at the aesthetic display of material culture, as it would divest the objects of their meaning and significance (Dupaigne 2006; Price 2007).
15. Although she did not explain why, I would assume that being the most numerous and significant, the African and Oceanic collections were curated and displayed by Viatte and Nouvel (see also Price 2007).

Glossary

Aotearoa. New Zealand, the land of the long white cloud (Maori)
Atua. God (Maori)
goulong mask. Cone-shaped mask (Bislama)
Hapu. Sub-tribe (Maori)
hei tiki. Carved pendant, usually a greenstone representing a person (Maori)
hui. Meeting (Maori)
huia. Native New Zealand bird, now extinct (Maori)
ipu whenua. Afterbirth container (Maori)
iwi. Tribe (Maori)
kaihautu. Leader, captain of the canoe (Maori)
kapa haka. Performing arts (Maori)
karakia. Blessing ceremony (Maori)
karanga. Ceremonial call (Maori)
karapuna. Ancestors (Maori)
kastom. Pre-colonial culture, derived from English word "custom" (Bislama)
kaumatua. Elder (Maori)
Malvatumauri. Council of Chiefs (Bislama)
mana. Prestige, authority, power (Maori)
marae. Meeting space (Maori)
Matariki. The Pleiades (Maori)
matauranga. Knowledge systems (Maori)
mauri. Life force (Maori)
moa. Giant flightless bird, now extinct (Maori)
moana. Sea (Maori)
nakamal. Meeting house (Bislama)
nasara. Ceremonial space (Bislama)
nawita. Octopus (Bislama)
Pakeha. New Zealanders of European descent (Maori)
Papatuanuku. Earth Mother (Maori)

pataka. Raised storehouse (Maori)

paua. Sea ear (Maori)

pepeha. Tribal sayings (Maori)

poi. Light ball on a string used in female dances and songs (Maori)

pounamu. Greenstone (Maori)

powhiri. Welcoming ceremony (Maori)

rakau whakapapa. Genealogy stick (Maori)

sandroing. Sand-drawing (Bislama)

tangata. People (Maori)

tangata tiriti. People of the Treaty of Waitangi (Maori)

tangata whenua. People of the land (Maori)

taonga. Treasure (Maori)

tauihi. Canoe prow (Maori)

Te Reo Maori. Maori language (Maori)

tikanga. Custom (Maori)

toi moko. Tattooed head (Maori)

waharoa. Gateway (Maori)

waiata. Song (Maori)

wairua. Spirit (Maori)

waka. Canoe (Maori)

waka taua. War canoe (Maori)

whakapapa. Genealogy (Maori)

whare. House (Maori)

wharenui. Meeting house (Maori)

wharepuni. Storehouse (Maori)

whenua. Earth, land, placenta (Maori)

References

Aikawa, N.
    2009 From the Proclamation of Masterpieces to the Convention for the Safeguarding of Intangible Heritage. *In* Intangible Heritage. L. Smith and N. Akagawa, eds. Pp. 13–44. New York: Routledge.
    2004 An Historical Overview of the Preparation of the UNESCO International Convention for the Safeguarding of the Intangible Cultural Heritage. Museum International 56:137–149.

Alivizatou, M.
    2011 Intangible Heritage and Erasure: Rethinking Cultural Preservation and Contemporary Museum Practice. International Journal of Cultural Property 18(1):37–60.
    2008a The Politics of "Arts Premiers": Some Thoughts on the Musée du Quai Branly. Museological Review 13:44–56.
    2008b Contextualising Intangible Cultural Heritage in Heritage Studies and Museology. International Journal of Intangible Heritage 3:42–54.
    2007 The UNESCO Programme for the Proclamation of Masterpieces of the Oral and Intangible Heritage of Humanity: A Critical Examination. Journal of Museum Ethnography 19:34–42.

Amato, S.
    2006 Quai Branly Museum: Representing France after Empire. Race & Class 47(4):46–65.

Ames, M.
    2006 Counterfeit Museology. Museum Management and Curatorship 21(3):171–186.
    1999 How to Decorate a House: The Re-Negotiation of Cultural Representations at the University of British Columbia. Museum Anthropology 22(3):41–51.
    1992 Cannibal Tours and Glass-Boxes: The Anthropology of Museums. Vancouver: University of British Columbia Press.

Appadurai, A., and C. Breckenridge
    1992 Museums are Good to Think: Heritage on View in India. *In* Museums and Communities: The Politics of Public Culture. I. Karp, C. Mullen Creamer, and S. D. Lavine, eds. Pp. 34–55. Washington: Smithsonian Institution Press.

Atalay, S.
    2006 No Sense of the Struggle: Creating a Context for Survivance at the NMAI. Special issue, "Critical Engagements with the National Museum of the American Indian," A. Lonetree, ed., American Indian Quarterly 30(3–4):597–618.

Basu, P.
2007 Highland Homecomings: Genealogy and Heritage Tourism in the Scottish Diaspora. London: Routledge.
Bauer, A. A.
2009 The Terroir of Culture: Long-term History, Heritage Preservation and the Specificities of Place. Heritage Management 2(1):81–104.
Belich, J.
2001 Paradise Reforged: A History of the New Zealanders from the 1880s to the Year 2000. Honolulu: University of Hawai'i Press.
Bennett, T.
2004 Pasts beyond Memory: Evolution, Museums, Colonialism. London: Routledge.
1995 The Birth of the Museum: History, Theory, Politics. London: Routledge.
Berry, S.
2006 Voice and Objects at the NMAI. Review roundtable, National Museum of the American Indian. Public Historian 28(2):62–67.
Bezombes, S.
2006 L'ethnologue, le musée et le multimédia: Produire et exposer le patrimoine immatériel au musée du quai Branly. Electronic document, http://www.reciproque.net/wp-content/uploads/pdf/Article_SBE.pdf, accessed April 12, 2010.
Bharucha, R.
2000 Beyond the Box: Problematising the "New Asian Museum." Third Text 52:11–19.
Bhatti, S.
2012 Translating Museums: A Counterhistory of South Asian Museology. Walnut Creek: Left Coast Press.
Blake, J.
2006 Commentary on the 2003 UNESCO Convention on the Safeguarding of Intangible Cultural Heritage. Leicester: Institute of Art and Law.
Blanc, P.
2006 Le jardin vertical. In Le musée du quai Branly. A. Lavalou and J. P. Robert, eds. Pp. 106–107. Paris: Le Moniteur.
Boast, R.
2011 Neocolonial Collaboration: Museum as Contact Zone Revisited. Museum Anthropology 34(1): 56–70.
Bolton, L.
2007 Resourcing Change: Fieldworkers, the Women's Culture Project and the Vanuatu Cultural Centre. In The Future of Indigenous Museums: Perspectives from the Southwest Pacific. N. Stanley, ed. Pp. 23–37. New York: Berghan Books.
2006 The Museum as Cultural Agent: The Vanuatu Cultural Centre Extension Worker Programme. In South Pacific Museums: Experiments in Culture. C. Healy and A. Witcomb, eds. Pp. 1–13. Melbourne: Monash University Press.
2003 Unfolding the Moon: Enacting Women's Kastom in Vanuatu. Honolulu: University of Hawai'i Press.
2000 Review of Kilim Taem. The Contemporary Pacific 12(2):561–563.
1999 Introduction. Oceania 70(1):1–8.
Bouchenaki, M.
2004 Editorial. Museum International 56:6–10.
Bourdieu, P., and A. Darbel
1989 The Love of Art: European Art Museums and their Public. C. Beattie and N. Merriman, trans. Cambridge: Polity Press.
Bowdler, S.
1988 Repainting Australian Rock Art. Antiquity 62:517–523.

Bowen, J. R.
   2000   Should We Have a Universal Concept of "Indigenous Peoples" Rights? Ethnicity and Essentialism in Twenty-first Century. Anthropology Today 16(4):12–16.
Boylan, P.
   2006   The Intangible Heritage: A Challenge and an Opportunity for Museums and Museum Professional Training. International Journal of Intangible Heritage 1:54–65.
Brown, M.
   2002   Representing the Body of a Nation: The Art Exhibitions of New Zealand's National Museum. Third Text 16(3):125–139.
Brown, M. F.
   2005   Heritage Trouble: Recent Work on the Protection of Intangible Cultural Property. International Journal of Cultural Property 12(1):40–61.
   2004   Heritage as Property. In Property in Question: Value Transformation in the Global Economy. K. Verdery and C. Humphrey, eds. Pp. 49–68. Oxford: Berg.
   1998   Can Culture Be Copyrighted? Current Anthropology 39(2):193–222.
Butler, B.
   2007   Return to Alexandria: An Ethnography of Cultural Heritage Revivalism and Museum Memory. Walnut Creek: Left Coast Press.
   2006   Heritage and the Present Past. In Handbook of Material Culture. C. Tilley, W. Keane, S. Kuechler-Fogden, M. Rowlands, and P. Spyer, eds. Pp. 463–479. London: Sage.
Byrne, D.
   2009   A Critique of Unfeeling Heritage. In Intangible Heritage. L. Smith and N. Akagawa, eds. Pp. 229–252. London: Routledge.
   1995   Buddhist Stupa and Thai Social Practice. World Archaeology 27(2):266–281.
   1991   Western Hegemony in Archaeological Heritage Management. History and Anthropology 5:269–276.
Carpio, M. V.
   2006   (Un)disturbing Exhibitions: Indigenous Historical Memory at the NMAI. Special issue, "Critical Engagements with the National Museum of the American Indian," A. Lonetree, ed., American Indian Quarterly 30(3–4):619–631.
Chirac, J.
   2006   Preface. In Musée du quai Branly: Museum Guide Book. Pp. 6–7. Paris: Musée du quai Branly.
Choay, F.
   2006   Branly: Un nouveau luna park était-il nécessaire? Urbanisme 350:1–6.
   2001   The Invention of the Historic Monument. L. M. O'Connell, trans. Cambridge: Cambridge University Press.
Chrisafis, A.
   2006   Chirac Leaves Controversial Legacy with Monument to African and Asian Culture. The Guardian, April 7.
Churchill, N.
   2006   Dignifying Carnival: The Politics of Heritage Recognition in Puebla, Mexico. International Journal of Cultural Property 13(1):1–24.
Clavir, M.
   2002   Preserving What Is Valued: Museums, Conservation, and First Nations. Vancouver, BC: University of British Columbia Press.
Cleere, H.
   2001   Uneasy Bedfellows: Universality and Cultural Heritage. In Destruction and Conservation of Cultural Property. R. Layton, P. Stone, and J. Thomas, eds. Pp. 22–29. London: Routledge.
   1995   Cultural Landscapes as World Heritage. Conservation and Management of Archaeological Sites 1:63–68.

Clément, G.
  2006 Le jardin des graminées. *In* Le musée du quai Branly. A. Lavalou and J. P. Robert, eds. Pp. 102–103. Paris: Le Moniteur.
Clifford, J.
  2007 Quai Branly in Process. October 120:3–23.
  2004 Looking Several Ways: Anthropology and Native Heritage in Alaska. Current Anthropology 45(1):5–30.
  1997 Routes: Travel and Translation in the Late 20th Century. Cambridge: Harvard University Press.
  1991 Four Northwest Coast Museums: Travel Reflections. *In* Exhibiting Culture: The Poetics and Politics of Museum Display. I. Karp and D. Lavine, eds. Pp. 212–254. Washington: Smithsonian Institution Press.
  1988 The Predicament of Culture: Twentieth-Century Ethnography, Literature, and Art. Cambridge: Harvard University Press.
Clifford, J., and G. E. Marcus, eds.
  1986 Writing Culture: The Poetics and Politics of Ethnography. Berkeley: University of California Press.
Conil-Lacoste, M.
  1994 The Story of a Grand Design: UNESCO 1946–1993. Paris: UNESCO Publishing.
Conn, S.
  2006 Heritage vs History at the National Museum of the American Indian. Review round-table, National Museum of the American Indian. Public Historian 28(2):68–73.
Coody Cooper, K., and N. I. Sandoval, eds.
  2006 Living Homes for Cultural Expressions: North American Native Perspectives on Creating Community Museums. Washington: National Museum of the American Indian Editions.
Coombes, A. E.
  1994 Reinventing Africa: Museums, Material Culture and Popular Imagination in Late Victorian and Edwardian England. London: Yale University Press.
Cowen, T.
  2002 Creative Destruction: How Globalization is Changing the World's Cultures. Princeton: Princeton University Press.
Cruickshank, J.
  1992 Oral Tradition and Material Culture: Multiplying Meanings of "Words" and "Things." Anthropology Today 8(3):5–9.
Davis, P.
  1999 Ecomuseums: A Sense of Place. London: Leicester University Press.
de Jong, F.
  2007 A Masterpiece of Masquerading: Contradictions of Conservation in Intangible Heritage. *In* Reclaiming Heritage: Alternative Imaginaries of Memory in West Africa. F. de Jong and M. Rowlands, eds. Pp. 161–184. Walnut Creek: Left Coast Press.
de Jong, F., and M. Rowlands, eds.
  2007 Reclaiming Heritage: Alternative Imaginaries of Memory in West Africa. Walnut Creek: Left Coast Press.
de l'Etoile, B.
  2007a Le goût des autres : De l'exposition coloniale aux arts premiers. Paris: Flammarion.
  2007b L'oubli de l'héritage colonial. Le Débat 147:91–100.
Deacon, H., L. Dondolo, M. Mrubata, and S. Prosalendis
  2004 The Subtle Power of Intangible Heritage: Legal and Financial Instruments for Safeguarding Intangible Heritage. Cape Town: HSRC Publishers.
Degli, M., and M. Mauzé
  2000 Arts premiers: Le temps de la reconnaissance. Paris: Gallimard.

Derlon, B.
2007 Des "fétiches à clous" au Grand Verre de Duchamp: Une nouvelle théorie anthropologique de l'art. Le Débat 147:124–135.
Desvallées, A.
2008 Quai Branly: Un mirroir aux alouettes? A propos d'ethnographie et d'arts premiers. Paris: L'Harmattan.
Désveaux, E.
2006 The Singularity of Amerindian Objects. In Musée du quai Branly: Museum Guide Book. Pp. 238–240. Paris: Musée du Quai Branly.
2002 Le musée du quai Branly au miroir de ses prédécesseurs. Ethnologies: Musées/Museums 24(2):219–227.
Dias, N.
2008 Cultural Difference and Cultural Diversity: The Case of the Musée du Quai Branly. In Museums and Difference. D. J. Sherman, ed. Pp. 124–154. Bloomington and Indianapolis: Indiana University Press.
2007 Le musée du quai Branly: Une généalogie. Le Débat 147:65–79.
Duncan, C.
1995 Civilizing Rituals: Inside Public Art Museums. London: Routledge.
Dupaigne, B.
2006 Le scandale des arts premiers: La véritable histoire du musée du quai Branly. Paris: Mille et Une Nuit.
Durie, M.
1998 Te Mana Te Kawanatanga: The Politics of Maori Self-Determination. Oxford: Oxford University Press.
Early, J., and P. Seitel
2002 No Folklore without the Folk. Smithsonian Talk Story 21:19–21.
Fabian, J.
1983 Time and the Other: How Anthropology Makes its Object. New York: Columbia University Press.
Fisher, M.
2004 Indian Museum's Appeal, Sadly, Only Skin-Deep. The Washington Post, September 21.
Geismar, H.
2003 Markets, Museums and Material Culture: Presentations and Prestations in Vanuatu, Southwest Pacific. Ph.D. dissertation, University of London.
Geismar, H., and C. Tilley
2003 Negotiating Materiality: International and Local Museum Practices at the Vanuatu Cultural Centre and National Museum. Oceania 73:170–188.
Gell, A.
1998 Art and Agency: An Anthropological Theory. Oxford: Clarendon Press.
Gibbons, F.
2006 Musée de Bogus Art. The Guardian, July 3.
Gibson, S.
2003 Te Papa and New Zealand's Indian Communities: A Case Study about Exhibition Development. Tuhinga 14:61–75.
Gob, A., and N. Drouguet
2003 La Muséologie: Histoire, Développements, Enjeux Actuels. Paris: Armand Colin.
Goldsmith, M.
2003 "Our Place" in New Zealand Culture: How the Museum of New Zealand Constructs Biculturalism. Ethnologies Comparées 6, http://alor.univ-montp3.fr/cerce/r6/m.g.s.htm, accessed July 5, 2007.
Gosden, C.
1999 Archaeology and Anthropology: A Changing Relationship. London: Routledge.

Gruber, J.
  1959 Ethnographic Salvage and the Future of Anthropology. American Anthropologist 61:379–389.
Hafstein, V.
  2009 Intangible Heritage as a List: From Masterpieces to Representation. *In* Intangible Heritage. L. Smith and N. Akagawa, eds. Pp. 93–111. Abingdon: Routledge.
  2004 The Making of Intangible Cultural Heritage: Tradition and Authenticity, Community and Humanity. Ph.D. dissertation, University of California, Berkeley.
Hafstein, V., and R. Bendix
  2009 Culture and Property: An Introduction. Ethnologia Europaea 39(2):5–10.
Hakiwai, A.
  2005 The Search for Legitimacy: Museums in Aotearoa, New Zealand—A Maori Perspective. *In* Heritage, Museums and Galleries: An Introductory Reader. D. Corsane, ed. Pp. 154–162. London: Routledge.
Hamilakis, Y., and A. Anagnostopoulos, eds.
  2009 Archaeological Ethnographies. Special double issue, Public Anthropology 8(2–3). London: Maney.
Handler, R., and E. Gable
  1997 The New History in an Old Museum: Creating the Past at Colonial Williamsburg. Durham: Duke University Press.
Hannerz, U.
  2003 Being There... and There... and There! Reflections on Multi-Site Ethnography. Ethnography 4(2):201–216.
  1998 Transnational Research. *In* Handbook of Methods in Cultural Anthropology. H. R. Bernard, ed. Pp. 235–256. Walnut Creek: AltaMira Press.
Hanson, A.
  1989 The Making of the Maori: Cultural Invention and Its Logic. American Anthropologist 91(4):890–902.
Harrison, S.
  1999 Identity as a scarce resource. Social Anthropology 7:239–251.
Harvey, D.
  2001 Heritage Pasts and Heritage Presents: Temporality, Meaning, and the Scope of Heritage Studies. International Journal of Heritage Studies 7(4):319–338.
Hassan, F.
  2007 The Aswan High Dam and the International Rescue Nubia Campaign. African Archaeological Review 24:73–94.
Henare, A.
  2005 Museums, Anthropology and Imperial Exchange. Cambridge: Cambridge University Press.
  2004 Rewriting the Script: Te Papa Tongarewa the Museum of New Zealand. Social Analysis 48(1):55–63.
Hendry, J.
  2005 Reclaiming Culture: Indigenous People and Self-Representation. New York: Palgrave MacMillan.
  2003 An Ethnographer in the Global Arena: Globography Perhaps? Global Networks 3(4):497–515.
Herle, A.
  2003 Objects, Agency and Museums: Continuing Dialogues between the Torres Strait and Cambridge. *In* Museums and Source Communities: A Routledge Reader. L. Peers and A. K. Brown, eds. Pp. 194–207. London: Routledge.
Herle, A., and S. Rouse, eds.
  1998 Cambridge and the Torres Strait: Centenary Essays on the 1898 Expedition. Cambridge: Cambridge University Press.

Hill, L.
    2004 A Home for the Collections. *In* Spirit of a Native Place: Building the National Museum of the American Indian. D. Blue Spruce, ed. Pp. 116–131. Washington: National Museum of the American Indian.
Hobsbawm, E., and T. Ranger, eds.
    1983 The Invention of Tradition. Cambridge: Cambridge University Press.
Holtorf, C.
    2006 Can Less Be More? Heritage in the Age of Terrorism. Public Archaeology 5(2):101–110.
    2001 Is the Past a Non-Renewable Resource? *In* The Destruction and Conservation of Cultural Property. R. Layton, P. Stone, and J. Thomas, eds. Pp. 286–295. London: Routledge.
Hooper-Greenhill, E.
    2000 Museums and the Interpretation of Visual Culture. London: Routledge.
    1992 Museums and the Shaping of Knowledge. London: Routledge.
Howarth, J.
    2004 New York City in Indian Possession. *In* Spirit of a Native Place: Building the National Museum of the American Indian. D. Blue Spruce, ed. Pp. 132–149. Washington: National Museum of the American Indian.
Hubert, J., and C. Fforde
    2005 The Re-Burial Issue in the Twenty-first Century. *In* Heritage, Museums and Galleries: An Introductory Reader. D. Corsane, ed. Pp. 107–121. London: Routledge.
Huffman, K. W.
    1996 The Fieldworkers of the Vanuatu Cultural Centre and their Contribution to the Audiovisual Collections. *In* Arts of Vanuatu. J. Bonnemaison, K. W. Huffman, and D. Tryon, eds. Pp. 290–293. Honolulu: University of Hawai'i Press.
Hylland-Eriksen, T.
    2003 Between Universalism and Relativism: A Critique of the UNESCO Concept of Culture. *In* Culture and Rights: Anthropological Perspectives. J. K. Cowen, M. B. Dembour, and R. Wilson, eds. Pp. 127–148. Cambridge: Cambridge University Press.
ICOM
    2007 ICOM Statutes. Electronic document, http://icom.museum/statutes.html#3, accessed December 10, 2008.
Isaac, G.
    2008 Technology Becomes the Object: The Use of Electronic Media at the National Museum of the American Indian. Journal of Material Culture 13(3):287–310.
Jacknis, I.
    2006 A New Thing? The NMAI in Historical and Institutional Perspective. Special issue, "Critical Engagements with the National Museum of the American Indian," A. Lonetree, ed., American Indian Quarterly 30(3–4):511–542.
Jacobson, L., ed.
    2006 Review Roundtable: The National Museum of the American Indian. The Public Historian 28(2):46–90.
James, P.
    2005 Building a Community-Based Identity at Anacostia Museum. *In* Heritage, Museums and Galleries: An Introductory Reader. D. Corsane, ed. Pp. 339–356. London: Routledge.
Jolly, M.
    2001 On the Edge? Deserts, Oceans, Islands. The Contemporary Pacific 13(2):417–466.
    1994 Kastom as Commodity: The Land-Dive as Indigenous Rite and Tourist Spectacle. *In* Kastom–Culture–Tradition: Developing Cultural Policy in Melanesia. L. Lamont and G. White, eds. Pp. 131–144. Suva: Institute of Pacific Studies.

Jolly, M.
    1993 Women of the Place: Kastom, Colonialism and Gender in Vanuatu. Chur: Harwood Academic Publishers.
Jolly, M., and N. Thomas, eds.
    1992a The Politics of Tradition in the Pacific. Special issue, Oceania 62(4).
    1992b Introduction. Special issue, Oceania 62(4):241–248.
Joy, C.
    2011 The Politics of Heritage Management: From UNESCO to Djenné. Walnut Creek: Left Coast Press.
Kaeppler, A.
    1994 Paradise Regained: The Role of Pacific Museums in Forging National Identity. In Museums and the Making of "Ourselves": The Role of Objects in National Identity. F. Kaplan, ed. Pp. 19–44. London: Leicester University Press.
Karp, I., C. Mullen Creamer, and S. D. Lavine, eds.
    1992 Museums and Communities: The Politics of Public Culture. Washington: Smithsonian Institution Press.
Kasarherou, E.
    2007 Small Island Countries and the Challenges of Dealing with Cultural Diversity. Paper presented at the Concurrent Session of the ICOM Cross Cultural Task Force on "Transformations: Museums and Cultural Diversity," ICOM General Conference, Vienna, August 19–24.
Keesing, R. M.
    1989 Creating the Past: Custom and Identity in the Contemporary Pacific. The Contemporary Pacific 1(1–2):19–42.
    1982 Kastom in Melanesia: An Overview. Special issue, "Reinventing Traditional Culture: The Politics of Kastom in Island Melanesia," Mankind 13(4):297–301.
Keesing, R. M., and R. Tonkinson, eds.
    1982 Reinventing Traditional Culture: The Politics of Kastom in Island Melanesia. Special issue, Mankind 13(4).
Kerchache, J.
    1990 Pour que les chefs d'œuvres du monde entier naissent libres et égaux. Libération, March 15.
Kerchache, J., J.-L. Paudrat, and L. Stephan
    1988 L'Art Africain. Paris: Mazenod.
Kimmelman, M.
    2006 A Heart of Darkness in the City of Light. The New York Times, July 2.
King, M.
    1985 The Penguin History of New Zealand. Auckland: Penguin.
Kirshenblatt-Gimblett, B.
    2004 Intangible Heritage as a Metacultural Production. Museum International 56:52–65.
Konare, A. O.
    1995 The Creation and Survival of Local Museums. In Museums and the Community in West Africa. C. Ardouin and E. Arinze, eds. Pp. 5–10. Washington: Smithsonian Institution Press.
Kreps, C.
    2011 Changing the Rules of the Road: Post-colonialism and the New Ethics of Museum Anthropology. In The Routledge Companion to Museum Ethics: Redefining Ethics for the Twenty-first Century Museum. J. Marstine, ed. Pp. 70–84. Abingdon: Routledge.
    2009 Indigenous Curation, Museums, and Intangible Heritage. In Intangible Heritage. L. Smith and N. Akagawa, eds. Pp. 193–208. Abingdon: Routledge.
    2007 The Theoretical Future of Indigenous Museums: Concept and Practice. In The Future of Indigenous Museums: Perspectives from Southwest Pacific. N. Stanley, ed. Pp. 223–234. New York: Berghahn Books.

2005 Indigenous Curation as Intangible Heritage: Thoughts on the Relevance of the 2003 UNESCO Convention. Theorizing Cultural Heritage 1(2):3–8.

2003 Liberating Culture: Cross-cultural Perspectives on Museums, Curation, and Heritage Preservation. London: Routledge.

Kuechler, S.

2002 Malanggan: Art, Memory, and Sacrifice. Oxford: Berg.

Kuper, A.

2003 The Return of the Native. Current Anthropology 44(3):389–402.

Kurin, R.

2007 Safeguarding Intangible Cultural Heritage: Key Factors in Implementing the 2003 Convention. International Journal of Intangible Heritage 2:9–20.

2004a Museums and Intangible Heritage: Culture Dead or Alive? ICOM News 57(4):7–9.

2004b Les problématiques du patrimoine culturel immatériel. In Le Patrimoine Culturel Immatériel: Les Enjeux, Les Problématiques, Les Pratiques. Pp. 59–67. Paris: Babel, Maison des Cultures du Monde.

Labadi, S., and C. Long, eds.

2010 Heritage and Globalisation. Abingdon: Routledge.

Latour, B., ed.

2007 Le Dialogue des Cultures: Actes des Rencontres Inaugurales du Musée du Quai Branly (21 Juin 2006). Paris: Babel.

Lavalou, A., and J. P. Robert, eds.

2006 Le Musée du Quai Branly. Paris: Le Moniteur.

Leach, J.

2003 Owning Creativity: Cultural Property and the Efficacy of Custom on the Rai Coast of Papua New Guinea. Journal of Material Culture 8(2):123–143.

Lenz, M. J.

2004 George Gustav Heye. In Spirit of a Native Place: Building the National Museum of the American Indian. D. Blue Spruce, ed. Pp. 86–115. Washington, DC: National Museum of the American Indian.

Levell, N.

2000 Oriental Visions: Exhibitions, Travel and Collecting in the Victorian Age. London: The Horniman Museum.

Lévi-Strauss, C.

1952 Race et Histoire. Paris: UNESCO.

Lindholm, C.

2008 Culture and Authenticity. London: Blackwell.

Lindstrom, L., and G. M. White

1994 Culture–Kastom–Tradition: Developing Cultural Policy in Melanesia. Suva: The University of South Pacific.

Linnekin, J.

1992 On the Theory and Politics of Cultural Construction in the Pacific. Oceania 62(4):249–63.

Lira, S., and R. Amoeda, eds.

2010 Constructing Intangible Heritage. Barcelos: Green Lines Institute for Sustainable Development.

Londres-Fonseca, M.

2002 Intangible Cultural Heritage and Museum Exhibitions. ICOM UK News 63:8–9.

Lonetree, A., ed.

2006a Critical Engagements with the National Museum of the American Indian. Special issue, American Indian Quarterly 30(3–4).

2006b Missed Opportunities: Reflections on the NMAI. Special issue, "Critical Engagements with the National Museum of the American Indian," American Indian Quarterly 30(3–4):632–645.

Lowenthal, D.
    1998 The Heritage Crusade and the Spoils of History. Cambridge: Cambridge University Press.
    1985 The Past is a Foreign Country. Cambridge: Cambridge University Press.
Lujan, J.
    2005 A Museum of the Indian, not for the Indian. American Indian Quarterly 29(3–4): 510–516.
Luke, T.
    2002 Inventing the Southwest: The Fred Harvey Company and Native American Art. In Museum Politics: Power Plays at the Exhibition. Pp. 82–99. Minneapolis: University of Minnesota Press.
MacCannel, D.
    1992 Empty Meeting Grounds: The Tourist Papers. London: Routledge.
MacDonald, S.
    2006 Expanding Museum Studies: An Introduction. In A Companion to Museum Studies. S. MacDonald, ed. Pp. 1–12. Oxford: Blackwell.
    2003 Museums, National, Postnational, and Transcultural Identities. Museum and Society 1(1):1–16.
    2002 Behind the Scenes at the Science Museum. Oxford: Berg.
Marcus, G. E.
    1995 Ethnography In/Of the World System: The Emergence of Multi-sited Ethnography. Annual Review of Anthropology 24:95–117.
Marcus, G. E., and M. J. Fischer
    1986 Anthropology as Cultural Critique: An Experimental Moment in the Human Sciences. Chicago: University of Chicago Press.
Martin, L. R.
    2004 The Potomac. In National Museum of the American Indian: Smithsonian Institution, Washington, DC: Map and Guide. Pp. 34–35. Washington, DC: National Museum of the American Indian.
Martin, S.
    2007 Un musée pas comme les autres. Le Débat 147:5–22.
Matsuura, K.
    2004 Preface. Museum International 56:4–5.
McBryde, I.
    1997 The Ambiguities of Authenticity: Rock of Faith or Shifting Sands? Conservation and Management of Archaeological Sites 2:93–100.
McCarthy, C.
    2007 Exhibiting Maori: A History of Colonial Cultures of Display. Oxford: Berg.
Mead, S. M.
    1983 Indigenous Museums in Oceania. Museum 138:98–101.
Meskell, L.
    2002 Negative Heritage and Past Mastering in Archaeology. Anthropological Quarterly 75(3):557–574.
Message, K.
    2006 New Museums and the Making of Culture. Oxford: Berg.
Mitchell, J.
    2002 Roads, Recklessness and Relationships: An Urban Settlement in Postcolonial Vanuatu. Ph.D. dissertation, University of York, Ontario.
Molotsky, I.
    1989 Smithsonian Votes Plan for an American Indian Museum. The New York Times, January 31.

Morphy, H.
  1992 Aesthetics in a Cross-cultural Perspective: Some Reflections on Native American Basketry. Journal of the Anthropological Society of Oxford 23(1):1–16.
Mowaljarlai, D., P. Vinnicombe, G. K. Ward, and C. Chippindale
  1988 Repainting of Images on Rock in Australia and the Maintenance of Aboriginal Culture. Antiquity 62:690–696.
Munjeri, D.
  2009 Following the Length and Breadth of the Roots: Some Dimensions of Intangible Heritage. In Intangible Heritage. L. Smith and N. Akagawa, eds. Pp. 131–150. Abingdon: Routledge.
  2004 Tangible and Intangible Heritage: From Difference to Convergence. Museum International 56:12–19.
Murphy, B.
  2007 Resolution No. 3: Informing Museums on Intellectual Property Issues. ICOM News (3–4):9.
Museum Association
  1998 Definition of the Museum. Electronic document, http://www.museumsassocia-tion.org/about/frequently-asked-questions, accessed February 14, 2011.
Myers, F.
  2002 Painting Culture: The Making of the Aboriginal High Art. Durham: Duke University Press.
Nas, P.
  2002 Masterpieces of Oral and Intangible Culture: Reflections on the UNESCO World Heritage List. Current Anthropology 43(1):139–143.
Nash, S. E., and C. Colwell-Chanthaphonh, eds.
  2010 NAGPRA after Two Decades. Special issue, Museum Anthropology 33(2).
National Museum of New Zealand Te Papa Tongarewa
  2006 Museum of New Zealand Te Papa Tongarewa Annual Report 2005/2006. Electronic document, http://tepapa.govt.nz/SiteCollectionDocuments/AboutTePapa/LegislationAccountability/AnnualReport_0506.pdf, accessed February 19, 2012.
Nederveen Pieterse, J.
  2004 Globalization and Culture: Global Melange. Maryland: Rowman & Littlefield Publishers.
  1997 Multiculturalism and Museums: Discourse about Others in the Age of Globalisation. Theory, Culture & Society 14(4):123–146.
Niezen, R.
  2003 The Origins of Indigenism: Human Rights and the Politics of Identity. Berkeley: University of California Press.
Nora, P.
  1989 Between Memory and History: Les Lieux de Memoire. Special issue, "Memory and Counter-Memory," Representations 26:7–24.
Nouvel, J.
  2006 Présence–absence: Ou la dématérialisation sélective. In Le Musée du Quai Branly. A. Lavalou and J. P. Robert, eds. P. 40. Paris: Le Moniteur.
O'Regan, G.
  1997 Bicultural Developments in Museums in Aotearoa: What is the Current Status? Wellington: Museum of New Zealand.
Oliver, P.
  2001 Re-Presenting and Representing the Vernacular: The Open-Air Museum. In Consuming Tradition, Manufacturing Heritage: Global Norms and Urban Forms in the Age of Tourism. N. Alsayyad, ed. Pp. 191–211. London: Routledge.

Oliver, W. H.
2004   Te Papa: Taking Shape. *In* Icons Nga Taonga from the Museum of New
       Zealand Te Papa Tongarewa. R. Anderson, P. Brownsey, J. Davidson, S.
       Mallon, H. Smith, I. Wedde, and B. Williams, eds. Pp. ix–xiii. Wellington: Te
       Papa Press.
Peers, L., and A. K. Brown, eds.
2003   Museums and Source Communities: A Routledge Reader. London: Routledge.
Peltier, P.
2002   Aboriginal Ceiling Paintings: Presentation. Electronic document, http://www.
       quaibranly.fr/uploads/media/doc-2508.pdf, accessed December 12, 2008.
2000   Les Musées: Arts ou Ethnographie? *In* Du musée colonial au musée des cultures
       du monde: Actes du colloque organisé par le Musée National des Arts d'Afrique
       et d'Océanie et le Centre Georges Pompidou, 3-6 Juin 1998. D. Taffin, ed. Pp.
       205–218. Paris: Maisonneuve.
Penny, H. G.
2002   Objects of Culture: Ethnology and Ethnographic Museums in Imperial Germany.
       Chapel Hill: University of North Carolina Press.
Philibert, J. M.
1986   The Politics of Tradition: Towards a Generic Culture in Vanuatu. Mankind
       16(1):1–12.
Phillips, R.
2007   Exhibiting Africa after Modernism: Globalization, Pluralism, and the
       Persistent Paradigms of Art and Artefact. *In* Museums After Modernism:
       Strategies of Engagement. G. Pollock and J. Zemans, eds. Pp. 80–103.
       Oxford: Blackwell.
2005   Replacing Objects: Historical Practices for the Second Museum Age. The
       Canadian Historical Review 86(1):83–110.
2003   Community Collaboration in Exhibitions: Introduction. *In* Museums and
       Source Communities: A Routledge Reader. L. Peers and A. K. Brown, eds. Pp.
       155–170. London: Routledge.
2002   Where is "Africa"? Re-Viewing Art and Artifact in the Age of Globalization.
       American Anthropologist 104(3):944–952.
Price, S.
2010   Return to the Quai Branly. Museum Anthropology 33(1):11–21.
2007   Paris Primitive. Chicago: University of Chicago Press.
1989   Primitive Art in Civilized Places. Chicago: University of Chicago Press.
Regenvanu, R.
2005   The Changing Face of "Custom" in Vanuatu. People and Culture in Oceania
       20:37–50.
2003   The Vanuatu Cultural Centre. Handout accompanying lecture, Institute of
       Archaeology, University College London, October 28.
1999   Afterward: Vanuatu Perspectives on Research. Oceania 70(1):98–100.
1996   Transforming Representations: A Sketch of the Contemporary Art Scene in
       Vanuatu. *In* Arts of Vanuatu. J. Bonnemaison, K. W. Huffman, and D. Tryon, eds.
       Pp. 309–317. Honolulu: University of Hawai'i Press.
Rivière, G. H.
1989   La muséologie selon George-Henri Rivière: Cours de muséologie/ Textes et
       témoignages. Paris: Dunod.
Rosoff, N.
2003   Integrating Native Views into Museum Procedures: Hope and Practice at
       the National Museum of the American Indian. *In* Museums and Source
       Communities: A Routledge Reader. L. Peers and A. K. Brown, eds. Pp. 72–80.
       London: Routledge.

Rothstein, E.
2004a Museum with an American Indian Voice. New York Times, September 21.
2004b Who Should Tell History: The Tribes or the Museum? New York Times, December 21.
Roulet, S.
2006 Jean Nouvel's Musée du Quai Branly. New European Architecture 10:62.
Rowlands, M.
2004 Cultural Rights and Wrongs: Uses of the Concept of Property. *In* Property in Question: Value Transformation in the Global Economy. K. Verdery and C. Humphrey, eds. Pp. 207–226. Oxford: Berg.
2002 Heritage and Cultural Property. *In* The Material Culture Reader. V. Buchli, ed. Pp. 105–114. Oxford: Berg.
Rowlands, M., and B. Butler
2007 Conflict and Heritage Care. Anthropology Today 23(1):1–2.
Ruggles, D. F., and H. Silverman, eds.
2009 Intangible Heritage Embodied. New York: Springer.
Sahlins, M.
1999 Two or Three Things That I Know about Culture. Journal of the Royal Anthropological Institute 5(3):399–421.
Saito, H.
2005 Protection of Intangible Cultural Heritage in Japan. Paper presented at the Sub-regional Experts Meeting in Asia on Intangible Cultural Heritage: Safeguarding and Inventory Making Methodologies, Bangkok, December 13–15. Electronic document, http://www.accu.or.jp/ich/en/pdf/c2005subreg_Jpn2.pdf, accessed December 13, 2006.
Sandell, R., ed.
2002 Museums, Society, Inequality. London: Routledge.
Schumpeter, J. A.
2010 [1942] Capitalism, Socialism, and Democracy. London: Taylor & Francis.
Seitel, P., ed.
2001 Safeguarding Traditional Cultures: A Global Assessment of the 1989 UNESCO Recommendation on the Safeguarding of Traditional Culture and Folklore. Washington, DC: UNESCO.
Shelton, A. A.
2009 The Public Sphere as Wilderness: Le Musée du quai Branly. *In* Museum Anthropology 32:1–16.
2003 Curating African Worlds. *In* Museums and Source Communities: A Routledge Reader. L. Peers and A. K. Brown, eds. Pp. 181–193. London: Routledge.
2000 Museum Ethnography: An Imperial Science. *In* Cultural Encounters: Representing Otherness. E. Hallam and B. V. Street, eds. Pp. 155–193. London: Routledge.
Simpson, M.
1996 Making Representations: Museums in the Post-colonial Era. London: Routledge.
Smith, L.
2006 Uses of Heritage. London: Routledge.
Smith, L., and N. Akagawa
2009 Intangible Heritage. Abingdon: Routledge.
Smith, L., and M. Waterton
2009 "The Envy of the World?" Intangible Heritage in England. *In* Intangible Heritage. L. Smith and N. Akagawa, eds. Pp. 289–302. Abingdon: Routledge.
Somé, R.
2003 Le musée à l'ère de la mondialisation: Pour une anthropologie de l'altérité. Paris: L'Harmattan.

Speiser, F.
    1996   [1923] Ethnology of Vanuatu: An Early 20th Century Study. D.Q. Stephenson, trans. Honolulu: University of Hawai'i Press.
Stanley, N., ed.
    2007   The Future of Indigenous Museums: Perspectives from Southwest Pacific. New York: Berghahn Books.
    1998   Being Ourselves for You. London: Middlesex University Press.
Stocking, G. W., ed.
    1985   Objects and Others: Essays on Museums and Material Culture. Madison, WI: The University of Wisconsin Press.
Sullivan, L. E., and A. Edwards
    2004   Stewards of the Sacred. Washington, DC: American Association of Museums.
Svensson, T. G.
    2008   Knowledge and Artifacts: People and Objects. Museum Anthropology 31(2):85–104.
Taffin, D., ed.
    2000   Du musée colonial au musée des cultures du monde: Actes du colloque organisé par le Musée National des Arts d'Afrique et d'Océanie et le Centre Georges Pompidou, 3-6 Juin 1998. Paris: Maisonneuve et Larose.
Tapsell, P.
    2011   "Aroha Mai: Whose Museum?" The Rise of Indigenous Ethics within Museum Contexts: A Maori-Tribal Perspective. *In* The Routledge Companion to Museum Ethics: Redefining Ethics for the Twenty-first Century Museum. J. Marstine, ed. Pp. 85–111. Abingdon: Routledge.
    1998   Taonga: A Tribal Response to Museums. Ph.D. dissertation, Oxford University.
Taylor, C.
    1992   Multiculturalism and "The Politics of Recognition." Princeton: Princeton University Press.
Thomas, N.
    1999   Possessions: Indigenous Art/ Colonial Culture. London: Thames and Hudson.
    1997   In Oceania: Visions, Artifacts, Histories. Durham: Duke University Press.
    1994   Colonialism's Culture: Anthropology, Travel, and Government. Cambridge: Polity Press.
    1991   Entangled Objects: Exchange, Material Culture and Colonialism in the Pacific. Cambridge: Harvard University Press.
Titchen, S.
    1996   On the Construction of "Outstanding Universal Value": Some Comments on the Implementation of the 1972 UNESCO World Heritage Convention. Conservation and Management of Archaeological Sites 1(4):235–242.
Todorov, T.
    1999   The Conquest of America: The Question of the Other. Norman: University of Oklahoma Press.
Tonkinson, R.
    1982a   Kastom in Melanesia: Introduction. Special issue, "Reinventing Traditional Culture: The Politics of Kastom in Island Melanesia," Mankind 13(4):302–305.
    1982b   National Identity and the Problem of Kastom in Vanuatu. Special issue, "Reinventing Traditional Culture: The Politics of Kastom in Island Melanesia," Mankind 13(4):306–315.
Trigger, B. G.
    2006   A History of Archaeological Thought. 2nd edition. Cambridge: Cambridge University Press.
Truscott, M. C.
    2000   "Intangible Values" as Heritage in Australia. ICOMOS News 10(1):4–11.

Tryon, D.
  1999   Ni-Vanuatu Research and Researchers. Oceania 70(1):9–15.
Tuhiwai Smith, L.
  1999   Decolonizing Methodologies: Research and Indigenous Peoples. Dunedin: University of Otago Press.
UNESCO
  2006   Masterpieces of the Oral and Intangible Heritage of Humanity: Proclamations 2001, 2003 and 2005. Electronic document, http://unesdoc.unesco.org/images/0014/001473/147344e.pdf, accessed February 14, 2012.
  2004   Second Proclamation of Masterpieces of the Oral and Intangible Heritage of Humanity. Electronic document, http://unesdoc.unesco.org/images/0013/001363/136370eb.pdf, accessed February 14, 2012.
Vergo, P., ed.
  1989   The New Museology. London: Verso.
Viatte, G.
  2006a L'invention muséologique. In Le musée du quai Branly. A. Lavalou and J. P. Robert, eds. Pp. 26–31. Paris: Le Moniteur.
  2006b The Collections and the Museographic Itinerary. In Musée du Quai Branly: Museum Guide Book. Pp. 24–29. Paris: Musée du Quai Branly.
  2006c Tu fais peur, tu émerveilles: Musée du quai Branly acquisitions 1998/2005. Paris: Musée du quai Branly.
Vogel, S.
  2007   Des ombres sur la Seine: L'art africain, l'obscurité et le musée du quai Branly. Le Débat 147:178–192.
Volkert, J., L. R. Martin, and A. Pickworth, eds.
  2004   National Museum of the American Indian: Map and Guide. Washington, DC: National Museum of the American Indian.
Watson, S., ed.
  2007   Museums and Their Communities. London: Routledge.
Were, G.
  2007   Musée du Quai Branly: The Future or Folly. Electronic document, http://blogs.nyu.edu/projects/materialworld/2007/05/musee_du_quai_branly_the_futur.html, accessed May 20, 2008.
  2005   Thinking through Images: Kastom and the Coming of Baha'is to Northern New Ireland, Papua New Guinea. Journal of the Royal Anthropological Institute 11:659–676.
West, R. W.
  2007   From the Director. National Museum of the American Indian Newsletter Spring 2007: 17.
West, R. W., ed.
  2000   The Changing Presentation of the American Indian: Museums and Native Cultures. Washington, DC: University of Washington Press.
Whiteley, P. M.
  2002   Archaeology and Oral Tradition: The Scientific Importance of Dialogue. American Antiquity 67(3):405–415.
Williams, P.
  2005   A Breach on the Beach: Te Papa and the Fraying of Biculturalism. Museum and Society 3(2):81–97.
Wood, P.
  2005   Community Consultation: Te Papa and New Zealand Indian Communities—The Other Side of the Coin. Tuhinga 16:127–135.
Yim, D.
  2004   Living Human Treasures and the Protection of Intangible Cultural Heritage: Experiences and Challenges. ICOM News 57(4):10–12.

Zagala, S.
  2004   Vanuatu Sand Drawing. Museum International 56:32–35.
Zimmerman, L.
  2010   "WHITE PEOPLE WILL BELIEVE ANYTHING!" Worrying about Authenticity, Museum Audiences, and Working in Native American-Focused Museums. Museum Anthropology 33(1):33–36.

PUBLIC DOCUMENTS

ICOMOS
  1994   *The Nara Document on Authenticity.*
  1964   *The Venice Charter: International Charter for the Conservation and Restoration of Monuments and Sites.*
  1954   *Convention for the Protection of Cultural Property in the Event of Armed Conflict—Hague Convention.*
  1931   *The Athens Charter for the Restoration of Historic Monuments.*
ICOMOS Australia
  1999   *The Burra Charter.*
New Zealand Government
  1992   Museum of New Zealand Te Papa Tongarewa Act 1992.
UN
  2007   *United Nations Declaration on the Rights of Indigenous Peoples.*
  1992   *United Nations Draft Declaration on the Rights of Indigenous Peoples.*
UN/ECOSOC
  1995   *Principles and Guidelines for the Protection of the Heritage of Indigenous Peoples.*
UNEP
  1992   *Convention on Biological Diversity.*
UNESCO
  2005   *Convention on the Protection and Promotion of the Diversity of Cultural Expressions.*
  2003   *Convention for the Safeguarding of the Intangible Cultural Heritage.*
  2001   *Universal Declaration on Cultural Diversity.*
  2001   *Convention for the Protection of Underwater Cultural Heritage.*
  1989   *Recommendation on the Safeguarding of Traditional Culture and Folklore.*
  1972   *Convention Concerning the Protection of the World Cultural and Natural Heritage*
  1970   *Convention on the Means of Prohibiting and Preventing the Illicit Import, Export and Transfer of Cultural Property.*
U.S. Congress
  1990   *Native American Grave Protection and Repatriation Act.*
  1989   *National Museum of the American Indian Act.*
Vanuatu Parliament
  1988   *Vanuatu National Cultural Council Act [Cap 186].*

INTERNET RESOURCES

Caribbean Currents, Horniman Museum, www.caribbean-currents.co.uk, accessed June 15, 2008.
Creusot-Montceau Ecomuseum, www.ecomusee-creusot-montceau.com, accessed July 10, 2010.

Folkways Recordings, CFCH, www.folkways.si.edu, accessed January 19, 2011.
Fondation Chirac, www.fondationchirac.eu, accessed February 12, 2011.
Global Sound, CFCH, www.smithsonianglobalsound.org, accessed February 10, 2010.
Horniman Museum, www.horniman.ac.uk, accessed February 10, 2011.
ICOMOS, www.international.icomos.org, accessed January 20, 2011.
Indigenous Geography, NMAI, www.indigenousgeography.si.edu, accessed February 2, 2011.
International Journal of Intangible Heritage, www.ijih.org, accessed January 12, 2011.
Live Earth, www.liveearth.org, accessed January 23, 2009.
Musée du quai Branly, www.quaibranly.fr, accessed February 12, 2011.
National Museum of New Zealand Te Papa Tongarewa, www.tepapa.govt.nz, accessed February 13, 2011.
National Museum of the American Indian, www.nmai.si.edu, accessed February 12, 2011.
Ralph Regenvanu's website, www.ralphregenvanu.org, accessed February 5, 2009.
UNESCO, www.unesco.org, accessed January 20, 2011.
Vanuatu Cultural Centre, www.vanuatuculture.org, accessed February 9, 2011.
World Heritage Centre, http://whc.unesco.org, accessed January 20, 2011.
World Intellectual Property Organisation, www.wipo.org, accessed January 15, 2011.

Index

About the Author

Marilena Alivizatou holds a PhD in Museum and Heritage Studies from University College London. She has worked as teaching fellow in museum studies at UCL's Institute of Archaeology, coordinating courses in collections management and care, collections curatorship, and critical museology. Her research and teaching interests are in the areas of intangible heritage, participatory museology, culture and development, and alternative approaches to museum curation. m.alivizatou@gmail.com

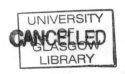

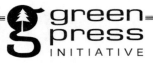